Novel Approaches to the Treatment of Alzheimer's Disease

ADVANCES IN BEHAVIORAL BIOLOGY

Recent Volumes in this Series

Volume 23   THE AGING BRAIN AND SENILE DEMENTIA
Edited by Kalidas Nandy and Ira Sherwin

Volume 24   CHOLINERGIC MECHANISMS AND PSYCHOPHARMACOLOGY
Edited by Donald J. Jenden

Volume 25   CHOLINERGIC MECHANISMS: Phylogenetic Aspects, Central and
Peripheral Synapses, and Clinical Significance
Edited by Giancarlo Pepeu and Herbert Ladinsky

Volume 26   CONDITIONING: Representation of Involved Neural Functions
Edited by Charles D. Woody

Volume 27   THE BASAL GANGLIA: Structure and Function
Edited by John S. McKenzie, Robert E. Kemm,
and Lynette N. Wilcock

Volume 28   BRAIN PLASTICITY, LEARNING, AND MEMORY
Edited by B. E. Will, P. Schmitt, and
J. C. Dalrymple-Alford

Volume 29   ALZHEIMER'S AND PARKINSON'S DISEASES: Strategies
for Research and Development
Edited by Abraham Fisher, Israel Hanin, and Chaim Lachman

Volume 30   DYNAMICS OF CHOLINERGIC FUNCTION
Edited by Israel Hanin

Volume 31   TOBACCO SMOKING AND NICOTINE: A Neurobiological Approach
Edited by William R. Martin, Glen R. Van Loon, Edgar T. Iwamoto, and
Layten Davis

Volume 32   THE BASAL GANGLIA II: Structure and Function—Current Concepts
Edited by Malcolm B. Carpenter and A. Jayaraman

Volume 33   LECITHIN: Technological, Biological, and Therapeutic Aspects
Edited by Israel Hanin and G. Brian Ansell

Volume 34   ALTERATIONS IN THE NEURONAL CYTOSKELETON IN
ALZHEIMER' DISEASE
Edited by George P. Perry

Volume 35   MECHANISMS OF CEREBRAL HYPOXIA AND STROKE
Edited by George Somjen

Volume 36   NOVEL APPROACHES TO THE TREATMENT OF ALZHEIMER'S DISEASE
Edited by Edwin M. Meyer, James W. Simpkins, and Jyunji Yamamoto

A Continuation Order Plan is available for this series. A continuation order will bring delivery of each new volume immediately upon publication. Volumes are billed only upon actual shipment. For further information please contact the publisher.

Novel Approaches to the Treatment of Alzheimer's Disease

Edited by

Edwin M. Meyer, and
James W. Simpkins
University of Florida
Gainesville, Florida

and

Jyunji Yamamoto
Taiho Pharmaceuticals, Ltd.
Tokushima, Japan

PLENUM PRESS • NEW YORK AND LONDON

Library of Congress Cataloging-in-Publication Data

Suncoast Workshop on the Neurobiology of Aging (1st : 1989 : Saint
  Petersburg, Fla.)
    Novel approaches to the treatment of Alzheimer's disease / edited
  by Edwin M. Meyer and James W. Simpkins and Jyunji Yamamoto.
       p.   cm. -- (Advances in behavioral biology ; v. 36)
    "Proceedings of the First Annual Suncoast Workshop on the
  Neurobiology of Aging, held February 26-March 1, 1989, in St.
  Petersburg, Florida"--T.p. verso.
    Includes bibliographical references.
    ISBN 0-306-43402-4
    1. Alzheimer's disease--Chemotherapy--Congresses.
  2. Acetycholine--Receptors--Effect of drugs on--Congresses.
  3. Neuropharmacology--Congresses.   I. Meyer, Edwin M.
  II. Simpkins, James W. III. Yamamoto, Jyunji. IV. Title.
  V. Series.
    [DNLM: 1. Alzheimer's Disease--drug therapy--congresses.
  2. Psychotropic Drugs--pharmacology--congresses.   WM 220 S957n
  1989]
  RC523.S86   1989
  616.8'31061--dc20
  DNLM/DLC
  for Library of Congress   89-26615
                                                      CIP

Center for the
Neurobiology of Aging

CNA

University of Florida

Proceedings of the First Annual Suncoast Workshop on
the Neurobiology of Aging, held February 26–March 1, 1989,
in St. Petersburg, Florida

© 1989 Plenum Press, New York
A Division of Plenum Publishing Corporation
233 Spring Street, New York, N.Y. 10013

This book is dedicated
to the memory of the
Honorable Claude Pepper,
whose crusade for the
rights and welfare of the
elderly inspired us all.

PREFACE

Alzheimer's disease afflicts up to 1 in 5 people over the age of 65 years and causes untold suffering of the patient and their family. The cause of this disease is unknown; indeed, evidence increasingly suggests that there may be multiple Alzheimer-type syndromes with different etiologies, analogous to different types of psychosis. Currently there are no means to prevent the disease, slow its progress or reverse its neurodegenerative consequences. With few exceptions, clinical trials of a variety of compounds have resulted in patient responses that are disappointing with respect to both the proportion of responders and the magnitude of the responses. Novel approaches to the treatment of Alzheimer's disease are clearly warranted.

For this reason, we organized the First Suncoast Workshop on the Neurobiology of Aging in St. Petersburg, Florida, which took place from February 26-March 1, 1989. This workshop focused on novel treatments and models for Alzheimer's disease and represented a cooperative venture among academia, government and industry, both in its participants and sponsorship. The Center for the Neurobiology of Aging at the University of Florida, the National Institute on Aging and Taiho Pharmaceutical Corporation in Japan sponsored the workshop in which scientists from the North America, Europe, Japan and other parts of Asia participated.

While not an official proceedings of the Suncoast Workshop, this text does reflect the breadth and depth of the research presented there. A few additional chapters were received from investigators who could not attend the workshop but who wished to augment the book. The text is divided into sections that deal with animal and clinical models for Alzheimer's disease, novel treatment strategies based on a new generation of cholinergic agents, neurotrophic agents that prevent or even reverse neurodegeneration, grafting neural tissue into the brain, other types of therapeutic approaches, and novel approaches to improve the delivery of drugs to the brain. Collectively, this text reflects an advanced level of thought on a variety of related strategies aimed at treating neurodegenerative diseases such as Alzheimer's disease.

In a field moving this quickly, it is imperative that new data and hypotheses be published as quickly as possible. Towards this end, we are indebted to Melanie Yelity and the others at Plenum Press who expedited the publication of this book in so many ways.

The organization of this workshop and the production of this text required the cross-continental efforts of many people. We are particularly grateful for the continuing intellectual, organizational and financial support of the following individuals at Taiho Pharmaceutical Company in Japan: Mr. Satoru Nakagami, who was so enthusiastic in his support of the Workshop; Dr. Takashi Suzui; and Dr. Katsuo Toide. Some of our best suggestions for organizing the workshop came from Dr. Ronald Micetish, President of Synphar, a North American affiliate of Taiho Pharmaceuticals. Our co-editor, Dr. Jyunji Yamamoto, graciously agreed to write a separate Preface for this volume.

This text would have been impossible without Janice E. Goodson. Ms. Goodson's devotion to the project far exceeded our expectations; her professional touch was evident in every workshop-related activity, ranging from the organization and advertisement of the workshop over a year ago through the editing of the last submitted manuscript. Special contributions to the text were made by the following individuals: Dr. Jennifer Poulakos, Dr. Suzanne Evans, and Judy Adams

Finally, we wish to acknowledge the support of the administration of the University of Florida, College of Medicine and College of Pharmacy, as well as the Office of the Vice President, J. Hillis Miller Health Science Center. Their support for this project and for the other activities of the Center for the Neurobiology of Aging daily facilitates our multidisiplinary approach to the problems of the aging brain, including Alzheimer's Disease. We believe that the knowledge base reflected in this text and the willing participation of eminent scientists from around the world, will similarly enhance our future workshops on novel treatments for Alzheimer's Disease.

Edwin M. Meyer
and
James W. Simpkins
Gainesville, Florida

Date: August 14, 1989

AN OPINION FROM JAPAN

Science, being an historically accumulated product, walks on one step after another with the achievements of scientists from each generation, with no possibility of leap-frogging even one of the steps. It is no easy task to know the historical background of scientific progress, and there are many cases in which scientists cannot become so enlightened. At the time of its advancement and development, science is confronted with many difficulties; how to solve these difficulties hangs on the shoulders of each generation, as a mission.

Each generation must also deal with the advancement of pharmacological products, which goes all the way from scientific research to social needs. Major social and medical problems in recent years are the age-related neurological disturbances Alzheimer's disease, dementia and senility, and researchers are burdened with the responsibility of tackling these problems squarely. Development of very highly advanced drugs such as those promoting memorization/learning capacities or inhibiting the aging process will be in greater demand in the future; further, scientific technologies in general have been progressing steadily and surely, along with individually specialized areas and techniques for dissemination of information. Under these evolving circumstances, solutions will almost undoubtedly involve group efforts and not those of any single investigator.

The question here is how effectively research works in different specialized disciplines to solve problems in as short a time period as possible. For this purpose, it will be desirable to develop a new research system with the capacity to promote joint research and design components in various forms as required.

Nowadays in Japan, the number of researchers and research-institutions studying the brain are steadily increasing. This state of affairs can also be commonly applicable to many countries in the world. The world abounds with people who have a variety of ideas. While cultures indigenous to each country exist, scientific differences will result. Combining these different sciences will make it possible to give rise to newer lines of research, widening the door open to a newer platform of prospects, which is really marvellous in itself.

I have in mind always to watch my own contribution to science and humanity.

J. Yamamoto, Ph.D.
Director of Alzheimer's Disease Research
Taiho Pharmaceuticals, LTD

CONTENTS

SECTION I. DRUGS THAT ACT AT CHOLINERGIC RECEPTORS

A Functionalized Congener Approach to Muscarinic Ligands   1
K. A. Jacobson, B. J. Bradbury and J. Baumgold

AF102B: A Novel M1 Agonist as a Rational Treatment Strategy in   11
Alzheimer's Disease
A. Fisher, R. Brandeis, I. Karton, Z. Pittel, S. Dachir, M. Sapir, Y.
Grunfeld, A. Levy and E. Heldman

Muscarinic Receptors, Phosphoinositide Hydrolysis and Neuronal   17
Plasticity in the Hippocampus
F. T. Crews, N. J. Pontzer and L. J. Chandler

Effects of Cholinergic Drugs on Extracellular Levels of Acetylcholine and   25
Choline in Rat Cortex, Hippocampus and Striatum Studied byu Brain Dialysis
K. Toide and T. Arima

Delayed Matching-to-Sample in Monkeys as a Model for Learning and Memory   39
Deficits: Role of Brain Nicotinic Receptors
W. J. Jackson, K. Elrod and J. J. Buccafusco

Muscarinic and Nicotinic Receptors in Alzheimer's Disease: Rationale for   53
Cholinergic Drug Treatment
P. A. Lapchak, D. M. Araujo and R. Quirion

SECTION II. CNS-ACTIVE NEUROTROPHIC FACTORS

Potential Pharmacological Use of Neurotrophic Factors in the Treatment of   63
Neurodegenerative Diseases
F. Hefti

The Use of Reaggregating Cell Cultures and Immortalized Central Nervous   71
System Cells to Study Cholinergic Trophic Mechanisms
B. H. Wainer, H. J. Lee, J. D. Roback, and D. N. Hammond

Approaches to Gene Therapy in the CNS: Intracerebral Grafting of Fibroblasts   95
Genetically Modified to Secrete Nerve Growth Factor
M. B. Rosenberg, M. H. Tuszynski, K. Yoshida, T. Friedmann and F. H. Gage

Exogenous Nerve Growth Factor Stimulates Choline Acetyltransferase Activity   103
in Basal Forebrain of Axotomized and Aged Rats
L. R. Williams, K. S. Jodelis, M. R. Donald and H. K. Yip

Neuronotrophic Factors, Gangliosides and Their Interaction: Implications in   117
the Regulation of Nervous System Plasticity
S. D. Skaper, A. Leon and G. Toffano

Suppression of Active Neuronal Death by Immune Interferon   127
E. M. Johnson Jr., D. P. Martin, B. K. Levy and J. Y. Chang

Basic Fibroblast Growth Factor, an Example of a Multifunctional   133
Trophic Factor with Neurotrophic Activity
P. A. Walicke

Growth Factor and Lymphokine Effects on Brain Cholinergic Systems   153
D. M. Araujo, P. A. Lapchak, J.-G. Chabot and R. Quirion

Metabolic Support of Neural Plasticity: Implications for the Treatment of   165
Alzheimers Disease
J. E. Black and W. T. Greenough

SECTION III. ADDITIONAL NOVEL TREATMENT STRATEGIES: IMPROVED BRAIN DELIVERY, HORMONES, AND IMMUNOLOGY

Brain-Enhanced Delivery of Anti-Dementia Drugs   173 ·
M. E. Brewster, C. Robledo-Luiggi, A. Miyakeb, E. Pop and N. Bodor

Development of a Pyrrolidinone Derivative (Cyclic GABA) for Modulating   185
Brain Glutamate Transmission
K. Matsuyama, C. Miyazaki and M. Ichikawa

A Brain-Enhanced Chemical Delivery System for Gonadal Steroids: 197
Implications for Neurodegenerative Diseases
J. W. Simpkins, M. H. Rahimy and N. Bodor

Immunologic Approach to Therapy in Alzheimer's Disease   213
V. K. Singh and R. P. Warren

The Influence of ACTH 4-9 Analog upon Avoidance Learning in Normal and   221
Brain Damaged Rats
W. F. McDaniel, M. S. Schmidt, F. I. Chirino Barcelo and B. K. Davis

SECTION IV. MODELS FOR DRUG-DEVELOPMENT: CHOLINERGIC HYPOFUNCTION

Transneuronal Neurochemical and Neuropathological Changes Induced by
Nucleus Basalis Lesions: A Possible Degenerative Mechanism in Alzheimer's
Disease   235
G. W. Arendash, G. J. Sengstock, G. Shaw and W. J. Millard

Presynaptic Markers of Cholinergic Function in Cortex Following Ibotenic   255
Acid Lesion of the Basal Forebrain
M. Downen, K. Sugaya, S. P. Arneric and E. Giacobini

Cholinergic-Neuropeptide Y Interactions in the Rat Cerebralcortex: Towards a 269
Model for the Trans-synapticEffects of Cholinergic Transmission
J. J. Poulakos, G. W. Arendash, W. J. Millard, N. N. Sjak-Shie and E. M.
Meyer

The Effects of Nucleus Basalis Lesions in the Rat on One Way Passive and   279
Active Avoidance, Two Way Avoidance and Lashly III Maze Learning: An Animal
Model for SDAT
P. N. Strong and G. W. Arendash

SECTION V. MODELS FOR DRUG DEVELOPMENT: OTHER NEUROCHEMICAL AND BEHAVIORAL CHANGES

NMDA Receptors, Aging and Alzheimer's Disease   293
K. J. Anderson, D. T. Monaghan and J. W. Geddes

An Excitotoxic Model of Alzheimer's Disease: NMDA Lesions and Initial Neural 303
Grafting Results
D. A. Turner and W. Q. Dong

Excitotoxin Mediated Neuronal Loss and the Regulation of Excitatory Amino   319
Acid Release in the Aging Brain
R. Dawson Jr., M. J. Meldrum and D. R. Wallace

EEG Power Spectra and Brain Function   329
J. Yamamoto

Postmortem Stability of RNA Metabolism in Human Brain: Studies of the   347
Nondemented Conrol and Alzheimer's Disease Cases
E. M. Sajdel-Sulkowska, H. J. Manz and C. A. Marotta

A Model System Demonstrating Parallels in Animal and Human Aging: 355
Extension to Alzheimer's Disease
D. S. Woodruff-Pak, R. G. Finkbiner and I. R. Katz

Computer-Simulated Everyday Memory Testing for Clinical Trials in
Memory Disorders of Aging
G. J. Larrabee and T. H. Crook III

373

INDEX

383

A FUNCTIONALIZED CONGENER APPROACH TO MUSCARINIC LIGANDS

Kenneth A. Jacobson,* Barton J. Bradbury,* and Jesse Baumgold

*Laboratory of Chemistry, NIDDK, and Laboratory of Molecular
and Cellular Neurobiology, Section on Membrane Biochemistry
NINDS, NIH, Bethesda, MD 20892

INTRODUCTION

Most clinically available cholinergic drugs (eg. the agonist pilocarpine, 1, and the antagonist atropine, 2, Figure 1) are non-selective in
their interaction with muscarinic receptor subtypes. The recent cloning,
sequencing, and expression of five separate genes for muscarinic receptors
(1-4), has raised the possibility of developing novel organic compounds that
act as agonists or antagonists at one of these subtypes. Selective compounds could be therapeutically useful in treating a variety of diseases,
including Alzheimer's disease, cardiac disease, neurogenic bladder, and
certain sleep disorders. Futhermore, such specific compounds, by virtue of
their subtype selectivity, should be devoid of many of the side effects of
currently used compounds.

FUNCTIONALIZED CONGENERS: A STRATEGY FOR THE DESIGN OF NOVEL DRUGS

In view of the above, a goal is to develop novel and selective muscarinic agonists and antagonists. We have used a functionalized congener
approach in the design of new muscarinic ligands.

By the functionalized congener approach (5), an insensitive site on the
structure of a pharmacophore is identified by structure-activity studies and
utilized for attachment of a chemically reactive chain, designed not to
preclude receptor binding of the derivative (Figure 2). This chain may vary
in length and composition, depending on the requirements at a particular
receptor to achieve high selectivity and/or affinity. At the terminal
position of the chain is a chemically functional group (hence the designa-
tion "functionalized" congener). This distal functional group may be an
amine, carboxylic acid, or other group that is easily coupled covalently to
a complementary group on another molecule ("carrier"). Thus, this functional group serves as general attachment site for derivatization, resulting
in conjugates that retain affinity for the receptor and that may have additional desired chemical or pharmacological properties depending on the
attached "carrier." The structure activity relationships at this distal
site may be utilized to design additional analogs having enhanced pharmacological properties (6). In general, the affinity of a drug for a receptor
may be increased using this strategy.

1

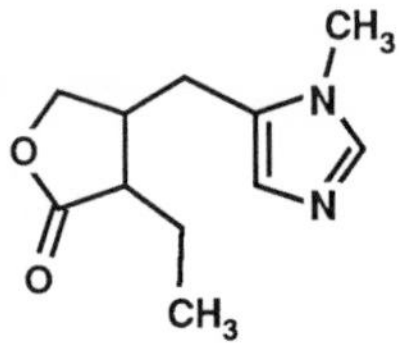

1 Pilocarpine

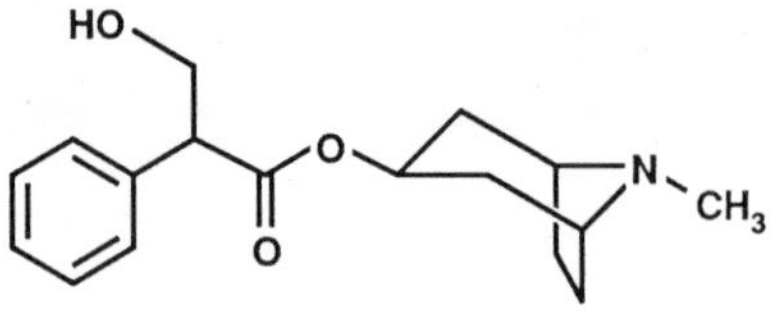

2 Atropine

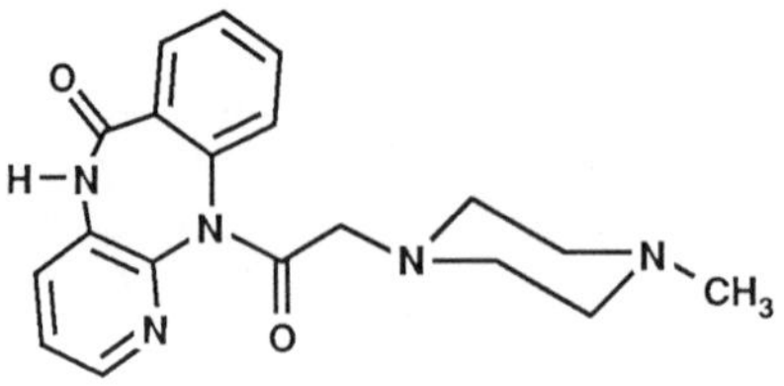

3 Pirenzepine

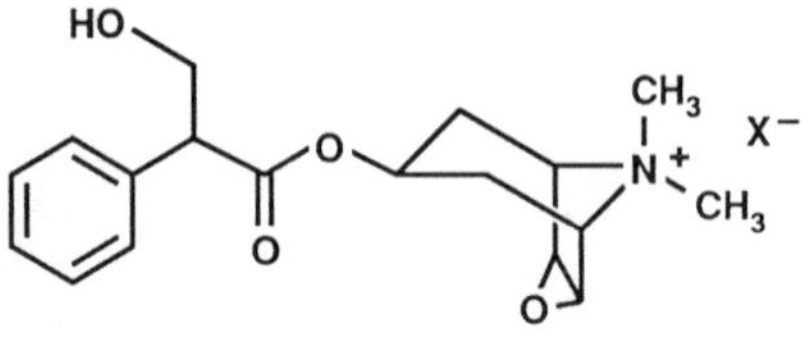

4 NMS

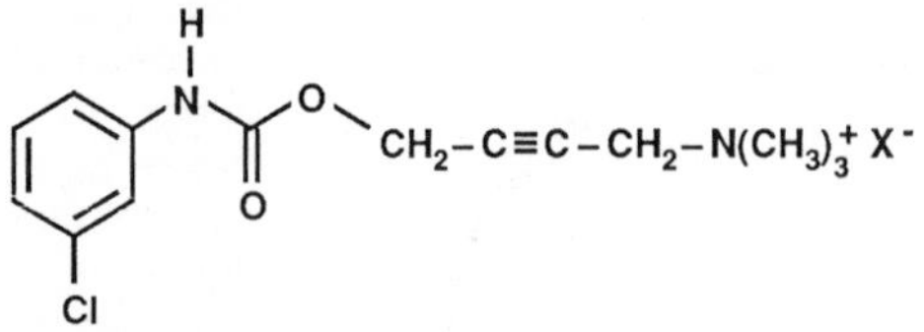

5 McN-A-343

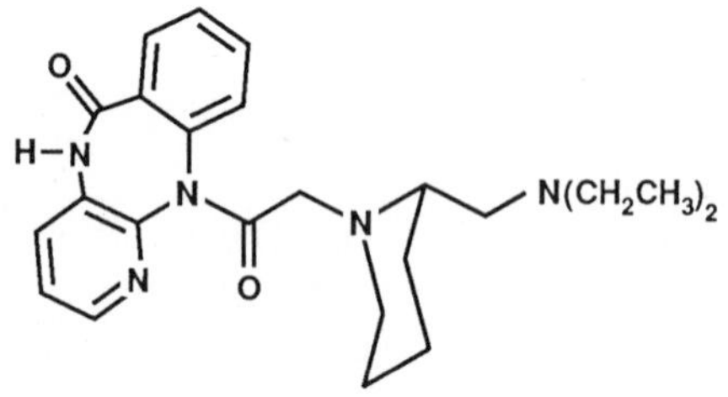

6 AF-DX-116

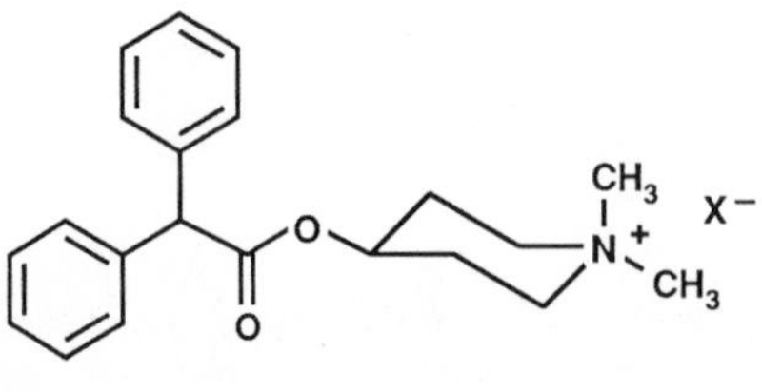

7 4-DAMP

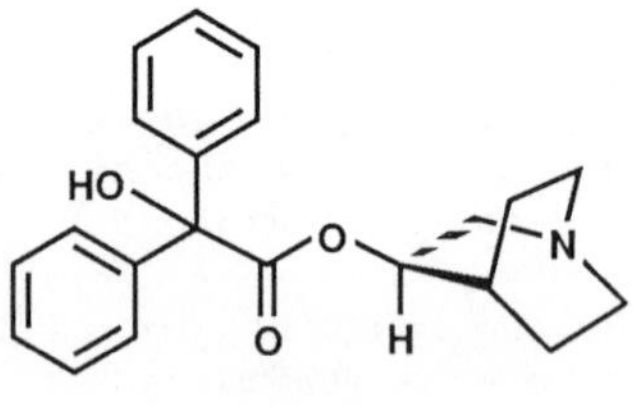

8 R-(-)-QNB

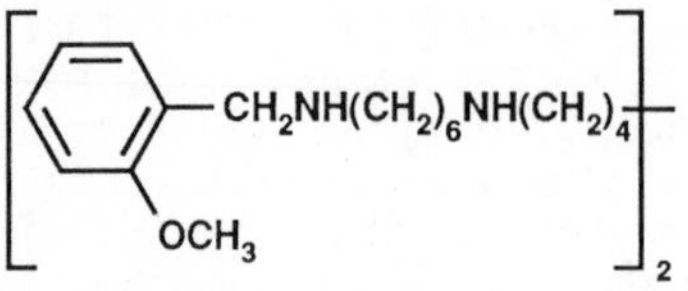

9 Methoctramine

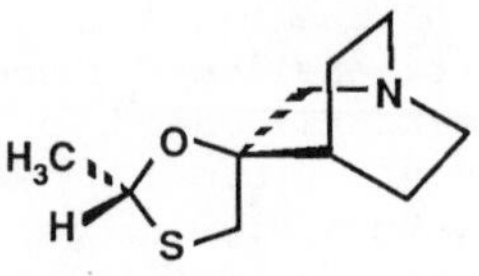

10 cis-AF102B (R,R isomer shown)

Figure 1. Structures of muscarinic ligands

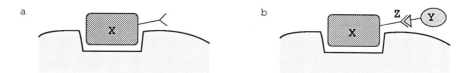

Figure 2. a. Functionalized congener (x) bound to receptor-site.
          b. Functionalized congener covalently coupled to carrier group
          (y) through amide or other linkage (z).

In order for this approach to succeed, the binding site on the receptor must not impose strict steric constraints at the point of derivatization on the ligand.

A further benefit of developing selective and potent receptor ligands that are chemically functionalized is the development of specialized receptor probes (7), detected by radioactive, spectroscopic, or other means. A prosthetic group to serve as a reporter group is attached at the distal functional site (Figure 2b). An example of such a prosthetic group for radiolabeling is the p-aminophenylacetyl group (8), which is a substrate for ^{125}I incorporation.

We have developed series of functionalized congeners for A_1- and A_2-adenosine receptors. A carboxyl or amino group was placed at a newly created distal site on an adenosine (agonist) or xanthine (antagonist) derivative. These functionalized purines (abbreviated XAC and ADAC for A_1 sites, and APEC for A_2 sites) were useful both as synthetic intermediates and as prototypical affinity receptor probes (8). A distal amino group was observed to enhance potency and/or selectivity for certain agonists and antagonists. Moreover, this functional group was covalently condensed with reporter groups for probing the receptor binding interaction and characterization of A_1-adenosine receptors by radioactive and spectroscopic methods (7).

PHARMACOLOGICAL MODELS FOR MUSCARINIC RECEPTOR SUBTYPES

Previously, muscarinic receptors were divided into two subtypes, M_1 and M_2, based on sensitivity for the antagonist pirenzepine (3, Figure 1). Pirenzepine is an anti-ulcer agent that inhibits the binding (9) of the antagonist [^{3}H]N-methylscopolamine (NMS, 4) to membranes from cerebral cortex (M_1) with an affinity that is 25-fold higher than its affinity for membranes from atria (M_2). Difficulties with the M_1/M_2 classification included the presence of a receptor of intermediate affinity (9), which was often classed together with the low affinity receptor (both being unresponsive to the specific agonist McN-A-343 (10), 5). Furthermore, it was not possible to correlate the two subtypes consistently with intracellular responses.

It is now apparent that each of these two pharmacological classes contains heterogeneous receptor protein populations, encoded by distinct genes. Bonner, Brann, and coworkers (1) at NIH, screening a rat brain complementary DNA library; Peralta, Capon, and coworkers (2), screening a human brain cDNA library; Numa and coworker (3); and other groups have identified and cloned separate genes for four separate subtypes. The subtypes are designated m1 - m4 in the notation of Bonner. The notation of Peralta uses HM1 through HM4 for the analogous receptors, except that HM3 corresponds to m4, and HM4 to m3. Thus, for screening new muscarinic agents for selectivity it is desirable to compare the potency of such agents at each distinct subtype through binding and functional assays.

Table 1 lists the muscarinic receptor subtypes, their location, and second messengers. Particular genetically-defined muscarinic subtypes are preferentially coupled to second messenger systems, including the stimulation of phosphoinositide (PI) turnover (ml and m3), the inhibition of cyclic AMP accumulation (m2 and m4), and other intracellular signals. Thus, selectivity of a muscarinic agonist for one of the second messengers is a result of selective binding to receptor subtypes. From amino acid sequence information, there is a high degree of homology (roughly 80%) between ml and m3 and between m2 and m4 muscarinic receptors. It is no coincidence there are also pharmacological similarities between the same pairs of receptor subtypes. Baumgold and White (11) and others (1,12-14) have found that muscarinic agonists stimulate PI turnover, but do not inhibit cyclic AMP production in SK-N-SH cells (neuroblastoma transformed line). In NG108-15 cells (neuroblastoma-glioma hybrid cells), the opposite occurs, i.e., inhibition of cyclic AMP accumulation with no effect on PI turnover. These cell types, which contain primarily or exclusively single muscarinic subtypes, may be used for screening new analogs for selectivity. SK-N-SH cells contain m3 receptors, and NG108-15 cells contain m4 receptors. These assignments have been corroborated by probing Northern blots with oligonucleotide probes to each of the receptor subtypes (2 and unpublished).

Table 1. Muscarinic Receptor Subtypes

"New" Subtype	"Old" Subtype Correlation[3]	Pirenzepine Affinity	2nd Messenger Response	Tissue Location[3]
m1	M_1	high	PI metab $\uparrow$	brain, exocrine
m2	M_2 cardiac	low	cAMP $\downarrow$	atrium, brain, smooth muscle
m3	M_2 glandular	intermed.	PI metab $\uparrow$	brain, exocrine smooth muscle
m4	M_1	intermed./high	cAMP $\downarrow$	brain

STRUCTURE ACTIVITY STUDIES AT MUSCARINIC RECEPTORS

Antagonists

In view of the problems associated with the M_1/M_2 classification system, selective agents for subclassification have been sought. AF-DX 116 (6, Figure 1) is an antagonist, structurally related to pirenzepine, that displays a higher affinity for cardiac M_2 receptors than for M_2 receptors in brain, smooth muscle, or bladder (15). The M_1 antagonist 4-DAMP, 7, prefers receptors in the ileum and glands versus ganglionic and cardiac receptors (15,16). A number of derivatives of quinuclidinyl benzilate, QNB, 8, (17, 18) are M_1-selective antagonists of sub-nanomolar affinity. The polymethylene tetramine, methoctramine, 9 (19), is a highly cardiac selective antagonist.

Agonists

The rigid analog AF102B, 10, developed by A. Fisher and collaborators, has been characterized as an M_1 selective agonist (20). McN-A-343, 5, also is selective for pirenzepine high affinity receptors as a partial agonist (10). At M_2 receptors, one of the most potent class of agonists is the

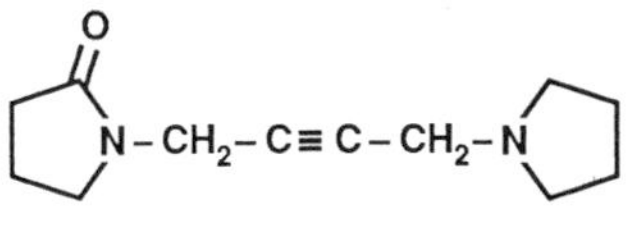

11 Oxotremorine

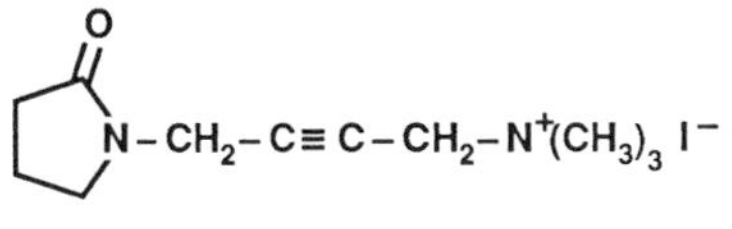

12 Oxo-M

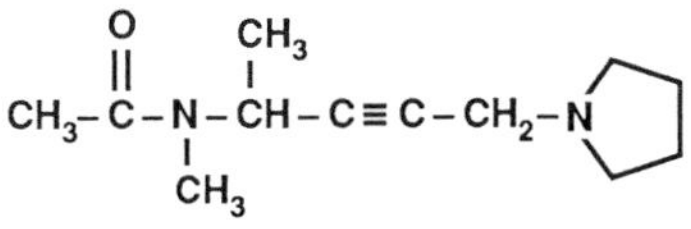

13 BM 5

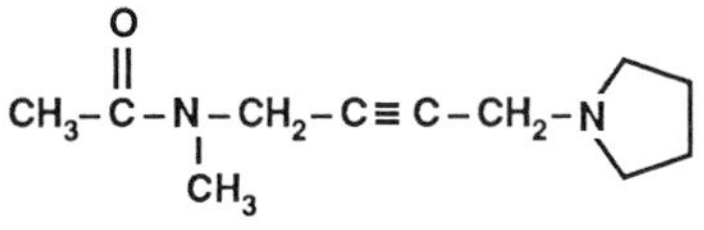

14 UH 5

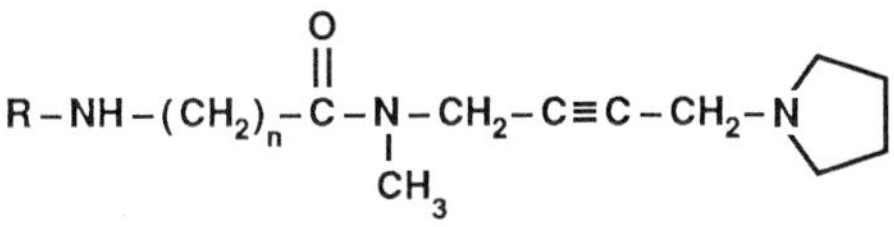

15 R = H		a n = 1
		b n = 2
16 R = CH$_3$CO		c n = 3
		d n = 4
17 R = C$_6$H$_5$CO		e n = 5
		f n = 6
18 R = (CH$_3$)$_3$COCO		g n = 7

R–NH–(CH$_2$)$_n$–C–N–CH$_2$–C≡C–CH$_2$–N

Figure 3. Structures of oxotremorine and analogs

acetylene amines (Figure 3) related to oxotremorine, 11. Oxotremorine (21)
is a nearly symmetrical molecule, having a pyrrolidine ring (charged in the
protonated state) and a pyrrolidone ring bridged by a 2-butynyl chain.
Oxotremorine-M, 12, in which the pyrrolidine ring has been replaced with a
quaternary trimethyl amine, is a full agonist (22) at muscarinic receptors.
Many of the recent structure activity studies for oxotremorine analogs have
been carried out by Ringdahl and coworkers (21,23). An analog in which the
pyrrolidone ring has been opened, N-methyl-N-(4-pyrrolidino-2-butynyl)acet-
amide (UH 5), 14, has been identified as a potent agonist (24). Addition of
a methyl group to the butynyl moiety, adjacent to the pyrrolidone ring,
results in the analog BM 5, 13 (25). BM 5 has been characterized as an agonist at post-synaptic muscarinic receptors and an antagonist at pre-synap-
tic muscarinic receptors (26).

Alzheimer's disease, one of the therapeutic targets of this study, is
associated with a premature decrease in the density of receptors for a
number of neurotransmitters in the brain. In particular, a profound degeneration of presynaptic central muscarinic pathways in the cholinergic basal
forebrain system has been observed (27, 28). These pathways originate in
the nucleus basalis and in other regions. The postsynaptic muscarinic
receptors are thought to be mainly intact (28) and amenable to pharmacological manipulation. Therefore, many attempts have been made at treating Alzheimer's patients with cholinergic compounds, with mixed success. One
reason for difficulties with the cholinergic approach to treatment of Alzheimer's disease may be that most muscarinic agonists stimulate both pre-
and postsynaptic receptors. Agonist action at presynaptic muscarinic receptors may be counter-productive since it inhibits the release of acetylcholine in the remaining fibers. It has been suggested that muscarinic
agents like BM 5, which are presynaptic antagonists and postsynaptic agonists (26), are potentially useful in treating Alzheimer's dementia (29).

We have derivatized acetylenic amines related to oxotremorine using the functionalized congener approach (30). The muscarinic agonist UH 5, 14 (Figure 3), first synthesized in 1966 (24), contains an acetyl group, which was probed as a site for derivatization through the preparation of compounds 15-18.

In order to determine whether this acetyl group constitutes a site at which chains of varying length and composition are tolerated in receptor binding, a series of alkyl amino derivatives, 15a-g, was synthesized. The amine-derivatized chain in each case consisted of an n-alkyl chain of length 1-7 methylene units, terminating in the chemically reactive amino group. Several standard acyl modifications of the amino group were included, in order to evaluate the effects of charged vs. uncharged and hydrophilic vs. hydrophobic groups and the effects of bulky substituents at varying distances (in the extended conformation) from the main pharmacophore. Thus N-acetyl, 16, and certain N-benzoyl, 17, substituents were prepared. For each chain length, the N-t-butyloxycarbonyl derivative, 18, the synthetic precursor of the free amine, was also tested for biological activity.

This series of modifications, in which the acetyl group of 14 was extended formalistically to long, functionalized chains, suggested the synthesis of a common intermediate, N-methyl-4-(1-pyrrolidinyl)-2-butynamine, 19. 19 is a secondary amine which was acylated with urethane protected ω-amino acids to yield 18. The protecting groups were removed in acidic conditions without affecting the acetylenic group, to yield 15.

RESULTS

We have examined BM 5, 13, and new muscarinic agents, synthesized by the functionalized congener approach (see above), for effects on second messengers and by ligand binding techniques in cell membranes. Biological activity in SK-N-SH and NG108-15 cells were examined through the stimulation of PI turnover and inhibition of cyclic AMP accumulation, respectively, and compared to the activity of oxotremorine-M, 12. Inhibition of binding of [^{3}H]NMS in membranes derived from each cell type was examined as a measure of the affinity of antagonists for that receptor subtype. The degree of inhibition of binding of [^{3}H]N-methylscopolamine (NMS) by agonists is perhaps not directly comparable with the data for antagonists, due to the receptor conformational changes induced by agonists.

BM 5 was found to be a selective agonist (14) at muscarinic receptors linked to the inhibition of production of cyclic AMP as a second messenger system (IC$_{50}$ = 0.4 ± 0.1 µM). The metabolism of PI was not affected by BM 5, even at high concentrations. Thus, BM 5 displayed selectivity as an m4 (versus m3) agonist. Moreover, BM 5 was active at m2 receptors (also linked to adenylate cyclase) and inactive at m1 receptors.

Figure 4a shows a comparison of the activities of the butynyl amines synthesized in the inhibition of cyclic AMP accumulation in NG108-15 cells. All of the derivatives were inactive or nearly inactive in the stimulation of PI turnover in SK-N-SH cells, yet, several members at a concentration of 100 µM inhibited cyclic AMP accumulation. This activity was displayed primarily by the free amine derivatives and only by the shorter members of the homologous series (particularly chain lengths of one and two methylenes, conjugates of glycine and ß-alanine, respectively). Thus, compounds 15a and 15b are weak, but selective (versus activity at m3 receptors) m4 agonists.

Relative affinity obtained in competitive binding experiments in cell

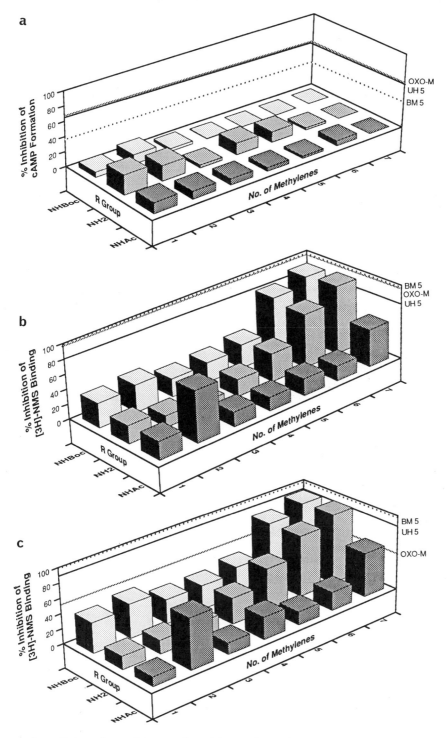

Figure 4.   Potencies of butynyl amide analogs in a functional assay (a) at
m4 receptors in NG108-15 cells and in binding assays at (b) m4
receptors (NG108-15 cell membranes) and at (c) m3 receptors (SK-
N-SH cell membranes). Compounds tested correspond to 15 (NH₂),
16 (NHAc), and 18 (NHBoc), all a-g (structures given in Figure
3), present at a concentration of 100 µM.

7

membranes using [^{3}H]NMS as a radioligand are shown in Figures 4b and 4c. The data are expressed as percent displacement of [^{3}H]NMS at a constant concentration of the agent (100 μM). Strikingly, the apparent affinity increases in direct relation to the chain length - the longer members of the series compete well for [^{3}H]NMs sites. The longest member of the amine series, containing seven methylene units (15g), displaces [^{3}H]NMs slightly more effectively than does oxo-M. Since these derivatives bearing longer chains display no biological activity in either cyclic AMP accumulation or PI assays, they are putative antagonists.

Compound 15c, a derivative of gamma-aminobutyric acid was condensed with a second urethane protected amino acid. The "di(amino acid)" conjugates of 15c coupled to Boc-glycine and Boc-B-alanine were devoid of agonist activity and displayed partial selectivity for m3 receptors in binding assays. This finding was in contrast to results for most of the putative antagonists, which were non-selective for m3 versus m4 receptors in binding assays.

CONCLUSIONS

Certain long-chain derivatives related to oxotremorine are muscarinic antagonists. For these antagonists the affinity at m3 and m4 receptors increases with chain length. Conjugates of glycine and of ß-alanine, compounds 15a and 15b, respectfully, are weak, but selective agonists at m4 receptors. We will explore other sites on butynyl amine molecules for functionalization, in an effort to enhance muscarinic agonist potency and selectivity.

REFERENCES

1. Bonner, T. I., Buckley, N. J., Young, A. C. and Brann, M. R. (1987) Identification of a family of muscarinic acetylcholine receptor genes.Science 237: 527-532.
2. Peralta, E. G., Ashkenazi, A., Winslow, J. W., Smith, D. H. , Ramachandran, J. and Capon, D. J. (1987) Distinct primary structures, ligand-binding properties and tissue-specific expression of four human muscarinic acetylcholine receptors. EMBO J. 6: 3923-3929.
3. Maeda, A., Kubo, T., Mishina, M. and Numa, S. (1988) Tissue distribution of mRNAs encoding muscarinic acetylcholine receptor subtypes. FEBS Lett. 239: 339-342.
4. Bonner, T. I., Young, A. C., Brann, M. R. and Buckley, N. J. (1988) Cloning and expression of human and rat m5 muscarinic acetylcholine receptor genes. Neuron 1: 403-410.
5. Jacobson, K. A., Ukena, D., Kirk, K. L., and Daly, J. W. (1986a) [3H]Xanthine amine congener of 1,3-dipropyl-8-phenylxanthine: an antagonist radioligand for adenosine receptors. Proc. Natl. Acad. Sci. USA 83: 4089-4093.
6. Jacobson, K. A., Kirk, K. L., Padgett, W. L., and Daly, J. W. (1986b) A functionalized congener approach to adenosine receptor antagonists: amino acid conjugates of 1,3-dipropylxanthine. Mol. Pharmacol. 29: 126-133.
7. Jacobson, K. A., Ukena, D., Padgett, W., Kirk, K. L., Daly, J. W. (1987) Molecular probes for extracellular adenosine receptors. Biochem. Pharmacol. 36: 1697-1707.
8. Barrington, W., Jacobson, K. A., Hutchison, A. J., Williams, M., and Stiles, G. (1989) Identification of the A2 adenosine receptor binding subunit by photoaffinity crosslinking. Proc. Natl. Acad. Sci. USA, in press.
9. Hammer, R., Berrie, C. P., Birdsall, N. J. M., Burgen, A. S. V., and Hulme, E. C. (1980) Pirenzepine distinguishes between different subclasses of muscarinic receptors. Nature 283: 90-92.

10. Eglen, R. M. and Whiting, R. L. (1986) Muscarinic receptor subtypes: a critique of the current classification and a proposal for a working nomenclature. J. Auton. Pharmac. 5: 323-346.

11. Baumgold, J. and White, T. (1989) Coupling and pharmacological characteristics of muscarinic receptors from SK-N-SH human neuroblastoma cells: comparison with those from NG108-15 cells. Biochem. Pharmacol. 38: 1605-1616.

12. Peralta, E. G. , Ashkenazi, A. , Winslow, J. W. , Ramachandran, J. and Capon, D. J. (1988) Differential regulation of PI hydrolysis and adenylyl cyclase by muscarinic receptor subtypes. Nature 334: 434-437.

13. Shapiro, R. ., Schere, N. M., Habecker, B. A., Subers, E. M., and Nathanson, N. M. (1988) Isolation, sequence and functional expression of the mouse Ml muscarinic acetylcholine receptor gene. J. Biol. Chem. 263: 18397-18403.

14. Baumgold, J. and Drobnick, A. (1989) An agonist that is selective for adenylate cyclase coupled muscarinic receptors. Mol. Pharmacol., submitted.

15. Doods, H. N. (1987) Selective muscarinic antagonist for peripheral muscarinic receptor subtypes. In: Pharmacology (eds: Rand, M.J. and Raper C.), Elsevier Science, New York, pp. 59-66.

16. Nilvebrant, L. and Sparf, B. (1988) Receptor binding profiles of some selective muscarinic antagonists. Eur. J. Pharmacol. 151: 83-96.

17. Rzeszotarski, W. J., McPherson, D. W.., Ferkany, J. W.., Kinnier, W. J., Noronha-Blob, L., and Kirdien-Rzeszotarski, A. (1988) Affinity and selectivity of the optical isomers of 3-quinuclidinyl benzilate and related muscarinic agonists. J. Med. Chem. 31: 1463-1466.

18. Chang, Y-F. (1988) Structure-binding relationship of quinuclidinyl benzilate analogs on N4TGl neuroblastoma muscarinic receptors. Neurochem. Res. 13: 455-462.

19. Melchiorre, C. (1988) Polymethylene tetramines: A new generation of selective muscarinic anatagonists. Trends Pharmacol. Sci. 9: 216-220.

20. Ono, S., Saito, Y., Ohgane, N., Kawanishi, G., and Mizobe, F.(1988) Heterogeneity of muscarinic autoreceptors and heteroreceptors in the rat brain: effects of a novel Ml agonist, AF102B. Eur. J. Pharmacol. 155: 77-84.

21. Ringdahl, B. and Jenden, D. J. (1983) Pharmacological properties of oxotremorine and its analogs. Life Sci. 32: 2401-2413.

22. Fisher, S. K., Klinger, P. D. and Agranoff, B. W. (1983) Muscarinic agonist binding and phospholipid turnover in brain. J. Biol. Chem. 258: 7358-7363.

23. Nilsson, B. J., Ringdahl, B. and Hacksell, U. (1988) Derivatives of the muscarinic agent N-methyl-N-(1-methyl-4-pyrrolidino-2- butynyl)acetamide. J. Med. Chem. 31: 577-582.

24. Bebbington, A., Brimblecombe, R. W. and Shakeshaft, D. (1966) The central and peripheral activity of acetylenic amines related to oxotremorine. Brit. J. Pharmacol. 26: 56-67.

25. Resul, B., Dahlbom, R., Ringdahl, B. and Jenden, D. J. (1982) N-Alkyl- N-(4-tert-amino-1-methyl-2-butynyl)carboxamides, a new class of potent oxotremorine antagonists. Eur. J. Med. Chem. 17: 317-322.

26. Casamenti, F., Cosi, C., and Pepeu, G. (1986) Effect of BM-5, a presynaptic agonist, on cortical acetylcholine release. Eur. J. Pharmacol 122: 288-290.

27. Whitehouse, P. J., Price, D. L., Struble, R. G., Clark, A. W., Coyle, J. T., and DeLong, M. R. (1982) Alzheimer's disease and senile dementia: los of neurons in the basal forebrain. Science 215: 1237-1239.

28. Kellar, K. J., Whitehouse, P. J., Martino-Barrows, A. M., Marcus, K., and Price, D. L. (1987) Muscarinic and nicotinic cholinergic binding sites in the Alzheimer's disease cerebral cortex. Brain Res. 436: 62-68.

29. Hershenson, F. M. and Moos, W. H. (1986) Drug development for senile cognitive decline. J. Med. Chem. 29: 1125-1130.

30. Bradbury, B., Baumgold, J., and Jacobson, K. A. (1989) Functionalized congener approach for the design of novel muscarinic agents. Synthesis an pharmacological evaluation of N-methyl-N-[4 -(1-pyrrolidinyl)-2- butynyl] amides. J. Med. Chem., submitted.

AF102B: A NOVEL Ml AGONIST AS A RATIONAL TREATMENT STRATEGY IN ALZHEIMER'S DISEASE

Abraham Fisher, Rachel Brandeis, Ishai Karton, Zipora Pittel, Shlomit Dachir, Michal Sapir, Y. Grunfeld, Aharon Levy and Eliahu Heldman

Israel Institute for Biological Research, P.O.Box 19, Ness-Ziona 70450, Israel

INTRODUCTION

Alzheimer's disease (AD), a progressive cerebral neurodegenerative disorder with no effective treatment as yet, is known to affect 5-7% of the population over age 65. This disorder is characterized by a progressive deterioration of cognitive and mnemonic abilities. Morphological, neurochemical and behavioral studies indicate a major degeneration of the central cholinergic .system in AD (1, 2). There is also evidence that noradrenergic, serotonergic, and somatostatin-like immunoreactivity are abnormal in AD, though to a lesser extent (for reviews see refs. 3 and 4). The contribution of the cholinergic dysfunction to the cognitive symptoms in AD is indicated by a direct correlation between loss of presynaptic cholinergic markers and mental test scores (1, 2). Postmortem evaluations of brains from patients with AD have revealed a select degeneration of cholinergic cells in the basal forebrain which project to the cerebral cortex and hippocampus (reviews 1-3). This degeneration is associated with a marked reduction of presynaptic cholinergic indices in these brain regions involved in cognitive processes (5). Somewhat conflicting results were reported regarding muscarinic receptors in AD. A loss of M2 muscarinic receptors was reported in a few studies (6-8 but see also 9, 10) while postsynaptic muscarinic receptors are relatively unchanged (6-9), decreased (10) or even upregulated (11).

Given presynaptic but not postsynaptic losses in AD, the demented state might be altered by treatment of cholinergic hypofunction. In principle, an increase in central cholinergic activity can be achieved via presynaptic or postsynaptic modulation. The greatest effort to date has been directed toward a so-called "replacement therapy" which should enhance cholinergic activity (for reviews see refs 12, 13). Such therapeutic strategies tried in the clinic include: a) precursors of acetylcholine, ACh, (e.g. choline, lecithin); b) enhancers of ACh release (e.g. 4-aminopyridine); c) inhibitors of acetylcholinesterase (e. g. physostigmine, tacrine); d) muscarinic agonists (e.g. arecoline, bethanecol, RS86, oxotremorine and pilocarpine); e) nootropic compounds believed to enhance cholinergic stimulation (e.g. piracetam, aniracetam and oxiracetam).

The outcome of the clinical trials ranked from lack of significant success to modest improvement (12, 13). The reasons for the modest effects in AD patients with the currently available cholinergic compounds remain obscure. Some could be attributed to the properties of the drugs tested such as: short duration of action, lack of selectivity for brain reglons involved In memory processes leading to central side-effects, adverse peripheral side-effects, variable penetration of the blood-brain barrier, and narrow therapeutic indices.

In order to obtain drugs with fewer disadvantages, Ml selective agonists have been suggested as a rational treatment strategy in AD (2, 12, 14). Such a candidate drug should have all or at least most of the following properties: a. selectivity for synapses involved in cognitive functions; b. positive effects on mnemonic processes; c. lack of peripheral and central side- effects; d. wide therapeutic index; e. passage through the blood- brain barrier; f. adequate pharmacokinetic profile and activity when taken orally; g. long duration of action; h. lack of or minimal tolerance when administered chronically.

Since ACh is a highly flexible molecule capable of attaining a number of conformations with the same energy, one can speculate that it is this conformational flexibility which enables this neurotransmitter to interact with all types of cholinergic receptors (e.g. Ml, M2, and further subtypes and nicotinic). In this context, we have hypothesized that a rational drug design of an Ml selective agonist could be via rigid analogs of ACh. This is based on the premise that the utmost rigidity limits the ability of ligands to adapt to minor differences in receptor structure and thereby provides selectivity towards a limited population of receptors. (±)-Cis-2-methyl-spiro(1,3-oxathiolane-5,3')quinuclidine (AF102B), a closely related analog of ACh embodying the "muscarinic pharmacophore" in a framework of utmost rigidity, is such a selective Ml agonist (14-16). The aim of this paper is to overview some of the properties of AF102B in vitro and in vivo and to show that this compound fulfills most of the conditions required for an ideal muscarinic drug aimed to treat AD.

RESULTS AND DISCUSSION

AF102B is a full muscarinic agonist as shown on the isolated guinea-pig ileum and trachea, being 87 and 1.3 fold less potent than ACh (16). One of the remarkable features of AF102B is its Ml selectivity. This was shown in a number of studies including:

1. **Binding studies.** These experiments were done with selective and non-selective radiolabelled ligands (in vitro, rat brain regions) and in comparison with muscarinic agonists such as: oxotremorine and carbachol (CCh) (mainly M2 agonists), McN-A-343 (a prototype Ml ganglionic stimulant), cis-AF30 and trans-AF30 (relatively selective ganglionic and central muscarinic agonists (17-19). The relative Ml selectivity was assayed using the radiolabelled ligands: ^{3}H-pirenzepine (^{3}H-PZ) an Ml selective antagonist (20), (-)-^{3}H-QNB (a mixed Ml and M2 antagonist), (21, 22); and (+)- ^{3}H-cis-dioxolane, a mixed Ml and M2 agonist with some preference for M2 receptors (23). In these studies, on rat forebrain or frontal cortex homogenates, AF102B showed preference for PZ-sensitive binding sites (16). In the same line, when evaluated on rat forebrain (rich in Ml receptors) vs. cerebellum homogenates (predominantly M2 receptors; see refs. 21, 24) respectively, AF102B had higher affinity for the first, as expected from a selective Ml probe (unpublished results). In fact, when compared with the other agonists in this study, AF102B is most selective for Ml receptor sites (15).

2. **Functional and neurochemical studies**. All foregoing experiments support the Ml selectivity of this compound. Thus in contrast to CCh, AF102B did not potentiate phosphoinositides (PI) hydrolysis nor did it inhibit adenylate cyclase (AC) activity in rat cerebral cortex in vitro; however, AF102B blocked CCh-induced activation of PI hydrolysis without altering CCh-induced inhibition of AC (15). This would imply that AF102B, as an Ml probe, is apparently more selective than PZ, since the later shows only a 15 fold preference for Ml sites (e.g. inhibition of CCh-induced stimulation of PI turnover) vs M2 sites (e.g. inhibition of CCh-induced inhibition of AC activity), (25). The remarkable Ml agonistic activity of AF102B was shown in the following studies: i) Both AF102B and McN-A-343 induced only PZ- sensitive depolarization of isolated rabbit superior cervical ganglion (26); ii) AF102B had preferential (40 fold) agonistic activity on potassium-evoked release of H-dopamine as compared to release ^{3}H-ACh in rat striatal and hippocampal synaptosomes, respectively (27). The Ml agonistic activity of AF102B in this study was attributed to the finding that muscarinic autoreceptors regulating ACh release and heteroreceptors controlling dopamine release were classified as M2 and Ml subtype, respectively, based on their affinities to PZ (28).

In line with the above mentioned findings, whole body autoradiography revealed that ^{3}H-AF102B (mice; 2.3mg/kg, iv) concentrates preferentially in brain regions rich in Ml receptors such as the cerebrum but significantly less in the cerebellum (predominantly M2 receptors). These findings together with pharmacokinetic studies reveal that, regardless of the route of administration, AF102B is capable of crossing the blood- brain barrier at a very short time after peripheral administration and has a rapid plasma absorption (unpublished results).

Since the etiology of AD is unknown, there is no perfect animal model capable of modelling all aspects of this neurological disoder. Under such limitations the evaluation of new drugs for the treatment of AD would require approximate animal models that mimic different aspects of this disease. Therefore, AF102B was evaluated, inter alia, in the following animal models:

i. **Ethylcholine aziridinium (AF64A)-induced cholinotoxicity (3 nmole/2 µl/ side, icv) in rats (29)**. AF64A induces a long-term presynaptic cholinergic hypofunction confined mainly to the hippocampus which mimics the cholinergic dysfunction in AD. In this model, AF102B (1-5 mg/kg, ip or po) consistenly restored cognitive impairments (inter alia) in a step-through passive avoidance (PA), a Morris water maze (MWM) and an 8-arm radial maze (RAM) task. Physostigmine (0.06 and 0.1 mg/kg, ip, for PA and MWM, RAM, respectively), was beneficial only in the PA test (15, 16, 30) for example.

ii. **Scopolamine model and aged rats.** In this context, cognitive dysfunctions induced by scopolamine in young human volunteers mimic some clinical manifestations of AD patients (31) and old rats can serve as a useful model for the study of behavioral aspects of brain aging in the human (32). In these animals, AF102B (3-5 mg/kg, ip) restored scopolamine-HBr (0.5 mg/kg, sc)-induced cognitive impairments in a PA task. Furthermore, AF102B (1 mg/kg, ip) attenuated aged (19-26 old months) rats associated cognitive impairments in MWM (reference memory) and RAM (working memory) task, respectively. Similar results using AF102B in a PA task were recently reported in AF64A- treated rats and in scopolamine-induced amnesia in mice (33).

AF102B has a wide therapeutic index since it restores cognitive impairments in these animal models at 50-100 fold lower doses than required to induce other unwanted central or peripheral cholinomimetic effects. The beneficial activity of AF102B in all these behavoral tests may be attributed to its unique Ml selectivity.

A prerequisite for a drug that has to be administered chronically is that it should not produce tolerance to its beneficial effects. In this regard, repetitive administration of AF102B (0.2 mg/ kg/ day, ip for three weeks) restored cognitive function in AF64A-treated rats in the MWM (working memory paradigm) without a diminuition of the effect of the agonist. This might be in line with the findings that, although AF102B is a full agonist on the guinea-pig ileum, no down-regulation of muscarinic receptors (assayed from Bmax and Kd using ^{3}H-QNB as the radioligand) from rat forebrain occured upon chronic daily administration of AF102B (po, 5-100 mg/kg; 14 and 90 days studies), (unpublished results). The absence of desensitization or tolerance in both binding and behavioral studies could be attributed to lack of stimulation of AF102B on PI turnover in the rat cerebral cortex. Two studies demonstrating a direct correlation between desensitization and PI turnover in rat brain are described briefly in order to support our hypothesis. Thus, PI turnover induced by full agonists (maximal stimulation of PI turnover; class A) was associated with the desensitization of electrophysiological responses following prolonged ejection periods of the compounds on hippocampal pyramidal cells. On the other hand partial agonists (poor stimulation of PI turnover; class B) produced stimulatory responses upon prolonged ejection without causing a desensitization (34). A recent study showed that muscarinic desensitization of cell-firing in rat hippocampus is related to large increases in PI hydrolysis. All muscarinic agonists tested stimulated firing to a similar extent, but the efficacy for stimulation of PI hydrolysis varied greatly. Decreases in firing rate (desensitization) occurred at a threshold of PI turnover except for oxotremorine (e.g. a class B agonist) which did not exhibit desensitization (35). Based on these reports and our results regarding AF102B, we can hypothesize that a rational drug design of Ml muscarinic agonists should focus especially on those compounds which are poor stimulators of PI turnover, since then no desensitization is expected to occur. In fact, AF102B can represent such a compound.

In conclusion, all these new features of AF102B, together with others previously reported, indicate that AF102B may be considered a rational candidate drug for treating AD and is presently under extensive development to achieve this important goal.

Acknowlededmement: This work was supported by Snow Brand, Tokyo, Japan.

REFERENCES

1. Bartus, R.T., Dean, R.L., Beer, B. and Lippa, A.S. (1982) The cholinergic hypothesis of geriatric memory dysfunction. Science 217: 408-417.
2. Whitehouse, P.J. (1986) Neuronal loss and neurotransmitter receptor alterations in Alzheimer's disease, In: Alzheimer's and Parkinson's Diseases: Strategies for Research and Development. (eds. Fisher, A., Hanin, I and Lachman, C.) Plenum Press, New York pp. 85-94.
3. Whitehouse, P. J. and Unnerstall, J.R. (1988) Neurochemistry of dementia. Eur. Neurol. 28 (suppl.): 36-41.
4. Rossor, M. N., and Iversen, L. L. (1986) Non-cholinergic neurotransmitter abnormalities in Alzheimer's disease. Br. Med. Bull. 42: 70-74.
5. Sims, N. R., Bowen, D. M., Allen, S. J., Smith, C. C. T., Neary, D., Thomas, D.J., and Davison, A.N. (1983) J. Neurochem. 40: 503-509.
6. Mash, D.C., Flynn, D.D. and Potter, L.T. (1985) Loss of M2 muscarine receptors in the cerebral cortex in Alzheimer's disease and experimental cholinergic denervation. Science 228: 115-117.
7. Araujo, D. M., Lapchak, P. A., Robitaille, Y., Gauthier, S., and Quirion, R. (1988) Differential alteration of various cholinergic markers in cortical and subcortical regions of human brain in Alzheimer's disease. J. Neurochem. 50: 1914-1923.
8. Rinne, J. 0., Lonnberg, P., Marjamaki, P. and Rinne, U. K. (1989) Brain muscarinic receptor subtypes are differently affected in Alzheimer's disease and Parkinson's disease. Brain Res. 483: 402-406.
9. Probst, A., Cortes, R., Ulrich, J., and Palacios, J. M. (1988) Differential modification of muscarinic cholinergic receptors in the hippocampus of patients with Alzheimer's disease: an autoradiographic study. Brain Res. 450: 190-201.
10. Smith, C. J., Perry, E. K., Perry, R. H., Candy, J. M., Johnson, M., Bonham, J. R., Dick, D.J., Fairbairn, A., Blessed, G., and Birdsall, N. J. M. (1988) Muscarinic cholinergic receptor subtypes in hippocampus in human cognitive disorders. J. Neurochem. 50: 847-856.
11. Waller, S.B., Ball, M.J., Reynolds, M.A. and London, E.D. (1986) Muscarinic binding and choline acetyltransferase in postmortem brains of demented patients. Can. J. Neurol. Sci. 53: 528-532.
12. Moos, W. H., Davis, R. E., Schwarcz, R.D. and Gamzu, E.R. (1988) Cognition. Med. Res. Rev. 8: 353-391.
13. Becker, R. E. and Giacobini, E. (1988) Mechanisms of cholinesterase inhibition in senile dementia of the Alzheimer type: clinical, pharmacological, and therapeutic aspects. Dev. Res. 12: 163-195.
14. Fisher, A., Karton, I., Heldman, I., Levy, A. and Grunfeld, I. (1986). Derivatives of quinuclidine. Israel Patent.
15. Fisher, A., Brandeis, R., Pittel, Z., Karton, I., Sapir, M., Dachir, S., Levy, A., Mizobe, F. and Heldman, E. (1987) AF102B: A new Ml agonist with potential application in Alzheimer's disease. Soc. Neurosci. (Abstr.) 13: 657.
16. Fisher, A., Brandeis, R., Pittel Z., Karton I., Sapir, M., Dachir, S., Levy, A. and Heldman E.(1989).(+)Cis-2-methyl-spiro(1,3-oxathiolane-5,3')quinuclidine (AF102B):a new Ml agonist attenuates cognitive dysfunctions in AF64A-treated rats. Neurosci. Lett., in press.

17. Fisher, A., Weinstock, M., Gitter, S. and Cohen, S. (1976) A new probe for heterogeneity in muscarine receptors: 2- Methyl-spiro(1,3-dioxolane-4,3')-quinuclidine. Eur. J. Pharmacol. 37: 329-338.
18. Palacios, J.M., Bolliger, G., Closse, A., Enz, A., Gmelin, G. and Malanowski, J. (1986) Th e p h a rm acological assessment of RS 86 (2-ethyl-8-methyl-2,8-diazaspiro-[4,5]-decan-1,3- dion hydrobromide). A potent, specific muscarinic acetylcholine receptor agonist. Eur. J. Pharmacol. 125: 45-62.
19. Pazos, A., Wiederhold, K.H. and Palacios, J.M. (1986) Central pressor effects induced by muscarinic receptor agonists: evidence for a predominant role of M2 receptor subtype. Eur. J. Pharmacol. 125: 63-70.
20. Hammer, R., Berrie, C.P., Birdsall, N.J.M., Burger, A.S.V. and Hulme, E.C. (1980) Pirenzepine distinguishes between different subclasses of muscarinic receptors. Nature 283: 90-92.
21. Tonnaer, J.A.D.M., Van Vugt, M.A., DeBoer, T.H. and DeGraaf, J.S. (1987) Differential interactions of muscarinic drugs with binding sites of [3H]pirenzepine and [3H]-quinuclidinyl benzilate in rat brain tissue. Life Sciences 40: 1981-1987.
22. Watson, M., Yamamura, H.I. and Roeske, W.R. (1986) [3H]Pirenzepine and [3H]quinuclidinyl benzilate binding to rat cerebral cortical and cardiac muscarinic cholinergic sites. I. Characterization and regulation of agonist binding to putative muscarinic subtypes J. Pharmacol. Exptl. Therap. 237: 411-418.
23. Closse, A., Bittiger, H., Langenegger, D. and Wanner, A. (1987) Binding studies with [3H]cis-methyldioxolane in different tissues. N. S. Arch. Pharmacol. 333: 372-377.
24. Potter, L.T., Flynn, D.D., Hanchett, H.E. and Kalinski, D.L.D. (1984) Independent Ml and M2 receptors: ligands, autoradiography and functions, In: Subtypes of Muscarinic Receptors. Trends Pharmacol.Sci. (suppl.) (eds. Hirschowitz B.I., Hammer, R., Giachetti, A., Keirns, J.J. and Levine, R.R.) Elsevier Science Publishers UK, (1984) pp. 22-31.
25. Gil, D.W. and Wolfe, B.B. (1985) Pirenzepine distinguishes between muscarinic receptor-mediated phosphoinositide breakdown and inhibitors of adenylate cyclase. J. Pharmacol. Exptl. Therap. 232: 608-616.
26. Mochida, S., Mizobe, F., Fisher, A., Kawanishi, G. and Kobayashi, H. (1988) Selective Ml muscarinic agonists McN-A-343 and AF102B cause dual effects on superior cervical ganglia of rabbits, Brain. Res. 45: 9-17.
27. Ono, S., Saito, Y., Ohgane, N., Kawanishi, G., and Mizobe, F. (1988) Heterogeneity of muscarinic autoreceptors and heteroreceptors in the rat brain: effects of a novel Ml agonist, AF102B. Eur. J.Pharmacol. 155: 77-84.
28. Marchi, M and Raiteri, M. (1985) On the presence in the cerebral cortex of muscarinic receptor subtypes which differ in neuronal localization, function and pharmacological properties. J. Pharmacol. Exptl. Therap. 235: 230-233.
29. Fisher, A. and Hanin, 1. (1986) Potential animal models for senile dementia of Alzheimer's type with particular emphasis on AF64A-induced cholinotoxicity. Ann. Rev. Pharmacol. Toxicol. 26: 161-181.
30. Brandeis, R., Pittel, Z., Lachman, C., Heldman, E., Luz, S., Dachir, S., Levy, A., Hanin, I. and Fisher, A. (1986) AF64A-induced cholinotoxicity: behavioral and biochemical correlates. In: Alzheimer's and Parkinson's Diseases: Strategies for Research and Development (eds: Fisher, A., Hanin, I. and Lachman, C.) Plenum Press, New York, pp. 469-477.
31. Drachman, D.A. and Leavitt, J.L. (1974) Human memory and the cholinergic system. A relationship to aging? Arch. Neurol. 30: 113-121.
32. Schuurman, T., Horvath, E., Spencer, D.G., Jr. and Traber, J. (1986) Old rats: an animal model for senile dementia In: Senile Dementias: Early Detection (eds. Bes A., Cahn, J., Hoyer, S., Marc-Vergnes, J.P. and Wisniewski, H.M.) John Libbey Eurotext, London, Paris pp. 624-630.
33. Nakahara, N., Iga, Y., Mizobe, F., and Kawanishi G. (1988) Amelioration of experimental amnesia (passive avoidance failure) in rodents by the selective Ml agonist AF102B. Japan. J. Pharmacol. 48: 502-506.

34. Lippa A.S., Crichett, D.J. and Joseph, J.A. (1986) Desensitization of muscarinic acetylcholine receptors: a possible relation to receptor heterogeneity and phosphoinositides. Brain Res. 366: 98-105.
35. Crews F.T., Pontzer, N.J. and Chandler, L.J. (1989) Muscarinic cholinergic neurotransmission: receptor subtypes and signal transduction. First Ann. Suncoast Workshop on the Neurobiology of Aging, St. Petersburg, Fl., USA, Feb 26-March 1.

MUSCARINIC RECEPTORS, PHOSPHOINOSITIDE HYDROLYSIS, AND NEURONAL PLASTICITY IN THE HIPPOCAMPUS

Fulton T. Crews, Norbert J. Pontzer and L. Judson Chandler

Department of Pharmacology and Therapeutics
Box J-267, J.H. Miller Health Center
University of Florida College of Medicine
Gainesville, FL 32610

Previous studies have suggested that muscarinic cholinergic receptors in the hippocampus are associated with memory processes. Antimuscarinic drugs, well known for their amnestic effects, support the cholinergic hypothesis of memory (Bartus et al,, 1982). Several biochemical and electrophysiological responses to muscarinic agonist stimulation have been described in the hippocampus, including reduction of a calcium-dependent potassium current (IK_{ca}) that is responsible for after-hyperpolarization (AHP) (Bernado and Prince, 1982), reduction of a time- and voltage-dependent non-inactivating potassium current termed the M-current (IK_m) (Halliwell and Adams, 1982), inhibition of cyclic-AMP (Olianas et al., 1983), stimulation of cyclic-GMP (Snyder et al., 1984), and stimulation of phosphoinositide (PI) turnover (Gonzales and Crews, 1985; Fisher and Bartus, 1985). This multiplicity of responses has obscured the relationship between biochemical and electrophysiological responses to muscarinic agonists. In addition, the relationship between muscarinic action on specific membrane ionic conductances, especially IK_m, and neuronal action potential generation, is not clear.

Muscarinic agonists have been subdivided into two groups according to their binding affinities and efficacy for stimulation of PI hydrolysis (Fisher et al., 1983). Carbachol and muscarine are representative of "type A" agonists that bind to two sites and are full agonists at stimulation of PI hydrolysis. Oxotremorine and pilocarpine are representative of "type B" muscarinic agonists that bind to a single site and are partial agonists for stimulation of PI hydrolysis. In agreement with a previous report by Fisher et al. (1983), we observed that carbachol best fit a 2 site model for PI hydrolysis (Figure 1). The existence of similar two-site interactions for both binding and biochemical response suggest that carbachol acts on two separate sites to stimulate PI turnover, while partial agonists like oxotremorine, probably act at only a single site. Both of these receptors are likely to be postsynaptic to the cholinergic innervation (Fisher et al, 1980).

Muscarinic agonists probably increase neuronal excitability by inhibiting IK_{ca}, IK_m, and a more recently described voltage-insensitive "leak" potassium current (Madison et al., 1987). Inactivation of IK_{ca} by both carbachol and oxotremorine would increase action potential discharge rates by reducing accommodation (Madison and Nicoll, 1984).

Carbachol inactivates IK_{ca} with an EC_{50} of about 0.3 mM and a maximal effect at about 5 mM (Madison et al, 1987). This is similar to the concentration range over which we observe both carbachol stimulated cell firing and the high potency component of PI hydrolysis. Thus, it is likely that inactivation of IK_{ca} is at least partly responsible for the increase in firing rates produced by low concentrations of carbachol. Like carbachol, oxotremorine also inactivates IK_{ca} and the "leak" potassium current (Dutar and Nicoll, 1988a, 1988b). However, oxotremorine does not decrease the IK_m. Taken together, these findings suggest that increased neuronal firing induced by both full and partial muscarinic PI agonists is due to agonist stimulation at a muscarinic site that inhibits IK_{ca} and/or the "leak" current.

The similarity in the concentration-response curves for muscarinic stimulated firing rate and PI hydrolysis (when the high affinity component of the full PI agonist two-site fit is used) suggests that there may be a relation between the two responses. Since phorbol esters have been reported to inhibit IK_{ca} (Baraban et al., 1985; Malenka et al., 1986), it is possible that DAG, formed during receptor mediated PI hydrolysis, could increase cell firing by inhibiting IK_{ca}. However, due to oxotremorine's low efficacy for PI hydrolysis, the ability of oxotremorine to inhibit IK_{ca} has been interpreted as evidence against a causal role for PI hydrolysis in IK_{ca} inhibition (Dutar and Nicoll, 1988b). Since sequences of muscarinic receptor mRNA suggest that all subtypes interact with G-proteins, direct G-protein interaction with IK_{ca} mediated by the high potency muscarinic receptor cannot be ruled out (see Figure 3).

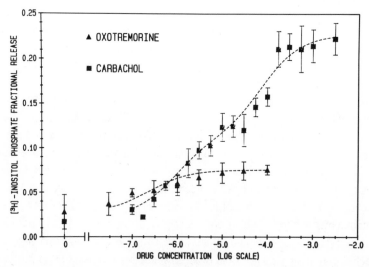

Figure 1. *Comparison of the concentration-response relationship for carbachol and oxotremorine stimulated phosphoinositide hydrolysis in hippocampal slices. Slices were prelabeled with [³H]inositol, and phosphoinositide hydrolysis expressed as the fraction of total incorporated [³H]inositol that accumulated as inositol phosphates after 60 min of stimulation in the presence of 8 mM lithium. Nonlinear curve fitting of the data to one and two site models showed that carbachol best fits a two-site model and was a full agonist, while oxotremorine was a partial agonist and best fits one site.*

Although the functional effect of a reduction in IK_m has not yet been elucidated, our data suggest that sufficient inhibition of this current may decrease firing rates. The overlap of the IK_m voltage activation-inactivation range with spike threshold, and its non-transient nature, imply a powerful ability to alter cell firing rate by affecting neuronal membrane repolarization. Madison et al. (1987) reported that carbachol blocks IK_m with an EC_{50} of about 5 mM and a maximal effect at about 30 mM. This is within the concentration range in which we observe desensitization (Figure 2). Thus, the closeness of the concentration-response curves for carbachol induced desensitization and inhibition of IK_m suggests that desensitization of cell firing may be due to muscarinic mediated blockade of IK_m. Oxotremorine, which does not inhibit IK_m (Dutar and Nicoll, 1988b) and does not desensitize, can block (Dutar and Nicoll, 1988a) and reverse (Dutar and Nicoll, 1988b) the actions of full muscarinic PI agonists on IK_m, and can block and reverse desensitization by carbachol (Pontzer and Crews, 1989). Thus, oxotremorine may pharmacologically distinguish a higher potency binding site associated with increased cell firing and inhibition of IK_{ca} from a lower potency binding site at which oxotremorine can block carbachol mediated desensitization of cell firing, inhibition of IK_m, and increases in PI hydrolysis.

Evidence suggests there is a PI hydrolysis threshold associated with decreased cell firing for those muscarinic agonists (e.g. carbachol) that produce desensitization (Pontzer and Crews, 1989). Oxotremorine, the weakest PI agonist, does not reach this threshold and does not desensitize. Bethanechol and arecoline barely reach the PI threshold and desensitize more slowly with increasing concentration than carbachol or muscarine. Lippa et al. (1986) have shown that similar desensitizing responses occur when full, but not partial, PI agonists are iontophoresed in the hippocampus of anesthetized rats *in vivo*. Thus, PI hydrolysis may mediate muscarinic inhibition of IK_m, and therby cause desensitization; i.e., decreased cell firing.

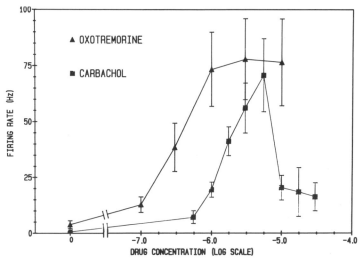

Figure 2. Comparison of the concentration-response relationships for carbachol and oxotremorine stimulated neuronal firing in the CA1 region of hippocampal slices. Drug additions were made in a cumulative manner to the buffer flowing through an interface chamber. Extracellular firing rate was measured 30 min after each drug addition when the responses had stabilized.

Although phorbol esters do not block the IK_m (Malenka et al, 1986), Ins(1,4,5)P3 may inactivate this conductance in a novel, calcium-independent, manner (Dutar and Nicoll, 1988a; Dutar and Nicoll, 1988b). Additional evidence that PI hydrolysis may mediate desensitization, is provided by studies showing that pirenzepine, a muscarinic antagonist acting through the M1 receptor, potently inhibits PI hydrolysis (Gonzales and Crews, 1984; Fisher and Bartus, 1985) and reverses carbachol desensitization (Pontzer and Crews, 1989). A further 10-fold increase in pirenzepine concentration can block cell firing, suggesting that pirenzepine can distinguish muscarinic receptor sites responsible for increased firing rates and desensitization. This pirenzepine sensitivity also suggests that the mRNA defined m1 is equivalent to the pharmacological M1 (Hammer et al., 1980) where oxotremorine-like drugs act as antagonists or weak partial agonists for stimulation of PI hydrolysis and inhibition of IK_m. Further support for our hypothesis that PI hydrolysis is associated with desensitization of firing rates is provided by experiments with lithium. Low concentrations of lithium disrupt the PI cycle by inhibiting inositol monophosphatases (Hallcher and Sherman, 1980). This could result in the accumulation of inositol monophosphate and depletion of free inositol in the CNS (Allison et al., 1976). Depletion of free inositol could reduce polyphosphoinositide synthesis, and thereby reduce IP_3 production. The reversal of carbachol mediated desensitization by lithium has a slow time-course which is consistent with a slow depletion of phosphoinositides and an ensuing decline in the production of DAG and IP_3. The ability of exogenous inositol to reverse lithium inhibition of desensitization clearly establishes the involvement of the phosphoinositide system in desensitization. It is also possible that desensitization could occur secondary to uncoupling of muscarinic stimulated PI hydrolysis. The ability of phorbol esters to desensitize muscarinic stimulated PI hydrolysis suggests that PKC could act in this manner (Gonzales et al., 1987). Carbachol induced partial desensitization has been reported in hippocampal slices (Lennox et al., 1988), but this desensitization occurs in the presence of lithium and is not rapidly reversed by the removal of carbachol or the addition of an antagonist, in contrast to the electrophysiological desensitization we observe.

Molecular biological techniques have found five subtypes of muscarinic receptors (Bonner et al., 1987; Barnard, 1988). Buckley et al. (1988) has shown that both m1 and m3 mRNA are highly expressed in rat hippocampal CA1. The molecular biological equivalents of both m1 (HM1) and m3 (HM4) have been found to stimulate PI hydrolysis (Peralta et al., 1988; Barnard, 1988). It is possible that one of these subtypes has a higher affinity for full agonist stimulated PI hydrolysis and is associated with increased neuronal firing rates. A second lower affinity muscarinic receptor could also stimulate PI hydrolysis. Carbachol and muscarine are full agonists at PI hydrolysis due to activation of both muscarinic subtypes, whereas oxotremorine appears to be an agonist at the higher affinity site and an antagonist at the second site.

Although both muscarinic receptors could couple to PI hydrolysis, this may occur through separate mechanisms. All of the agonists may act in a non-PI linked manner to decrease IK_{ca} directly (or through a G-protein) and/or the "leak" potassium current (Figure 3). The influx of calcium caused by the subsequent depolarization and action potential generation may partially stimulate PI hydrolysis through a calcium sensitive phospholipase C (Gonzales and Crews, 1985; Gonzales and Crews, 1988; Kendall and Nahorski, 1984). Partial agonists, especially oxotremorine, may act primarily through this mechanism, as would the high potency component of full agonists. A second lower affinity site may further increase PI hydrolysis, perhaps by direct receptor-guanine nucleotide-phospholipase coupling. This model is consistent with two phospholipase C enzymes, one guanine nucleotide sensitive, and the other calcium sensitive (Gonzales and Crews, 1985; Gonzales and Crews., 1988). Gurwitz and Sokolovsky (1987) found that oxotremorine stimulated PI hydrolysis is much more sensitive to tetrodotoxin than carbachol, further indicating a role for neuronal activation, and perhaps calcium influx, in stimulation of PI hydrolysis.

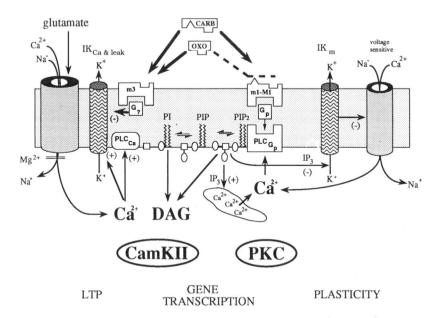

Figure 3. Schematic illustration of the interactions between the various receptors, second messengers and ion channels which may be involved in the induction of LTP and other aspects of neuronal plasticity. Although activation of NMDA receptors is necessary for the establishment of LTP in most systems, it is not sufficient because at resting membrane potential, Mg^{2+} blocks NMDA gated calcium flux. Simultaneous activation of NMDA receptors and receptors mediating depolarization, through second messengers or direct action on the ion channel, may also be required for the production of LTP. Stimulation of phospholipase C (PLC) by carbachol (Carb) acting on muscarinic receptors, or of quisqualate acting on glutaminergic receptors, produces the second messengers inositol 1,4,5 trisphosphate (IP_3) and diacylglycerol (DAG) that may in turn close potassium channels. Depolarization through closure of potassium channels, or opening of sodium/calcium channels, removes the Mg^{2+} block from NMDA gated calcium channels. Both depolarization induced calcium influx and IP_3 mediated calcium mobilization increase $[Ca^{2+}]i$, which could in turn further increase the activity of PLC and DAG. The high levels of $[Ca^{2+}]i$ and DAG that result from the feed-forward augmentation in these interacting systems, could lead to activation of protein kinase C (PKC) and calcium-calmodulin type II kinase (CamKII), which may in turn mediate long term changes in synaptic strength.

Glutamate receptors are thought to be involved in neuronal plasticity. Many studies dealing with LTP, and other forms of plasticity, have focused on the large calcium currents associated with NMDA receptor activation as a major factor in modifying synaptic transmission (Baudry and Lynch, 1980; Eccles, 1983; Jahr and Stevens, 1987). These currents are blocked by physiological levels of magnesium when the membrane is in the resting state; e.g. polarized. It has thus been hypothesized that there must be simultaneous activation of other receptors that depolarize the membrane in order to allow NMDA gated calcium flux to occur (Figure 3). Although the mechanisms involved in heterosynaptic control of calcium and phosphoinositide-linked second messengers remain to be elucidated, it is likely that the synergistic interactions between receptors causing depolarization and those causing direct, G-protein mediated, activation of PLC, may be needed to produce the pronounced excitation that triggers long term plasticity in the CNS (Figure 3) Our evidence that both quisqualate and carbachol stimulate neuronal excitation and produce a possible depolarization block. This would allow them to fulfill this function. Muscarinic and/or non-NMDA glutamatergic receptor activation may thus be important in LTP and memory. The membrane depolarization produced could both increase intracellular calcium and remove the magnesium block of NMDA gated calcium channels.

In conclusion, our findings suggest that two muscarinic sites are involved with changes in hippocampal CA1 cell firing rates and phosphoinositide hydrolysis. Oxotremorine is representative of agonists that bind to a single high affinity site, weakly stimulate PI hydrolysis, and increase firing rates at concentrations consistent with inhibition of IK_{ca}. Carbachol is representative of a group of agonists that bind to two muscarinic sites, stimulate PI hydrolysis with high and low potency components, increase firing rates in the range of the high potency site and desensitize firing responses in the range of the low-potency sites. Oxotremorine and low concentrations of pirenzepine antagonize carbachol stimulated PI hydrolysis, desensitization of firing rates and inhibition of IK_m, suggesting that these processes are mediated by a pharmacologically defined M1 site that may be identical to the mRNA defined m1 site. Since the mRNA defined m3 is also prominent in hippocampal CA1, and is linked to PI hydrolysis in cultured cells, this receptor may represent the high potency muscarinic site associated with increased neuronal cell firing and inhibition of IK_{ca}. The pharmacological distinctions between these sites could impact on muscarinic drugs of choice for treatment of Alzheimer's disease.

REFERENCES

Allison, J.H., M.E. Blisner, W.H. Holland, P.P. Hipps and W.R. Sherman (1976) Increased brain myo-inositol-1-phosphate in lithium treated rats. Biochem Biophys. Res. commun 71: 664-670.

Barbaran, J.M., S.H. Snyder and B.E. Alger (1985) Protein kinase C regulates ionic conductance in hippocampal pyramidal neurons: Electrophysiological effects of phorbol esters. Proc. Natl. Acad. Sci. USA. 82: 2538-2542.

Barnard, E.A. (1988) Separating receptor subtypes from their shadows. Nature 335: 301-302.

Bartus, R.T., Dean, R.L., Beer, B. and Lippa, A.S. (1982) The cholinergic hypothesis of geriatric memory dysfuction. Science 217:408-414.

Baudry, M. and Lynch, G. (1980) Regulation of hippocampal glutamate receptors: evidence for the involvement of calcium activated protease. Proc. Natl. Acad. Sci. U.S.A. 77:2298-2302.

Bernado, L.S. and D.A. Prince (1982) Cholinergic excitation of mammalian hippocampal pyramidal cells. Brain Res. 249: 315-331.

Bonner, T.I., N.J. Buckley, A. Young and M.R. Braun (1987) Identification of a family of muscarinic receptor genes. Science 237: 527-532.

Buckley, N.J., T.I. Bonner and M.R. Brann (1988) Localization of a family of muscarinic receptor mRNAs in rat brain J. Neurosci. 8: 4646-4652.

Dutar P. and R.A. Nicoll (1988b) Classification of muscarinic responses in hippocampus in terms of receptor subtype. J. Neurosci. 8: 4214-4224.

Dutar, P. and R.A. Nicoll (1988a) Stimulation of phosphatidlylinositol (PI) turnover may mediate the muscarinic suppression of the M-current in hippocampal cells. Neurosci. Lett. 85: 89-94.

Eccles, J.C. (1983) Calcium in long-term potentiation as a model for memory. Neurosci. 10:1071-1081.

Fisher, S.K. and R.T. Bartus (1985) Regional differences in the coupling of muscarinic receptors to inositol phospholipid hydrolysis in guinea pig brain. J. Neurochem. 45: 1085-1095.

Fisher, S.K., C.A. Boast and B.W. Agronoff (1980) The muscarinic stimulation of phospholipid labeling in hippocampus is independent of its cholinergic input. Brain Res. 189: 284-288.

Fisher, S.K., P.D. Klinger and B.W. Agranoff (1983) Muscarinic agonist binding and phospholipid turnover in brain. J. Biol. Chem. 258: 7358-7363.

Gonzales, R.A. and F.T. Crews (1984) Characterization of the cholinergic stimulation of phosphoinositide hydrolysis in rat brain slices. J. Neurosci. 4: 3120-3127.

Gonzales, R.A. and F.T. Crews (1985) Guanine nucleotides stimulate production of inositol triphosphate in rat cortical membranes. Biochem. J. 232: 799-804.

Gonzales, R.A. and F.T. Crews (1988) Guanine nucleotide and calcium-stimulated inositol phospholipid hydrolysis in brain membranes. J. Neurochem. 50: 1522-1528.

Gonzales, R.A., P.H. Greger, S.P. Baker, N.I. Ganz, C. Bolden, M.K. Raizada and F.T. Crews (1987) Phorbol esters inhibit agonist-stimulated phosphoinositide hydrolysis in neuronal primary cultures. Dev. Brain Res. 37: 59-66.

Gurwitz, D. and M. Sokolovsky (1987) Dual pathways in muscarinic receptor stimulation of phosphoinositide hydrolysis. Biochemistry 26: 633-638.

Hallcher, L.M. and W.R. Sherman (1980) The effect of lithium ion and other agents on the activity of myo-inositol-1-phosphate phosphatase from bovine brain. J. Biol. Chem. 225: 10896-10901.

Halliwell, J.V. and P.R. Adams (1982) Voltage-clamp analysis of muscarinic excitation in hippocampal neurons. Brain Res. 250: 71-92.

Hammer, R., C.P. Berrie, N.J.N. Birdsall, A.S.V. Burgen, and C. Hulme (1980) Pirenzine distinguishes between different subclasses of muscarinic receptors. Nature 283: 90-92.

Jahr, C.E. and Stevens, C.F. (1987) Glutamate activates multiple single channel conductances in hippocampal neurons. Science 325:522-525.

Kendall, D.A. and S.R. Nahorski (1984) Inositol phospholipid hydrolysis in rat cerebral cortical slices II. Calcium requirement. J. Neurochem. 42: 1388-1394.

Lennox, R.H., D. Hendley and J. Ellis (1988) Desensitization of muscarinic receptor-coupled phosphoinositide hydroysis in rat hippocampus: Comparison with the a-adrenergic response. J. Neurochem. 50: 558-564.

Lippa, A.S., D.J. Critchet and J.A.. Joseph (1986) Desensitization of muscarinic acetylcholine receptors: possible relationship to receptor heterogeneity and phosphoinositides. Brain Res. 366: 98-195.

Madison, D.V. and R.A. Nicoll (1984) Control of the repetitive discharge of rat CA1 pyramidal neurons in vitro. J. Physiol. 354: 319-331.

Madison, D.V., B. Lancaster and R.A. Nicoll (1987) Voltage-clamp analysis of cholinergic action in the hippocampus. J. Neurosci. 7: 733-741.

Malenka, R.C., D.V. Madison, R. Andrade and R.A. Nicoll (1986) Phorbol esters mimic some cholinergic actions in hippocampal pyramidal neurons. J. Neurosci. 6: 475-480.

Olianas, M.C., P. Onali, N.H. Neff and E. Costa (1983) Adenylate cyclase activity of synaptic membranes from rat striatum. Inhibition by muscarinic receptor agonists. Mol. Pharmacol. 23: 393-398.

Peralta, E.G., A. Ashkenazi, J.W. Winslow, J. Ramachandran and D.J. Capon (1988) Differential regulation of PI hydrolysis and adenylate cyclase by muscarinic receptor subtypes. Nature 334: 434-437.

Pontzer, N.J. and Crews, F.T. (1989) Desensitization of muscarinic stimulated hippocampal cell firing is related to phosphoinositide hydrolysis and inhibited by lithium. J. Neurosci. submitted.

Snyder, R.M. , M. McKinney, C. Forray and E. Richelson (1984) Neurotransmitter receptors mediate cyclic GMP formation by involvement of arachidonic acid and lipoxygenase. Proc. Natl. Acad. Sci. USA 81: 3905-3909.

EFFECTS OF CHOLINERGIC DRUGS ON EXTRACELLULAR LEVELS OF ACETYLCHOLINE
AND CHOLINE IN RAT CORTEX, HIPPOCAMPUS AND STRIATUM STUDIED BY BRAIN
DIALYSIS

Katsuo Toide and Takashi Arima

Section of Pharmacology, Biological Research Laboratory,
Taiho Pharmaceutical Co., Ltd.
224-2, Ebisuno, Hiraishi, Kawauchi-cho, Tokushima 771-01,
Japan

SUMMARY

The central effects of cholinergic drugs on the release of
acetylcholine (ACh) and changes in extracellular choline level were
investigated by the brain dialysis technique.

Scopolamine (0.5 mg/kg s.c.) markedly increased ACh release in the
frontal cortex, hippocampus and corpus striatum. Correspondingly, a
significant decrease of choline levels in the extracellular space was
observed in the three regions of brain. Oxotremorine (0.5 mg/kg i.p.)
displayed almost no effect upon ACh release in the frontal cortex,
however, a tendency toward inhibition of ACh release was observed in
both the hippocampus and corpus striatum. Conversely, oxotremorine
induced an increase of choline levels in both the frontal cortex and
hippocampus but not in the corpus striatum. Nicotine (0.5 mg/kg s.c.)
displayed a biphasic effect upon ACh release in both the frontal cortex
and hippocampus but not in the corpus striatum. No significant changes
in the choline levels of these three brain regions were observed after
administration of nicotine.

The present approach permits the direct detection of changes in
ACh and choline levels in the extracellular space of discrete brain
areas of experimental animals. These results indicate that the *in vivo*
brain dialysis technique applied to freely moving rats may be useful in
investigating cholinergic transmission via presynaptic terminals by
means of cholinergic drugs.

Key words: Brain dialysis; ACh and choline; Scopolamine; Oxotremorine;
            Nicotine; Discrete brain regions

INTRODUCTION

Since it was reported that the cholinergic neurons of the cerebral
cortex and hippocampus, regions that are closely associated with
memory, were markedly degenerated in Alzheimer's disease, information
has been accumulated that strongly suggests that degeneration of the

cholinergic neurons is concerned with the cause of this disease (1, 2, 3, 4). Scientific studies with postmortem brains from patients with Alzheimer's disease have shown that whereas cerebral tissue levels of postsynaptic receptors are nearly normal, the nerve terminals are so degenerated that the tissue content of ACh, CAT activity, and such presynaptic receptors as muscarinic and nicotinic receptors are depressed (4, 5, 6). In light of these findings, various kinds of compounds have been synthesized through use of radioactive ligands, such as one with strong affinity to muscarinic receptors, one that increases the concentration of synaptic ACh and one that stimulates ACh release from the nerve terminals. These compounds have been tested in animal experiments which have yielded plenty of suggestive evidence of beneficial effects. In clinical work as well ACh agonists have been evaluated for efficacy, resulting in the advent of compounds like AChE inhibitor, tetrahydroaminoacridine (THA) (7).

On the other hand, it should not be overlooked that experimental techniques have improved and progressed in the neurological studies of ethiopathologies of Alzheimer's disease in the pathological animal brain or postmortem human brain model. The approach on which we focus our attention in elucidating presynaptic function does not consist of removing the brain to determine the brain tissue levels of neurotransmitters but of brain dialysis. The latter technique consists of implanting a fine dialysis probe in each region of the brain in order to determine *in vivo* the levels of neurotransmitters in the extracelluar spaces in conscious and unrestrained animals (8, 9, 10, 11, 12, 13, 14, 15, 16, 17). Furthermore, an important advantage of this technique is that spontaneous motor activity as well as other behavioral changes can be measured simultaneously (13).

It is our intent in this study to find application for this technique in the development of a therapeutic for Alzheimer's disease by clarifying the action of ACh agonists and antagonist on chemical transmission through determination of ACh release from the nerve terminals and changes in the content of choline in the extracellular space.

MATERIAL AND METHODS

Brain Dialysis and Surgery

Male rats (230-260 g, Wistar strain) were anesthetized with pentobarbital sodium (40 mg/kg i.p.) and placed in a stereotaxic frame. The skull was exposed and holes were drilled for a unilateral dialysis probe which was placed into the left frontal cortex (coordinates: A +3.0, L -2.0, V -4.0 mm, relative to the bregma), the left hippocampus (coordinates: A -7.5, L -4.5, V -7.0 mm, relative to the bregma) and the left corpus striatum (coordinates: A 0, L -2.7, V -6.0 mm, relative to the bregma) according to König and Klippel (18).

A semipermeable regenerated cellulose tube was glued along a U-shaped stainless steel guide and lengths of 2.0 mm (frontal cortex) and 3.0 mm (hippocampus and corpus striatum) from the top were kept free, exposing the dialysis surface (Fig. 1). The device was fixed with dental cement and fastened with one screw onto the skull of the rat (Fig. 1). To exclude the effects of anesthesia the rats were first allowed time to recover; perfusion experiments were carried out between 26 and 48 hrs after surgery, during daylight hours. The dialysis tube was perfused at a constant rate of 2 µl/min with Ringer solution(147 mM NaCl, 4 mMKCl, 3.4 mMCaCl2, pH6.1) containing 10µM physostigmine sulfate.

The dialysis device has been indicated in our previous report (13), but it was essentially the same as that described by Damsma (10) with only slight modifications. This dialysis device was connected to the perfusion pump and to the injection valve of the HPLC system by means of polyethylene tubing (length 40 cm, inner diameter 0.1 mm). The motor driven injection valve of an autoinjector was controlled by an adjustable electronic timer. The sample loop (100 μl) was held in the load position for 15 min and automatically switched to the injection position for 20s. after which the cycle was repeated. One stainless steel cannula was connected to the perfusion pump by a polyethylene tube, and the outlet of the other cannula was connected to

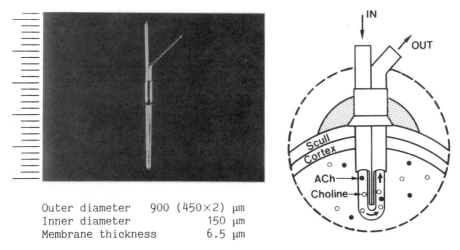

Outer diameter   900 (450×2) μm
Inner diameter   150 μm
Membrane thickness   6.5 μm

Fig. 1 U-typed probe and schema of dialysis probe in rat brain

the injection valve. In the present case, the internal standard, ethylhomocholine (EHC), delivered by the perfusion pump, was fed into the perfusate tube proximally to the injection valve (Fig. 2).

Assay of ACh and Choline

Assays of ACh and choline were performed as previously described by Toide (13) with minor modification of 1.03 mM sodium 1-decansulfonate.

Drugs and Chemicals

Physostigmine sulfate (Sigma) was added to the perfusion solution. Scopolamine hydrobromide (Sigma), oxotremorine sesquifumarate (Sigma) and nicotine tartrate (Tokyo Kasei) were dissolved in saline and injected in a volume of 1 ml/kg. Internal standard ethylhomocholine (EHC) was synthesized in our laboratory. Aqueous solutions were prepared from distilled water and all other chemicals were of analytical special grade.

RESULTS

Chromatography

Fig. 3 shows typical chromatograms of a standard samples containing 15 pmol of ACh, choline and EHC, and of brain perfusion samples. The EHC concentration in brain samples were 30 pmol. Both ACh and choline peaks are recognized in each of these brain regions, and the respective substances are well separated. To estimate the

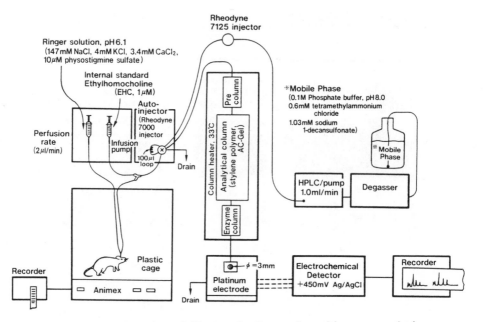

Fig. 2   Diagram of the perfusion and on-line connected analytical system

variation between different dialysis devices, the efficiency for five probes was determined *in vitro* at 2 µl/min. The average recoveries for ACh and choline were $24.8 \pm 1.3\%$ and $29.6 \pm 1.9\%$ (n=5, S.E.), respectively. Recent modifications in the design of the dialytic probe have resulted in improved performance, increased recovery rate and better reproducibility.

Fig. 4 shows the standard curves for ACh, choline and EHC. Each substance displays good linearity at concentrations between 10 and 100 pmol. The detection limits of ACh and choline were 60 and 30 fmol/injection, respectively.

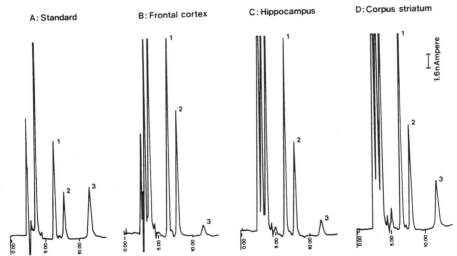

Fig. 3 Chromatograms of ACh, choline and EHC in the standard solution and in the dialysate from rat frontal cortex, hippocampus and corpus striatum. A; standard solution containing 15 pmol of ACh, choline and EHC. B and C; 30 pmol of EHC and 30 µl of perfusate with Ringer solution containing physostigmine.
1; Choline, 2; EHC, 3; ACh

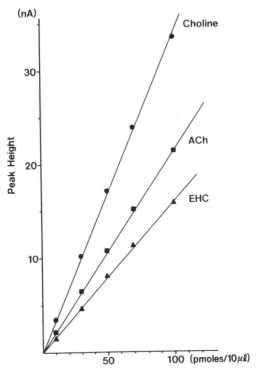

Fig. 4 Standard curves for ACh, choline and EHC

Table 1 Extracellular concentration of ACh and choline measured
by brain dialysis in the discrete regions of rat brain

Brain regions pmol/15 min	Frontal cortex	Hippocampus	Corpus striatum
ACh	1.40±0.29	2.28±0.22	5.40±1.02
Choline·	18.81±1.74	32.07±3.38	33.78±4.76

Dialysed ACh and choline levels represent pmol/15 min.
Data are mean ±S.E. values from 12 to 13 rat brains, respectively.

The average values for ACh and choline in the discrete regions of
rat brain indicated in Table 1.

Effects of Systematic Administration of Scopolamine on *in vivo* Dialysis
Levels of ACh and Choline in Frontal Cortex, Hippocampus and Corpus
Striatum

Fig. 5 shows the changes in ACh and choline levels in dialysates
of the discrete regions of brain of freely moving rats after
administration of scopolamine (0.5 mg/kg s.c.).

In the frontal cortex, scopolamine displayed a pronounced
enhancing effect upon the release of ACh between 30 and 75 min after
administration. This action upon ACh release was observed up to 105
min but when 120 min had elapsed the ACh levels had almost reverted to
the previous level. Corresponding to this action upon ACh release, a
significant decrease of choline level in extracellular space was
observed from 30 min up to 90 min after administration of scopolamine,
reflecting the changes in ACh concentration. However, the choline
level gradually reverted to the control level.

In the hippocampus, as in the frontal cortex, a pronounced
enhancing action upon ACh release was observed 30 min after
administration of scopolamine, and in fact a strong enhancing effect
was observed until 105 min after administration. Thereafter, the ACh
concentrations gradually began reverting to the control level. But,
even 120 min and the concentration was still approximately 2.5 times
that of the control level. Also, the observed choline level
corresponded with the changes in ACh levels exhibited a significant
inhibition from 30 min after administration of scopolamine. A potent
inhibitory action was observed between 45 and 105 min after
administration. In fact, this effect remained significant even after
120 min.

In the corpus striatum scopolamine significantly induced ACh
release. However, the pattern of the effects induced by scopolamine
was different from those observed in the other two regions. 30 min
after administration, the enhancing effect upon ACh release reached a
peak. Although concentration of ACh reverted gradually, it was still
high even after 120 min. Subsequently, choline level displayed a sharp
decrease 45 min after administration of the drug, although the onset of
this effect was slightly delayed as compared with those manifested in
the other brain regions. However, this action was maintained even
after a lapse of 120 min, and no sign of reversion to control levels
was observed within this period.

Effects of Systemic Administration of Oxotremorine on *in vivo* Dialysis Levels of ACh and Choline in Frontal Cortex, Hippocampus and Corpus Striatum

Fig. 6 shows the changes in ACh and choline levels after administration of oxotremorine (0.5 mg/kg i.p.).

Oxotremorine displayed almost no effect upon release of ACh in the frontal cortex, except for a slight tendency toward elevation of ACh levels 120 min after administration. Subsequently, a significant

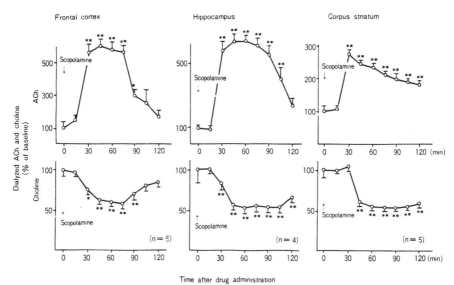

Fig. 5 Effect of scopolamine on the dialysate levels of ACh and choline in discrete regions of brain. The Ringer perfusion solution contained 10 μM physostigmine; the perfusion rate was 2 μl/min. Perfusate was collected for 1 hr (four 15-min fractions) before drug administration. The average ACh and choline contents in the four samples were taken as the baseline value for spontaneous release and extracellular level, respectively. Time zero on the abscissa corresponds to the time of injection of scopolamine (0.5 mg/kg s.c.). The data (mean and S.E.) represent the ACh and choline content for each 15-min fraction, expressed as a percentage of the average baseline ACh and choline. *P<0.05, **P<0.01 *vs* baseline by Dunnett's test. (Toide and Arima, *in press*)

increase in extracellular choline level was observed between 45 and 60 min. However, 120 min after administration of oxotremorine, a slight but significant decrease of choline levels was observed, presumably in response to changes in ACh concentration occurring during that period.

In the hippocampus following an enhancing effect upon release of ACh manifested between 15 and 30 min after administration of oxotremorine, a tendency toward inhibition of ACh release was observed from 45 to 60 min. Subsequently, the concentration of choline in the extracellular spaces displayed a significant increase between 30 and 75 min.

In the corpus striatum, a tendency toward lowered ACh levels in the extracellular spaces was noted during the period from 45 to 105 min. On the other hand, the choline level of the corpus striatum tended to decrease for 15 to 30 min after administration, and from about 60 min after administration, only a slight enhancing trend was observed.

Effects of Systemic Administration of Nicotine on *in vivo* Dialysis Levels of ACh and Choline in Frontal Cortex, Hippocampus and Corpus Striatum

Fig. 7 shows the changes in ACh and choline levels after administration of nicotine (0.5 mg/kg s.c.).

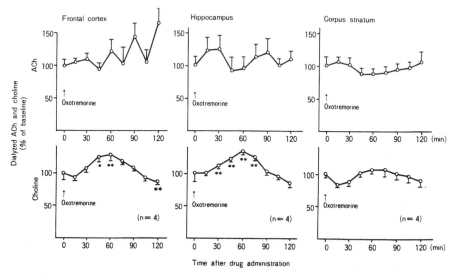

Fig. 6   Effect of oxotremorine on the dialysate levels of ACh and choline in discrete regions of brain. See legend in Fig. 6 for details. (Toide and Arima, *in press*)

In the frontal cortex, nicotine increased a transient yet significant ACh release 30 min after administration. However, after 45 min the ACh level reverted to the control value, but subsequently rose again during the period from 60 to 75 min after administration of nicotine. Thus, a biphasic action was observed. Choline concentration displayed a gradually increasing trend extending up to 120 min after administration of nicotine.

In the hippocampus as well, a significant enhanced ACh release was noted 30 min after administration of nicotine, but the ACh concentration reverted to the control level after 45 min. However, still later, about 90 min following administration of nicotine, it transiently yet significantly increased ACh levels as well, indicating a biphasic action. As for choline levels, these were virtually unaffected by nicotine. Thus, ACh changes in the hippocampus displayed a pattern quite similar to that observed in the frontal cortex.

In the corpus striatum, the response to nicotine was different from that displayed in either the frontal cortex or the hippocampus. That is, no transient rise in ACh content was observed during the initial period, but the ACh concentration tended to increase gradually over the entire period of 120 min after administration. The choline concentrations were slightly depressed to an extent corresponding to the changes in ACh.

DISCUSSION

In the field of neurochemical research, determination of neurotransmitters and their metabolites' content as well as enzyme activity in the brain have been investigated for the purpose of elucidating the functions of presynaptic terminals. On the other hand, receptor binding experiments using radio labelled ligands (this method has also been used in the case of presynaptic receptors) and adenylate cyclase systems as well as phosphatidyl inositide turnover systems, including Ca^{2+} mobilization as a signal transduction system have been investigated in studies of postsynaptic functions (19, 20). These research trends also indicate the importance to investigate chemical transmission as an index of neurotransmitter release from presynaptic nerve terminals in connection between pre- and postsynapse.

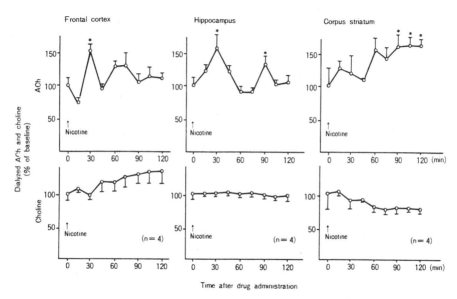

Fig. 7   Effect of nicotine on the dialysate levels of ACh and choline in discrete regions of brain. See legend in Fig. 6 for details. (Toide and Arima, *in press*)

In the central nervous system, cholinergic neurons are known to be involved in neural control from the septum to the hippocampus and from the nucleus basalis of Meynert and the diagonal band of Broca to the cerebral cortex, as well as existing in the intrinsic neurons of the corpus striatum. It is well known that the functions of the presynaptic cholinergic neurons in the hippocampus and cerebral cortex are impaired in Alzheimer's disease (5). Therefore, as a criterion of improvement of presynaptic function by drug therapy, it is very important to investigate ACh release from presynaptic cholinergic neurons simultaneously with the determination of ACh and choline levels and choline acetyltransferase activity in the presynaptic neurons.

Recently, the brain dialysis technique, employing a highly sensitive analytical method based upon high performance liquid chromatography, has made possible the measurement of ACh in the extracellular of freely moving rats (9, 10, 13), permitting the precise analysis of the effects of various drugs upon neurotransmission in the cholinergic system, using ACh release from nerve terminals.

The present research was concerned with the effects of the muscarinic antagonist scopolamine, the muscarinic agonist oxotremorine and the nicotinic agonist nicotine upon the activity of cholinergic nerve terminals in the frontal cortex, hippocampus and corpus striatum, using ACh release and changes in the choline content of the extracellular spaces.

Investigation of the effects of scopolamine administration (0.5mg/kg s.c.) upon ACh release and choline content in the extracellular spaces revealed a pronounced increase in the release of ACh from nerve terminals and a corresponding decrease in the extracellular concentrations of choline in each of the brain regions. The results of the present experiments disclosed that the intensity and duration of the effects of scopolamine varied in the three different brain regions. Comparison of effects upon ACh release showed an increase of 6.2 times in the hippocampus, 6.0 times in the frontal cortex and 2.8 times in the corpus striatum. Consolo et al. (9) had previously investigated the effects of scopolamine (0.34mg/kg s. c.) upon ACh release from the corpus striatum, and the results in the corpus striatum reported by those authors were almost identical with those obtained in the present study. It is well known that presynaptic muscarinic receptors modulate ACh release (22, 23, 24, 25). This enhancing effect of scopolamine upon ACh release seems attributed to a positive feedback mechanism due to an inhibitory action upon ACh autoregulation resulting from the blocking of presynaptic receptors, and presumably the observed decrease in choline content of the extracellular spaces results from enhanced synthesis of ACh in the nerve terminals. Some reports (26, 27, 28), performed *in vitro* experiments using ^{3}H-labelled choline, and indicated that scopolamine enhanced the uptake of choline by nerve terminals, which is consistent with the results obtained in our *in vivo* experiments.

Oxotremorine (0.5mg/kg i.p.) displayed no significant effects in the frontal cortex, where a slight tendency toward increased ACh release was observed two hours after administration. In the hippocampus, a slight increase was observed during the initial period after administration of the drug, but subsequently a mild transient inhibitory action upon ACh release was noted. In the corpus striatum, a moderate but sustained reduction in ACh levels was observed between 45 and 105 minutes after administration, suggesting an inhibitory action upon ACh release. An inhibitory effect upon ACh release was anticipated due to enhanced autoregulatory function resulting from the agonistic action of oxotremorine upon presynaptic receptors. Consolo et al. (9) reported that a transient inhibitory effect upon ACh release in the corpus striatum was manifested 20 minutes after administration of oxotremorine (0.53mg/kg i. p.), but the form of the reported effects differed somewhat from those observed in the present study. These discrepancies may be possibly due to differences in the rate of dialyzed time or intensity of desensitization. On the other hand, as regards the choline content of the extracellular spaces, significant increases were manifested in the frontal cortex and hippocampus about one hour after administration. These effects were presumably due to diminished turnover of ACh at the nerve terminals resulting from agonistic effects upon the pre- and/or postsynaptic receptors, inhibiting the uptake of choline, which constitutes the substrate for ACh synthesis. However, no changes in extracellular choline concentrations were observed in the corpus striatum, indicating differences among the brain regions with respect to the effects of the drug.

Nicotinic receptors are known to be present in the central as well as the peripheral nervous system, where presynaptic nicotine receptors serve to regulate the release of ACh (29, 30). Recent reports have indicated that not only muscarinic receptors but also presynaptic nicotinic receptors diminish in Alzheimer's disease, which is characterized by impaired cholinergic activity (4, 31, 32). Moreover, the clinical efficacy of nicotine with respect to Alzheimer's disease has been investigated, and some reports have indicated the effectiveness of such treatment (34). From the results of *in vivo* brain dialysis in the present study, although there were certain differences in pattern among the respective brain regions, enhancing effects upon ACh release were observed in the frontal cortex and hippocampus, which are intimately involved in memory function, suggesting an enhancing action of nicotine upon ACh-mediated neurotransmission. By contrast with the muscarinic agonist oxotremorine, reports of *in vivo* experiments have also indicated that this action of nicotine results from enhancement of ACh release mediated by presynaptic receptors (30, 31). On the other hand, prolonged exposure to nicotine has been reported to induce desensitization (35), and the biphasic action observed in the frontal cortex and hippocampus in the present experiments may presumably be attributed to desensitization effects. However, ACh-releasing effects were not observed virtually in the corpus striatum. As regards changes in choline content, choline concentrations displayed a tendency to increase in the frontal cortex and to diminish in the corpus striatum, but almost no effects were observed in the hippocampus, moreover, there were no corresponding changes in the release of ACh, as were observed in the case of scopolamine.

The above results appear to indicate that the muscarinic antagonist scopolamine, by its receptor blocking action, inhibits the autoregulatory function of ACh, thus providing a positive feedback mechanism which promotes the uptake of choline along with the enhancing effect upon release of ACh and, presumably, the concomitant turnover at the nerve terminals. As regards the muscarinic agonist oxotremorine, the changes induced by a negative feedback mechanism arising from agonist effects upon receptors were rather slight, but apparently the uptake of choline is impeded by an inhibitory action upon ACh release and, presumably, a resulting reduction in turnover at the nerve terminals, resulting in an increase in the choline concentration of the extracellular spaces. An enhancing effect of the nicotinic agonist nicotine upon the release of ACh from nerve terminals through the mediation of presynaptic receptors was observed in the frontal cortex and hippocampus. The results concerning the effects of the cholinergic agonists oxotremorine and nicotine in the frontal cortex and hippocampus revealed a different pattern of action from that observed in the corpus striatum. This was attributed to the manifestation of differences in drug effect owing to the predominance of intrinsic neurons in the corpus striatum. Moreover, differences in the manner of distribution of muscarinic receptors between the various brain regions have been reported (36), and likewise regional differences in distribution of nicotinic receptors have also been recognized (29, 37). The distribution of cholinergic receptors and the analysis of the effects upon ACh release mediated by these receptors constitutes an important subject for subsequent research.

In conclusion, the results of the present study suggest that *in vivo* brain dialysis provides an useful technique for the analysis of the nature of chemical neurotransmission by cholinergic neurons as well as the action of various drugs upon these neurons, using ACh release from nerve terminals and choline concentration in the extracellular spaces as indices of neuronal activity.

REFERENCES

1. Araujo, D.M., Lapchak, P.A., Robitaille, Y., Gauthier, S. and Quirion, R. (1988) Differential alteration of various cholinergic markers in cortical and subcortical regions of human brain in Alzheimer's disease. J. Neurochem. 50: 1914-1923.
2. Bartus, R.T., Dean III.R.L., Beer, B. and Lippa, A.S. (1982) The cholinergic hypothesis of geriatric memory dysfunction. Science 217: 408-417.
3. Haroutunian, V., Barnes, E. and Davis, K.L. (1985) Cholinergic modulation of memory in rats. Psychopharmacology 87: 266-271.
4. Whitehouse, P.J. (1987) Neurotransmitter receptor alterations in Alzheimer disease: A review. Alzheimer Dis. Assoc. Disord. 1: 9-18.
5. Coyle, J.T., Donald, L.P. and Delong, M.R. (1983) Alzheimer's disease: A disorder of cortical cholinergic innervation. Science 219: 1184-1190.
6. Reisine, T.D., Yamamura, H.I., Bird, E.D., Spokes, E. and Enna, S.J. (1978) Pre- and postsynaptic neurochemical alterations in Alzheimer's disease. Brain Res. 159: 477-481.
7. Summers, W.K., Majorski, L.V., Marsh, G.M., Tachiki, K. and Kling, A. (1986) Oral tetrahydroaminoacridine in long-term treatment of senile dementia, Alzheimer type. N. Engl. J. Med. 315:1241-1245.
8. Benveniste, H., Drejer, J., Schousboe, A. and Diemer, N.H. (1984) Elevation of the extracellular concentrations of glutamate and aspartate in rat hippocampus during transient cerebral ischemia monitored by intracerebral microdialysis. J. Neurochem. 43: 1369-1374.
9. Consolo, S., Wu, C.F., Fiorentini, F., Ladinsky, H. and Vezzani, A. (1987) Determination of endogenous acetylcholine release in freely moving rats by transstriatal dialysis coupled to a radioenzymatic assay: Effect of drugs. J. Neurochem. 48: 1459-1465.
10. Damsma, G., Westerink, B.H.C., De Vries, J.B., Van den Berg, C.G. and Horn, A.S. (1987) Measurement of acetylcholine release in freely moving rats by means of automated intracerebral dialysis. J. Neurochem. 48: 1523-1528.
11. Damsma, G., Biessels, P.T.M., Westerink, B.H.C., De Vries, J.B. and Horn, A.S. (1988) Differential effects of 4-aminopyridine and 2, 4-diaminopyridine on the *in vivo* release of acetylcholine and dopamine in freely moving rats measured by intrastriatal dialysis. European J. Pharmacol. 145: 15-20.
12 Hutson, P.H., Sarna, G.S., Kantamanei, B.D. and Curzon, G.(1985) Monitoring the effect of a tryptophan load on brain indole metabolism in freely moving rats by simultaneous cerebrospinal fluid sampling and brain dialysis. J. Neurochem. 44:1266-1273.
13. Toide, K. (1989) Effects of scopolamine on extracellular acetylcholine and choline levels and on spontaneous motor activity in freely moving rats measured by brain dialysis. Pharmacol. Biochem. Behav. 33:109-113.
14. Ungerstedt, U. (1984) Measurement of neurotransmitters release by intracranial dialysis, in Measurement of Neurotransmitter Release *In Vivo* (Mursden C.A., ed), John Wiley & Sons, Chichester. pp. 81-105.
15. Ungerstedt, U., Forster, Ch., Herreva-Marschitz, M., Hoffman, I., Jungnelius, U., Tossman, U., and Zetterström, T. (1982) Brain

dialysis - a new *in vivo* technique for studying neurotransmitter release and metabolism. Neurosci. lett (suppl.). 10: 493.

16. Westerink, B.H.C., Damsma, G., Rollema, H., De Vries, J.B. and Horn, A.S. (1987) Scope and limitations of *in vivo* brain dialysis: A comparison of its application to various neurotransmitter systems. Life Sci. 41: 1763-1776.

17. Zetterström, T. (1986) Pharmacological analysis of central dopaminergic neurotransmission using a novel *in vivo* brain perfusion method. Ph. D. Thesis, Karolinska Institutet, Stockholm, Sweden. pp. 1-45.

18. König, J.F.R. and Klippel, R.A. (1968) The rat brain: A stereotaxic atlas of the forebrain and lower parts of the brain stem. Williams & Wilkins, Baltimore.

19. Gilman, A.G. (1987) G proteins: Transducers of receptor-generated signals. Annu. Rev. Biochem. 56: 615-649.

20. Hokin, L.E. (1985) Receptors and phosphoinositide-generated second messengers. Annu. Rev. Biochem. 54: 205-253.

21. McGeer, E.G. (1981) Neurotransmitter systems in Aging and senile dementia. Prog. Neuro-Psychopharmacol. 5: 435-445.

22. Nordström, O. and Bartfai, T. (1980) Muscarinic autoreceptor regulates acetylcholine release in rat hippocampus: *in vitro* evidence. Acta Physiol. Scad. 108: 347-353.

23. Szerb, J.C., Hadhazy, P. and Dudar, J.D. (1977) Release of ^{3}H-acetylcholine from rat hippocampus slices: effect of septal lesion and of graded concentrations of muscarinic agonists and antagonists. Erain Res. 128: 285-291.

24. Kilbinger, H. (1984) Presynaptic muscarinic receptors modulating acetylcholine release. in: Receptor, again. eds. J.W. Lamble and A.C.Abbott (Elsevier science publishers, Amsterdam-New York-Oxford) p.174-179.

25. Meyer, E.M. and Otero, D.H. (1985) Pharmacological and ionic characterizations of the muscarinic receptors modulating [^{3}H] acetylcholine release from rat cortical synaptosomes. J. Neurosci. 5: 1202-1207.

26. Karlen, B., Lundgren, E., Lundin, J. and Holmstedt, B. (1979) Effect of physostigmine and atropine on acetylcholine turnover in mouse brain. Naunyn-Schmiedeberg's Arch Pharmacol. 808: 61-65.

27. Yamamura, H.I. and Snyder, S.H. (1973) High affinity transport of choline into synaptosomes of rat brain. J. Neurochem. 21: 1355-1374.

28. Richardson, P.J. (1986) Choline uptake and metabolism in affinity-purified cholinergic nerve terminals from rat brain. J. Neurochem. 46: 1251-1255

29. Morley, B.J. (1981) The properties of brain nicotine receptors. Pharmacol. Ther. 15: 111-122.

30. Rowell, P.P. and Winkler, D.L. (1984) Nicotinic stimulation of [^{3}H] acetylcholine release from mouse cerebral cortical synaptosomes. J. Neurochem. 43: 1593-1598.

31. Whitehouse, P.J., Martino, A.M., Anteaono, P.G., Lowenstein, P., Coyle, J.T., Price, D.L. and Kellar, K.J. (1986) Nicotine acetylcholine binding sites in Alzheimer's disease. Brain Res. 371: 146-151.

32. Shimohama, S., Taniguchi, T., Fujiwara, M. and Kameyama, M. (1985) Biochemical characterization of the nicotinic cholinergic receptors in human brain; binding of (−)-[^{3}H] nicotine. J. Neurochem. 45:604-610.

33. Newhouse, P.A., Sunderland, T., Tariot, P.N., Blumhardt, C.L., Weingartner, H. and Mellow, A. (1988) Intravenous nicotine in Alzheimer's disease: A Pilot study. Psychopharmacology 95: 171-175.

34. Schwartz, R.D. and Keller, K.J. (1985) *In vivo* regulation [^{3}H] acetylcholine recognition sites in brain by nicotine cholinergic drugs. J. Neurochem. 45: 427-433.

35. Beani, L., Bianchi, C., Nilsson, L., Nordberg, A., Romanelli, L. and Sivilotti, L. (1985) The effect of nicotine and cystein on ^{3}H-acetylcholine release from cortical slices of guinea pig brain. Naunyn-Schmiedeberg's Arch Pharmacol. 331: 293-296.

36. Birdsall, N.J.M. and Hulme, E.C. (1984) Presynaptic muscarinic receptors modulating acetylcholine release. in: Receptors, again. eds. J.W. Lamble and A.C. Abbott (Elsevier Science Publishers, Amsterdam-New York-Oxford) pp. 159-167.

37. Clark, P.B.S., Schwartz, R.D., Paul, S.M., Pert, C.B. and Pert, A. (1985) Nicotine binding in rat brain: autoradiographic comparison of [^{3}H] acetylcholine, [^{3}H] nicotine and [^{125}I]-alpha-bungarotoxin. J. Neurosci. 5: 1307-1315.

DELAYED MATCHING-TO-SAMPLE IN MONKEYS AS A MODEL FOR LEARNING AND

MEMORY DEFICITS: ROLE OF BRAIN NICOTINIC RECEPTORS

William J. Jackson[1], Karey Elrod[2] and Jerry J. Buccafusco[2,3]

[1]Department of Physiology and Endocrinology, [2]Department of
Pharmacology and Toxicology
Medical College of Georgia
and the [3]Veterans Administration Medical Center
Augusta, GA 30912

INTRODUCTION

The nervous system and behavioral repertoire of old world monkeys
resembles the human neuro-behavioral system more than any other laboratory
animal, except higher apes. In addition, spontaneous and conditioned
behavior exhibited by the monkey is more similar to that of the human than
any other laboratory animal[1]. Therefore, behavioral tasks which tap the
higher cognitive abilities of these nonhuman primates may provide
information more relevant to normal human aging and to the dementias. The
method most frequently employed to test the sophisticated cognitive
repertoire of these monkeys has been one or another variation of the
delayed response task. The delayed matching-to-sample (DMTS) task allows
the measurement of abilities which are relevant to human aging, such as
attention, strategy formation, reaction time in complex situations and
memory for recent events. Thus, comparisons to human behavioral situations
should involve less speculation than when lower animal subjects are
employed. Interestingly, a similar version of this task has been employed
to demonstrate cognitive impairment in Alzheimer's Disease patients[2]. The
advent of the personal computer age has facilitated the automation of
problem presentation and data collection associated with this task, and it
is now practical to analyze DMTS performance at a more detailed level.

Among the many neurochemical abnormalities demonstrated to occur in the
post mortem brains of Alzheimer's patients, is a loss of cholinergic
nicotinic receptor density[3-5]. This loss parallels a deficit in other
cholinergic markers and is consistent with the functional impairment
observed prior to death. While it is generally recognized that the brain
muscarinic receptor system plays an important role in learning and memory,
less is known about the role of the nicotinic system. In humans, nicotine
is known to not only improve the attentional component of information
processing in learning (acquisition), but also facilitates the input of
information to storage (retention) in the memory process[6]. Additionally,
selective blockade of central nicotinic receptors has been reported to
produce memory impairment in rodent animal models[7-10], and to slow cognitive
functioning in humans[11]. Thus, the loss of nicotinic receptors associated
with Alzheimer's disease may underlie, at least in part, the memory and/or

cognitive impairment observed in these patients. The purpose of these studies was to examine the effect of stimulation and blockade of nicotinic receptors in monkeys performing a DMTS task. Our initial experiments were performed in young adult animals, although subsequent preliminary experiments were also performed with aged (34-35 year old) animals.

METHODS

Five young adult <u>Macaca</u> <u>fascicularis</u> monkeys and two aged (>34 years old) monkeys were well-trained in a delayed matching-to-sample (DMTS) paradigm over a period of several months. Water was supplied on an unlimited basis, but monkeys received approximately 15% of their food during performance of the DMTS task. During our first series with the young animals, monkeys were placed in a restraining chair and the test drug administered i.m. (gastrocnemius muscle) in a volume of 0.3 ml. At 10 min after nicotine or vehicle (sterile, normal saline) injection the monkey was placed in a light- and sound-attenuated chamber to await the start of the testing session which was initiated by a computer. At this time a 2.8 mm

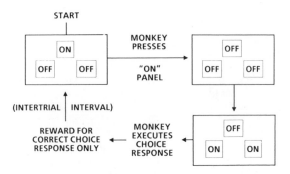

Figure 1. Schematic diagram of the delayed matching-to-sample behavioral paradigm performed by monkeys.

diameter red, blue or yellow colored circle was illuminated, representing the stimulus or sample key. The animal pressed the sample key, extinguishing the sample light. Following a pre-programmed delay period (0-60 sec) two choice lights located below the sample key were illuminated, one of which matched the previously presented sample light, while the other was one of the other two colors. The monkey executed a response by pressing one of the two choice keys which terminated the trial and 5 sec later re-initiated a new trial. A food reward pellet was provided for a correct (matching) choice. An incorrect (non-matching) choice was neither rewarded nor punished. Each session consisted of 108 such trials and lasted 30-45 min. A schematic diagram of the paradigm is illustrated in Figure 1.

During training sessions a set of 5 or 6 delays was randomized and presented in equal proportion. The longest delay period chosen for an individual monkey was that which consistently allowed correct choices to be significantly greater than chance (i.e., approximately 60%). During the ten months in which the first series were conducted, baseline data were consistent (Fig.2). In general, 3 levels of performance difficulties were exhibited by the animals. In order to simplify data analysis and reduce baseline variability, the data for each animal were separated into these 3 delay levels corresponding to the percentage correct values. The least difficult level of performance (Level 1) was a 0 sec delay period at which the animals averaged 94% correct responses. The moderately difficult level of performance (Level 2) consisted of delay periods of 5 to 10 sec at which

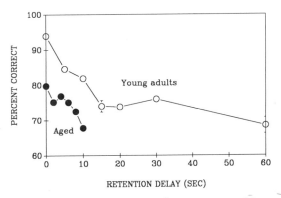

Figure 2. Baseline data for 4 young monkeys over a 10 month period, and 2 aged monkeys over a 2 month period (expressed as percent correct as a function of retention delay). Values represent the mean ± s.e.m. of 20-100 sessions. (Note: in some cases the standard error bar was smaller than the diameter of the symbol).

the monkeys averaged 80-85% correct responses. The most difficult level of performance (Level 3) consisted of delay periods of 15-60 sec at which the monkeys averaged 65-75% correct responses. Of the 5 animals employed, 1 animal's capabilities extended to delay periods of 20 sec, 3 animals performed to 30 sec and 1 animal performed to a delay of 60 sec. Values obtained for each performance level were averaged and recorded as the average percentage correct for the respective interval. Drug effects were calculated as the absolute change from baseline. A minimum drug "wash out" period of 2 days was allowed between sessions in which a drug was administered. During this period a return to baseline performance was established in each animal before again administering drugs.

In the second series of experiments, 4 of the 5 monkeys from the previous study were employed. Testing panels were constructed so that they could be attached directly to the front of the animal's home cage. This obviated the need for the restraining chair and test cubical, however, there was the potential problem of noise or distraction from other animals in the housing room. Four animals were tested simultaneously using a newly designed computer-automated training and testing system. This system allowed additional data collection features, including latency of response at each step of each matching problem, and percent correct for every possible combination of matching stimuli (position and color analysis) thus increasing the resolution of our behavioral analysis. Basically, the same protocol and experimental paradigm were employed as described for the first series. In this case the animal room was darkened, with the computer and operator isolated from the subjects.

Data were analyzed statistically using a one-way analysis of variance (ANOVA), and the Tukey honestly significant difference (HSD) procedure was used to determine confidence levels among sessions for main effects attaining the 0.05 level of confidence. In some cases an unpaired Student's t-test was employed as the post hoc test.

RESULTS

First Experimental Series

The results obtained from a representative monkey during the nicotine dose response experiment are illustrated in Figure 3. Values represent performance at delay level 3 (longer delay periods) only since nicotine was not found to produce a significant effect at delay level 1 or 2 (see Figure 4). A decrease in performance relative to baseline was observed with the lowest dose (1.25 μg/kg) of nicotine. Further increases in dosage yielded facilitation of performance, with the largest increase (26%) afforded by the 5 μg/kg dose. This dose response effect well exemplifies the inverted U dose response relationship commonly observed with cognitive enhancing agents. Subsequent re-administration of the "best dose" of nicotine (5 μg/kg) to the monkey again yielded enhancement (10%) of performance although not of the same magnitude as the prior injection of 5 μg/kg. Similar dose response effects were observed in the other four monkeys ($p < 0.05$).

Nicotine enhanced performance primarily at the longest delay intervals in each of the animals (Fig.4). The beneficial effect of nicotine occurred over a narrow dose window, usually between 1.25 and 5.0 μg/kg. Two of the monkeys did not respond to any of the 4 doses of nicotine. At first, these animals seemed insensitive to the drug, but when administered 0.625 and 7.5 μg/kg nicotine, respectively, each responded in a manner similar to the other monkeys. The values presented represent the mean of 3 experiments each at these doses for No. 2 and No. 4. For the other 3 monkeys, the most effective dose was repeated and found effective during 4-6 sessions each. On the average, nicotine increased performance at the longest delay interval by about 10 percentage points. The drug produced no significant effect on the shorter delay intervals. Any decline in the blood level of nicotine was not reflected by performance returning to baseline. Performance levels were maintained throughout the session. Also, tolerance was not apparent since re-administration of the best dose of nicotine produced the same or nearly the same enhancement of performance at some time during the study.

The effect of the centrally-acting nicotinic blocking drug, mecamyla-mine, was examined in the same subjects. The results of this experiment are depicted in Figure 5. While the two lower doses of mecamylamine (0.25

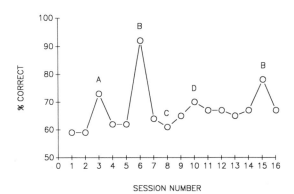

SESSION NUMBER

Figure 3. Dose response series to nicotine administration in one monkey at delay level 3. A = 2.5, B = 5.0, C = 1.25, D = 10 μg/kg. Doses were administered 10 min prior to initiating a testing session. All other sessions denote baseline performance between doses. Reproduced with permission from Pergamon Press[12].

and 0.50 mg/kg) had no significant effect on performance, the highest dose (2 mg/kg) produced a marked depression in performance with the effect most notable on the shorter delay intervals. Mecamylamine induced decreases in performance of 23%, 20%, and 10% at delay levels 1, 2 and 3, respectively (p<0.05). The next experiment was conducted to control for the potential peripheral effects of mecamylamine. Following administration of 2 mg/kg of the peripherally-acting nicotinic antagonist, hexamethonium, (the same dose at which mecamylamine exerted a significant effect on cognitive performance), signs of ganglionic blockade, particularly ptosis, were noted within several min. Despite the outward effects of the drug, no signifi-cant effect on performance during the testing session was noted (Fig. 6).

In the next series, animals received either 0.5 mg/kg of mecamylamine or 2 mg/kg hexamethonium (since neither one of these doses by themselves produced a significant effect on baseline performance) 15 min prior to each animal receiving its most effective dose of nicotine to examine the influence of antagonist pretreatment on the effects produced by nicotine administered 10 min later. The results of this experiment are illustrated in Figure 7. While hexamethonium pretreatment did not alter the ability of nicotine to enhance performance at the longest delay interval, mecamylamine pretreatment antagonized the beneficial effect of nicotine (p<0.05).

43

Second Experimental Series

Four animals from the first series were retrained to their original baseline performance (see Fig. 2) using the unrestrained technique described above in the Methods section. Numerous variables relating to the monkey's performance were collected; the variables related to one of three categories: (a) color preference, (b) position preference and (c) response latency. The data were tabulated in a matrix for each daily session. It

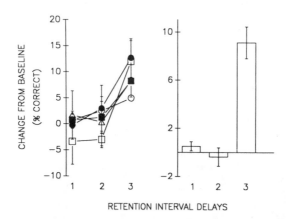

RETENTION INTERVAL DELAYS

Figure 4. Effect of the best dose of nicotine (0.625, 2.5, 5.0, or 7.5 μg/kg, i.m.) in five monkeys on their performance of a delayed matching-to-sample paradigm (expressed as the absolute change in percentage correct from baseline). Nicotine was administered 10 min prior to testing. In the line graph each symbol refers to data derived from an individual monkey (open circle = No.1, open triangle = No.2, closed circle = No.4, open square = No.7, closed square = No.8). Each value represents the mean of 4-6 replicates, except for No.2 and No.4, which represents the mean of 3 experiments each. The bar graph represents the mean of each animal's data averaged for the five monkeys. Vertical lines indicate the s.e.m. Retention intervals 1,2 and 3 refer to short, moderate and long delay intervals. The value for interval 3 was significantly greater than baseline. Reproduced with permission from Pergamon Press[12].

was therefore possible to separate two main components of the DMTS task, a test of memory recall and a cognitive component which tests the abstract conceptualization of "matching". Results obtained from this series confirm the results of Series 1 in that nicotine administration produced a significant enhancement of performance in the DMTS task. As with the earlier procedure (restraint and isolation during testing) the degree of enhancement was greatest for the longer (most difficult) delay intervals, with the magnitude of this enhancement (+10.5%), significantly greater than baseline performance. Drug vehicle administration (saline) did not significantly affect baseline performance. Also, there was no significant effect of nicotine on choice latencies (time elapsed during color choice selection), 3.8±0.64 and 3.9±0.57 sec, respectively for control and nicotine-treated; or trial latencies (time elapsed between the stimulus color presentation and the animal's starting the next trial), 2.7±0.32 and 3.5±0.91 sec, respectively. Position preference (left vs. right choice light) did not account significantly for the enhancement produced by

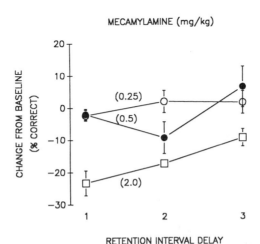

Figure 5. Effect of mecamylamine on performance of a delayed matching-to-sample paradigm by four monkeys (expressed as the absolute change in percentage correct from baseline). The numbers in parentheses refer to the dose of mecamylamine in mg/kg, i.m. Mecamylamine was administered 25 min prior to testing. The highest dose of mecamylamine produced a significant decrease in performance. Reproduced with permission of Pergamon Press[12].

nicotine in these young animals (Fig. 8). The most interesting finding, however, was that when animals were tested on the day following nicotine pretreatment, significant enhancement of performance was still observed for the longest delay interval (see Figs. 7 and 8). This chronic feature of nicotine's effects was unexpected, although our subjective impressions have always been that baseline performance in DMTS tends to increase when animals are receiving a dose regimen of nicotine. The mechanism for this delayed enhancement is not understood, but is clearly not related to significant levels of the drug in plasma or tissue. More likely, it is related to more long-term changes in neurotransmitter function following a single dose of nicotine.

Further analysis of the data from this new group indicates that monkeys have a significant color preference involved in their matching skills. When data were analyzed in terms of color preference it was determined that the least preferred color (color with which most mistakes in matching were made) was enhanced to the largest extent with nicotine (Fig. 8). In fact, performance was enhanced by over 30% when data were analyzed in this manner. The shift from a 10% overall enhancement to a 30% enhancement for the non-preferred color indicates that for the long delay interval, nicotine alters the color preference of the animal, towards a more balanced color preference. We are also training three aged (34-35 years old)

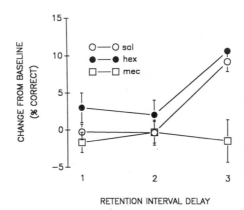

Figure 6. Effect of pretreatment with saline (SAL), 0.5 mg/kg mecamylamine (MEC) or 2 mg/kg of hexamethonium (HEX) prior to each animal receiving its best dose of nicotine on performance of a delayed matching-to-sample paradigm. Pretreatments were administered 15 min prior to nicotine which was administered 10 min prior to testing. Experiments were replicated in each animal 1-3 times. Mecamylamine pretreatment significantly inhibited the enhanced performance following nicotine at retention interval level 3 (p<0.05. Reproduced with permission of Pergamon Press[12].

monkeys in the DMTS task. It has proven much more difficult to train these animals and currently two are performing up to 5 or 10 sec delays at better than chance performance (see Fig. 2). Preliminary studies with nicotine in these animals have suggested the following: (1) That acute administration of nicotine produces a similar degree of enhancement in the DMTS task as with the young animals, except that the doses employed were higher (5-10 µg/kg vs. 2.5 µg/kg for old and young, respectively). (2) There continues to be an enhanced response observed 24 hours after the nicotine injection. (3) The old animals have a position (left/right) preference. (4) As with the color preference in the young monkeys, nicotine appeared to normalize the position preference in the aged monkeys. Color preference was not a major factor for the older monkeys. Our data with the aged animals are preliminary, however, and await further verification. While position vs. color preference may be a function of aging, it is also possible that it may be a function of the duration of training, since our older animals are just beginning drug trials.

DISCUSSION

The validity of the non-human primate performing a DMTS task as a model for human memory has been recently reviewed by Bartus,[13]. The fact that

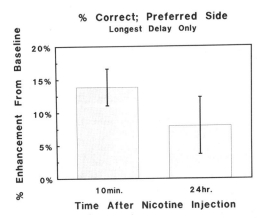

Figure 7. Delayed matching-to-sample performance by monkeys in the second series (unrestrained testing) analyzed in terms of delay interval 3 and the most preferred side (with which the subject, on average, performed the greatest number of problems correct). The 10 min point refers to testing 10 min after the best dose of nicotine; the 24 hr point refers to testing 24 hr after the best dose. In both cases the enhancement produced by nicotine was significant ($p < 0.05$).

aged monkeys perform this task with reduced efficiency compared with young animals is consistent with previous studies and serves to illustrate the sensitivity of the memory task to the age of the subject. Our experiments with nicotine clearly demonstrate a significant and reproducible facilitatory effect of the drug on performance of the DMTS task. Nicotine was most effective in enhancing the ability of animals to perform the longest delay intervals, that is, the most taxing with respect to recall. The lack of effect of nicotine at the shorter delay periods may relate to the fact that at shorter delay intervals, performance efficiency is already too high to observe significant improvement. This potential ceiling effect may also explain the results obtained when the highest dose of mecamylamine (2 mg/kg) was administered alone, in that there was more room for decrement in performance at the shorter delay periods. Nevertheless, the selective effect of the drugs on a specific delay interval indicates that altered performance was not related to drug effect on visual acuity, appetite or ingestive behavior.

Blockade of peripheral nicotinic receptors by hexamethonium failed to alter performance at any delay level. The lack of effect of hexamethonium indicates a central, not peripheral, effect of mecamylamine in producing the decrease in performance. Also, the inability of hexamethonium and the efficacy of mecamylamine to block the beneficial effects of nicotine, further substantiates the concept that the effect of nicotine and mecamylamine on performance are mediated through a central mechanism.

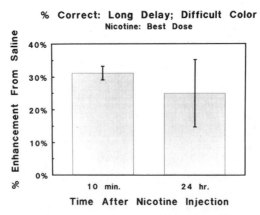

Figure 8. Delayed matching-to-sample performance by monkeys in the second series (unrestrained testing) analyzed in terms of delay interval 3 and the most preferred color (with which the subject, on average, performed the greatest number of problems correct). The 10 min point refers to testing 10 min after the best dose of nicotine; the 24 hr point refers to testing 24 hr after the best dose. In both cases the enhancement produced by nicotine was significant (p<0.05).

Delayed Matching involves two aspects: (1) the delay interval, which tests memory recall, and (2) a cognitive component, which tests the abstract conceptualization of "matching" and allows the subject to correctly match according to sameness, regardless of the stimuli involved. In the second nicotine series we investigated color and position preference with the hope that insight regarding effects of nicotine upon the conceptual component of matching could be provided. In regard to the first aspect of DMTS, recall as measured by length of delay interval, it may be important to remember that variations of the delayed response task are differentially sensitive to lesions in various brain regions. Thus the DTMS task is sensitive to different brain lesions than spatial tasks such as the AGED apparatus used by Bartus and colleagues,[14] or the DADTA apparatus[15]. There are apparently even differences between the DMTS task and the intuitively similar delayed non-matching to sample (DNMTS). For example, performance of the DTMS task is severely impaired by lesions of the prefrontal association areas, while monkeys with prefrontal damage perform as well as normals on the DNMTS task[16]. Conversely, the DNMTS task may be more sensitive than DMTS to the effects of temporal lobe damage[13]. Since the DNMTS task is currently being used more frequently than DMTS, it is worth making this point: The sensitivity of the DMTS task to prefrontal damage makes it a valuable tool, since frontal cortex appears to be particularly involved in age-related neurochemical and neuro-morphological changes. At the same time it is clear that the frontal cortex is only one part of a complex memory system involving at least the thalamus, basal ganglia, medial/anterior temporal lobe and the nucleus basalis. Performance of most variations of delayed response are severely impaired by advancing age, thus there is value to all these tasks; but the fact that there is differential sensitivity of the delayed response variations demonstrates the importance of multiple testing procedures in the overall search for memory enhancing drugs. It seems clear that age-related memory decrements result from changes in a variety of brain mechanisms. Similarly, a finer grained analysis of the classic variants, as evidenced by our analysis of position and color preference data, can also provide potentially valuable information.

In regard to the second, or conceptual aspect of DMTS, it is interesting that measuring color preference allowed us to account for the majority of long-delay enhancement associated with nicotine administration. The majority of the long-delay improvement associated with nicotine was due to increased percent correct of the non-preferred sample color. This finding strengthens our original hypothesis that nicotine enhances matching specifically during trials involved with the most difficult problems. In addition, the analysis of color preferences has raised an issue, which is worthy of speculation and perhaps further investigation. Specifically, the formation of color strategies reflect a category of cognitive ability, which not only is unique to primate species, but may be mediated by different neuronal substrates than those which mediate memory recall. Matching is a complex "conditional discrimination" problem[17] in which the significance of a discriminative stimulus is not invariant, but changes in relation to the stimulus context in which it appears. In that sense, DMTS is a task involving complex conditional discriminations. Discrimination in this sense does not mean inability to distinguish between stimuli, but rather the ability to abstract some common feature from a number of discriminable stimuli and to respond only to it. The ability to form concepts very likely relates to human declarative memory[18]. Squire and co-workers,[18] argued that human patients score well on tests originally designed as nonhuman primate tasks (such as matching) in proportion to the extent that they could verbalize the principle that determined which responses were rewarded. In the present study, the amount of stimulus control attached to each of the colors (as measured by color preferences) is a direct measure of the strength of the conceptual aspect of matching. It relates to the question of whether the cognition of each monkey involves the formation of efficient abstract concepts, or whether the monkey is responding on a more concrete level in which a "picture-memory" or stimulus-response type strategy is employed. A pronounced color or position preference would be compatible with such concrete cognition.

One measure of the strength of the matching concept is the transfer of training task, in which animals are tested for ability to transfer a previously learned concept to novel stimuli. In one demonstration of the unique ability of primates to transfer the matching concept, Jackson and Pegram,[19] used a test procedure almost identical to one described in this chapter. The findings demonstrated that monkeys transferred matching to novel sample color. This is in contrast to findings that pigeons (one of the rare non-primate species capable of matching from sample) do not transfer matching to a novel color[20]. These studies show that the behavioral control exerted by the sample reflects te ability to form a complex discrimination based upon the abstract conceptualization of matching. Tests of this type measure higher cognitive capabilities unique to primates, and as previously mentioned relate to human declarative memory. Such capabilities are Alzheimer's Disease, and thus an animal model capable of providing information about this form of higher cognitive ability could allow a valuable supplement to the information which is obtained from the monitoring of delay length.

In regard to the question of which neuronal systems are being stimulated or measured by the interaction between DMTS and nicotine, there are several points to be considered. First, the present data indicate a central substrate of the nicotine effects. Second, these forms of complex discrimination requirement appear to be the realm of the cortex. In the neurological examination, a classic test of cortical integrity is the two point discrimination test. This test requires patients to say whether they have been touched at one or two separated points on the skin. The patients in this case are asked to abstract to quality of singularity of duality, independent of the particular touch receptors stimulated. This abstraction requires multiple interconnections within and among sensory modalities and considerable plasticity among the connections. The only structure that has such characteristics in abundance is the cortex and thus it is not surprising that avstraction is only possible in those species with well developed neocortex. The particular sensitivity of the DMTS task has already been discussed. In addition, there are many studies indication that the transfer of concepts is dependent upon a properly functioning amygdala. Amygdalectomized monkeys, once trained to discriminated between large and small squares do not transfer the concept to large vs. small circles[21]. A similar failure of amygdalectomized monkeys to transfer a concept to novel situations have been described by many other studies involving non-human primates[22,23]. In contrast, lesions restrict to the amygdala do not alter delayed response capability. Instead, it apppears that a combination of lesions, involving the hippocampus and other structures of the anterior temporal lobe, must nec essarily be demanded before loss of delayed response performance is significantly interrupted[24,25]. It is known that lesions restricted to the hippocampus do not alter the transfer of matching to a novel stimulus (K.H. Pribram, personal communication; Jackson, umpublished data from 28 hippocampectomized monkeys). Thus, it appears that the two components of the matching (conceptual and recall) are subserved by different neuronal mechanisms, although both measure cognitive abilities which decrement in Alzheimer's Disease.

Finally, the possibility that activation of brain nicotinic receptors aged monkeys can also enhance performance in these animals is encouraging in the sense that this model is probably relevant to human memory/cognitive dysfunction. The possibility that nicotine did not reduce response latencies (if anything, there was a tendency to slightly increased latencies). Because of the toxicity of nicotine, it is not clear whether the drug could be useful as a treatment in human disease. The slightly better enhancement of DMTS by nicotine in the presence of selective nicotinic blockade (see Fig. 6) may be related to a reduction in the peripherally-mediated side effects of the agonist. Overall, our findings do suggest that central nicotinic receptors may be exploited pharmacologically in future treatments of human dementias.

ACKNOWLEDGEMENTS

This work was supported by the Smokeless Tobacco Research Council. The authors would also like to acknowledge the excellent technical assistance provided by Ms. Dianne Cox.

REFERENCES

1.   D.C. Rice, Primate research: relevance to human learning and development, Devel. Pharmacol. Ther. 10:314 (1987).
2.   E. Irle, J. Kessler, and H.J. Markowitsch, Primate learning tasks reveal strong impairments in patients with presenile or senile dementia of the alzheimer type, Brain Cogn. 6:429 (1987).
3.   D.D. Flynn and D.C. Mash, Characterization of 1-(3H)nicotine binding in human cerebral cortex: comparison between alzheimer's disease and the normal, J. Neurochem. 47:1948 (1986).
4.   P.J. Whitehouse and K.S. Au, Cholinergic receptors in aging and alzheimer's disease, Prog. Neuro Psychopharmacol. Biol. Psychiat. 10:656 (1986).
5.   P.J. Whitehouse and K.J. Kellar, Nicotinic and muscarinic cholinergic receptors in alzheimer's disease and related disorders, J. Neural Transm. (suppl.), 24:157 (1987).
6.   D.M. Warburton and K. Wesnes, Drugs as research tools in psychology: cholinergic drugs and information processing, Neuropsychobiology 11:121 (1984).
7.   L. Chiappeta and M.E. Jarvik, Comparison of learning impairment and activity depression produced by two classes of cholinergic blocking agents, Arch. Int. Pharmacodyn. Therap. 179:161 (1969).
8.   S.D. Glick and S. Greenstein, Differential effects of scopolamine and mecamylamine on passive avoidance behavior, Life Sci. 11:169 (1972).
9.   S.L. Dilts and C.A. Berry, Effect of cholinergic drugs on passive avoidance in the mouse, J. Pharmacol. Exper. Ther. 158:279 (1967).
10.   M.E. Goldberg, K. Sledge, M. Hefner, and R.C. Robichaud, Learning impairment after three classes of agents which modify cholinergic function, Arch. Int. Pharmacodyn. 193:226 (1971).
11.   I.P. Stolerman, T. Goldfarb, R. Fink, and M.E. Jarvik, Influencing cigarette smoking with nicotine antagonists, Psychopharmacology (Berlin) 28:247 (1973).
12.   K. Elrod, J.J. Buccafusco, and W.J. Jackson, Nicotine enhances delayed matching-to-sample performance by primates, Life Sci. 43:277 (1988).
13.   R.L.Dean and R.T. Bartus, Behavioral models of aging in nonhuman primates, in: Handbook of Psychopharmacology Vol. 10, L.L. Iverson, S.D. Iverson and S.H. Snyder, eds., Plenum Publishing Corp., New York (1988).
14.   R.T. Bartus and H.R. Johnson, Short-term memory in the rhesus monkey: disruption from the anti-cholinergic scopolamine, Pharmacol. Biochem. Behav. 5:539 (1976).
15.   K.H. Pribram, W.W. Gardner, G.L. Pressman and M. Bagshaw, An automated discrimination apparatus for discrete trial analysis (DADTA), Psycholog. Rep. 11:247 (1962).

16.   M. Mishkin, E.S. Prockop and H.E. Rosvold, One-trial object-discrimination learning in monkeys with frontal lesions, J. Comp. Physiological Psychol. 55:178 (1962).

17.   C.L. Hull, Principles of Behavior, Appleton, New York (1943).

18.   L.R. Squire, S. Zola-Morgan, and S.K. Chen, Human amnesia and animal models of amnesia: performance of amnesic patients on tests designed for the monkey, Behav. Neurosci. 102:210 (1988).

19.   W.J. Jackson and C.V. Pegram, Acquisition, transfer and retention of matching by rhesus monkeys, Psychol. Rep. 27:839 (1970).

20.   W.W. Cumming and R. Berryman, The complex discriminated operant: studies of matching-to-sample and related problems, in: Stimulus Generalization, D.I. Mostofsky, ed., Stanford University Press, Stanford, CA (1965).

21.   J.S. Schwartzbaum and K.H. Pribram, The effects of amygdalectomy in monkeys on transposition along a brightness continuum, J. Comp. Physiological Psychol. 53:396 (1960).

22.   M.H. Bagshaw and K.H. Pribram, Effect of amygdalectomy on transfer of training in monkeys, J. Comp. Physiological Psychol. 59:118 (1965).

23.   E. Hearst and K.H. Pribram, Appetitive and aversive generalization gradients in amygdalectomized monkeys, J. Comp. Physiological Psychol. 58:296 (1964).

24.   J.A. Horel, The neuroanatomy of amnesia, Brain 101:403 (1978).

25.   M. Mishkin, Memory in monkeys severely impaired by combined but not by separate removal of amygdala and hippocampus, Nature 273:297 (1978).

MUSCARINIC AND NICOTINIC RECEPTORS IN ALZHEIMER'S DISEASE:

RATIONALE FOR CHOLINERGIC DRUG TREATMENT

Paul A. Lapchak, Dalia M. Araujo*,
and Remi Quirion

Neuroanatomy Lab., Montreal Neurological Inst.
3801 University St., Montreal, Quebec, H3A 2B4 and
Douglas Hospital Res. Ctr., 6875 Lasalle Blvd
Verdun, Quebec, H4H 1R3

INTRODUCTION

Alzheimer's disease (AD) is characterized by an extensive degeneration of the cholinergic system in the human nucleus basalis of Meynert, neocortex and hippocampus (1-5), mainly based upon measures of choline acetyltransferase activity (ChAT). Cholinergic receptor populations (muscarinic and nicotinic) have also been studied in Alzheimer's disease; however the results of studies concerning muscarinic receptors are variable and inconsistent (1, 6-8). The variability may be due to the non-selective nature of the ligands used to measure muscarinic receptor populations. Alternatively, the discrepancy may be explained by the existence of multiple subtypes of muscarinic receptors in the CNS (see 5). Muscarinic receptors can be subdivided into a number of subtypes (M1-M3) which may be selectively labeled using ^{3}H-pirenzepine (M1), ^{3}H-ACh or ^{3}H-AF-DX 116 (M2), or ^{3}H-4DAMP (M3) (5, 9-12) In contrast to muscarinic receptors, results concerning the fate of neuronal nicotinic receptor populations in AD cortex are more consistent. These studies indicate that the density of nicotinic receptors, at least in cortical structures, is severely reduced in AD (3,5,13,14). It is essential to determine whether specific cholinergic receptor populations are affected in various regions of the AD brain in order to develop a strategy for the treatment of AD.

CHOLINERGIC MARKERS IN ALZHEIMER'S DISEASE

ChAT Activity

ChAT activity was measured in homogenates of AD brain (77.3 + 2.3 years of age, n=8) and compared to control brain tissue (70.1 + 3.3 years of age, n=9). The brain regions used were frontal cortex, hippocampus and striatum. There was a large decrease in ChAT activity in the frontal cortex (69%) and hippocampus (66%). In contrast, ChAT activity in the striatum was unaltered compared to control (Table 1).

TABLE 1. ChAT activity in control and AD brain.

	ChAt activity	(nmol/mg protein/h)
	Control	Alzheimer's
frontal cortex	5.2 ± 0.6	1.6 ± 0.2
hippocampus	13.4 ± 3.6	4.6 ± 1.2
striatum	40.5 ± 1.9	39.8 ± 4.3

Muscarinic Receptor Populations in Human Brain

To determine whether muscarinic M1 or M2 receptors were altered in AD, we used saturation analysis of ^{3}H-pirenzepine to M1 binding sites and ^{3}H-ACh binding to M2 binding sites. The maximal density (Bmax) of ^{3}H-pirenzepine (M1) binding sites was not altered in AD frontal cortex, but was slightly increased in AD hippocampus (25%) and striatum (33%). The affinity of ^{3}H-pirenzepine binding to M1 sites was not altered in diseased compared to control brains (Table 2). The Bmax for ^{3}H-ACh (M2) binding was significantly reduced in AD frontal cortex (49%) and hippocampus (56%) but was not changed in AD striatum. In addition, the affinity of M2 sites was not altered in AD (Table 2).

Nicotinic Receptors in Human Brain

Nicotinic binding sites were studied using saturation analysis of ^{3}H-methylcarbamylcholine (MCC) binding to homogenates of human brain. This ligand has previously been shown to bind to neuronal nicotinic receptors in mammalian brain (5, 8, 15-17). The density of ^{3}H-MCC binding sites was reduced in AD frontal cortex (68%) and hippocampus (61%) but not in AD striatum. The apparent affinity of ^{3}H-MCC binding sites was not significantly different in AD brain compared with normal brain tissue (Table 3).

TABLE 2. Muscarinic binding sites in control and AD brain. Results are expressed as the maximal binding capacity (Bmax) in fmol/mg protein and apparent affinity constant (Kd) in nM.

		^{3}H-pirenzepine (M1)		^{3}H-ACH (M2)	
		B_{max}	K_d	B_{max}	K_d
frontal	C	502 ± 25	17.0 ± 2.2	22.8 ± 1.4	5.6 ± 0.8
cortex	AD	378 ± 23	19.2 ± 4.0	11.6 ± 1.5	7.3 ± 2.1
hippocampus	C	287 ± 22	13.2 ±4.6	39.3 ± 3.0	7.7 ± 2.4
	AD	358 ± 20	20.2 ±4.8	17.1 ± 2.6	8.8 ± 2.7
striatum	C	491 ± 25	27.2 ± 4.0	39.6 ± 3.8	8.5 ± 3.9
	AD	651 ± 39	21.0 ± 4.1	42.3 ± 3.4	10.1 ± 4.7

TABLE 3. Nicotinic binding sites in control and AD brain

		^{3}H-MCC B_{max} (fmol / mg protein)	^{3}H-MCC K_d (nM)
frontal cortex	C	10.6 ± 2.8	11.9 ± 1.6
	AD	3.4 ± 1.1	9.1 ± 2.6
hippocampus	C	11.5 ± 2.4	7.5 ± 0.7
	AD	4.5 ± 1.3	6.4 ± 1.5
striatum	C	20.7 ± 2.6	10.0 ± 2.4
	AD	17.5 ± 3.5	11.5 ± 3.7

The present results indicate that muscarinic M2 receptors and nicotinic receptors are compromised in certain
regions of AD brains. The decrease in the density of M2 sites
and nicotinic sites in the AD frontal cortex and hippocampus
correlates with the decrease of ChAT activity in these brain
regions. In all cases, the positive correlation was
significant (r > 0.82). In contrast, there was no significant correlation between ChAT activity and M1 binding
sites in these brain regions. These correlations suggest that
nicotinic binding sites and M2 muscarinic binding sites may be
localized presynaptically to cholinergic terminals in the
frontal cortex and hippocampus. The exact function of these
receptors in human brain is not known, but they may represent
autoreceptors which regulate the release of acetylcholine.

Functional Role of Nicotinic Receptors in Mammalian Brain

Recent neurochemical findings indicate the widespread
existence of nicotinic autoreceptors on cholinergic terminals
in the mammalian brain (9, 16, 18). The rat CNS contains a
relatively low density of high affinity ^{3}H-MCC binding sites.
The hippocampus (14.9 ± 2.1 fmol/mg protein) contains a low
number of ^{3}H-MCC binding sites whereas both the striatum and
frontal cortex contain substantially higher amounts (23.3 ±
2.5 and 31.4 ± 4.4 fmol/ mg protein, respectively). The apparent affinity constant for these sites is 5.7-8.6 nM (9, 16,
17).

We have determined the effects of unlabeled MCC on the
release of endogenous ACh from brain slices of frontal cortex, hippocampus and striatum. MCC significantly increased
spontaneous ACh release from frontal cortical and hippocampal
slices but not from striatum (Table 4). The effect of MCC was
only apparent during incubation in the presence of normal
potassium Krebs medium but not in the presence of elevated
concentrations of potassium (25 or 50 mM). The MCC-induced
increased ACh release from cortex or hippocampus was abolished when slices were incubated in the presence of nicotinic
receptor antagonists (d-tubocurarine [DT] or dihydro-beta-
erythroidine [DBE]). Furthermore, the effect of MCC was calcium-dependent since MCC did not enhance ACh release when
brain slices were incubated in calcium-free medium (Table 4).

TABLE 4. Effect of MCC on spontaneous ACh release from rat
         brain slices

	Incubation Condition	ACh release (% control)
frontal cortex	MCC (10 µM)	177 ± 25
	MCC (10 µM), TTX (1 µM)	164 ± 12
	MCC (10 µM), Ca-free	98 ± 8
	MCC (10 µM), DT (1 µM)	102 ± 16
hippocampus	MCC (10 µM)	211 ± 33
	MCC (10 µM), TTX (1 µM)	191 ± 16
	MCC (10 µM), Ca-free	103 ± 13
	MCC (10 µM), DT (1 µM)	102 ± 3
striatum	MCC (0.1 nM to 10 mM)	98 to 120

To determine whether the MCC-induced increase in ACh release from cortex or hippocampus was due to an action on presynaptic nicotinic autoreceptors, we tested the effect of MCC
on spontaneous ACh release in the presence of the sodium
channel blocker, tetrodotoxin (TTX). This drug would block
impulse activity along an axon if MCC was acting distal to the
nerve terminal. The effect of MCC on ACh release from both
tissues was apparent even in the presence of TTX, suggesting
an action on nicotinic autoreceptors which are present at the
level of the terminal. Therefore, nicotinic autoreceptors are
present in certain regions of the rat brain (frontal cortex,
hippocampus, cerebellum) which, when activated by a nicotinic
drug (MCC, nicotine) or the endogenous ligand (ACh) result in
the enhancement of spontaneous ACh release which maintains an
elevated level of synaptic activity. It is conceivable that
this positive feedback mechanism may be exploited in order to
facilitate the release of ACh in vivo (see below).

Functional Role of Muscarinic-M2 Receptors in the Mammalian
Brain

Several studies have proposed that functional muscarinic
autoreceptors exist in the mammalian brain (9, 10, 19-23). The
identification of the subtype of muscarinic receptor involved
in the regulation of ACh release has been difficult due to the
lack of receptor subtype-selective probes, although it has
been suggested that M2 receptors may be involved in the
feedback regulation of ACh release. Recently, it has been
suggested that AF-DX 116 is a suitable ligand to study the M2-
muscarinic receptor (10, 12, 24-26). ^{3}H-AF-DX 116 binds to two
classes of muscarinic binding sites in homogenates of rat
frontal cortex, hippocampus and striatum. The characteristics
of these sites are such that one is of high affinity (Kd<
5nM)/low capacity (Bmax 30 - 63 fmol/mg protein) and the
second of lower affinity (Kd>65 nM) and higher capacity (Bmax
190 -260 fmol/mg protein).

We have determined the effects of unlabeled AF-DX 116 on
the spontaneous and potassium-evoked release of endogenous

ACh from rat brain slices. AF-DX 116 enhanced the potassium-evoked release of ACh from frontal cortex, hippocampus and striatum. The effect of the M2-selective antagonist AF-DX 116 was dose-dependent and occurred only when slices were incubated in medium containing elevated concentrations of potassium (25 mM): the effect of the non-selective antagonist atropine was similar to that of AF-DX 116 (hippocampal data shown in Table 5). The M1-selective antagonist pirenzepine and the M3-selective antagonist 4-DAMP were ineffective in altering spontaneous or evoked ACh release. In addition, AF-DX 116, like atropine, could effectively reverse the oxotremorine induced inibition of evoked ACh release. Neither pirenzepine nor 4-DAMP reversed the effects of oxotremorine.

In summary, the results described above indicate that presynaptic muscarinic autoreceptors appear to be of the the M2-subtype, as determined using the M2 antagonist AF-DX 116. These results suggest that the in vivo activation of M2 autoreceptors by ACh results in negative feedback control of evoked ACh release from cholinergic terminals in the frontal cortex, hippocampus and striatum. Therefore, this inhibitory feedback mechanism would modulate the level of ACh released and subsequently the extent of the postsynaptic signal in response to the quantity of ACh released. It is possible that the selective antagonism of muscarinic M2 autoreceptors may result in the enhancement of ACh release and thus have therapeutic applications (see below).

Pharmacological Basis for the use of Nicotinic and Muscarinic Drugs in Alzheimer's Disease

The positive correlation between ChAT activity and either nicotinic or muscarinic M2 receptors AD brains suggests that these two types of cholinergic receptors may be localized presynaptically to cholinergic terminals. If the activation of nicotinic receptors by nicotinic agonists or the blockade of muscarinic M2 receptors by a specific muscarinic antagonist results in an enhancement of ACh release from certain brain structures, then a treatment strategy may be developed which is beneficial to the AD patient. This treatment strategy would probably be useful in the early and middle

TABLE 5. Effect of muscarinic drugs on evoked ACh release from rat hippocampal slices

	Incubation Condition		ACh release (%control)
hippocampus	atropine (ATR)	(0.1 mM)	148 ± 8
	pirenzepine (PZ)	(0.1 mM)	97 ± 5
	AF-DX 116 (AF)	(0.1 mM)	152 ± 14
	4-DAMP	(0.1 mM)	110 ± 11
	oxo	(0.1 mM)	63 ± 6
	oxo (0.1 mM), ATR	(0.1 mM)	98 ± 7
	oxo (0.1 mM), PZ	(0.1 mM)	65 ± 6
	oxo (0.1 mM), AF	(0.1 mM)	98 ± 5
	oxo (0.1 mM), AF	(0.1 mM)	97 ± 12
	oxo (0.1 mM), 4-DAMP	(0.1 mM)	62 ± 6

stages of AD when the loss of nicotinic and muscarinic M2 receptors has not yet reached a maximum. Stimulation (nicotinic) or blockade (muscarinic) of cortical or hippocampal autoreceptor populations may increase ACh release, and perhaps ameliorate the memory dysfunctions associated with AD.

Administration of nicotine to animals is correlated with positive physiological responses such as improvement of learning, increase in information retention, increase in long-term information storage and the production of state dependent learning (27-29). Nicotine also serves as a positive reinforcer under certain experimental conditions (30). Studies testing the effects of nicotine (directly or indirectly via cigarette smoking) on human physiological responses have yielded mixed results. For instance, nicotine is a positive reinforcer (i.v.) (30), increases concentration and performance (cigarette puffs) (31), increases free recall and long-term recall (32) and also decreases intrusion error (33). However, the administration of nicotine is not without side effects. Administration of nicotine alters behavioral patterns and physiological functions. The effects of nicotine include an increase in anxiety-depression-fear (32,33). Physiological parameters are also altered by nicotine. Dose-dependent increases in pulse rate, systolic blood pressure and respiratory rate result from nicotine infusion (32).

These studies suggest that CNS nicotine receptors are important in regulating certain behavioral and physiological responses in man and animals. The administration of nicotinic agonists under controlled conditions may increase cognitive functions and possibly be useful in the treatment of the cognitive deficits associated with AD. The development of a successful treatment program with nicotine targeted against presynaptic nicotinic autoreceptors may be difficult considering the rapid desensitization phenomenon linked to nicotinic receptors (9). We have shown that nicotinic autoreceptor function in rats is severely compromised after multiple injections of nicotine, although the density of nicotinic receptors in cortex and hippocampus is markedly increased (9). It is interesting to note that long-term cigarette smoking in humans also results in the upregulation of the density of CNS nicotinic receptors (34). If this increase in receptor number in human brain is associated with the loss of autoreceptor function, then the administration of nicotine would not be beneficial to the AD patient. Alternatively, a treatment schedule could be devised which would guard against long-term receptor desensitization. The treatment of an AD patient with nicotine on an intermittent administration schedule is feasible and may be achieved with the use of nicotine gum. This method may produce presynaptic nicotinic receptor activation and increase ACh release in the CNS.

Muscarinic agonist (arecoline, bethanechol) therapies have been tested with little or no success in AD patients (33, 35, 36). These compounds have not been shown to significantly improve memory recall, learning or cognitive tasks suggesting that the postsynaptic action of these agonists on muscarinic receptors is not sufficient to increase cognitive function. The use of specific presynaptic muscarinic M2 anticholinergics may be useful in the treatment of AD if compounds could be developed which preferentially block M2 autoreceptors. This would cause an increase in ACh release from brain structures important in the formation of short and long term memory and learning processes. Finally, if this type of compound could be developed it could be used in combination with nicotinic agonists to enhance maximally ACh release from the remaining cholinergic terminals in the hippocampus and cortex of AD patients, which may result in significant cognitive improvement.

Acknowledgements

We wish to thank Colin Holmes for typesetting the manuscript. This work was supported by grants from MRC, Canada, , Quebec and FRSQ, Quebec.

References

1.   Hardy, J., Adolfsson, R., Alafuzoff, I., Bucht, G., Marcusson, J., Nyberg, P., Perdahl, E., Wester, P. and Winblad, B. (1985) Transmitter deficits in Alzheimer's disease. Neurochem. Int. 7: 545-563.
2.   Candy, J.M., Perry, E.K., Perry, R.H., Court, J.A., Oakley, A.E. and Edwardson, J.A. (1986) The current status of the cortical cholinergic system in Alzheimer's disease and Parkinson's disease. Prog. Brain Res. 70: 105-132.
3.   Quirion, R., Martel, J.C., Robitaille, Y., Etienne, P., Wood, P., Nair, N.P.V. and Gauthier, S. (1986) Neurotransmitter and receptor deficits in senile dementia of the Alzheimer type. Can. J. Neurol. Sci. 13: 503-510.
4.Plotkin, D.A. and Jarvik, L.F. (1986) Cholinergic dysfunction in Alzheimer's disease: cause or effect. Prog Brain Res. 65: 91-103.
5.   Araujo, D.M., Lapchak, P.A., Robitaille, Y., Gauthier, S. and Quirion, R. (1988) Differential alteration of various cholinergic markers in cortical and subcortical regions of human brain in Alzheimer's disease. J. Neuro- chem. 50: 1914-1923.
6.   Mash, D.C., Flynn, D.D. and Potter, L.T. (1985) Loss of M2 muscarine receptors in the cerebral cortex in Alzheimer's disease and experimental cholinergic denervation. Science 228: 1115-1117.
7.   Reinikinainen, K.J., Riekkinen, P.J., Halonoe, T. and Laakso, M. (1987) Decreased muscarinic receptor binding in cerebral cortex and hippocampus in Alzheimer's disease. Life Sci. 41: 453-461.
8.   Bowen, D.M., Allen, S.J., Benton, J.S., Goodhart, M.J., Haan, E.A., Palmer, A.M., Sims, N.R., Smith, C.C.T., Spillane, J.A., Esiri, M.M., Nearym D., Snowdon, J.S., Wilcock, G.K. and Davison, A.N. (1983) Biochemical assessment of serotonergic and cholinergic dysfunction and cerebral atrophy in Alzheimer's disease. J. Neuro- chem. 41: 266-272.
9.   Lapchak, P.A., Araujo, D.M., Quirion, R. and Collier, B. (1989) Effect of chronic nicotine treatment on nicotinic autoreceptor function and N-[3H]methylcarbamyl-choline binding sites in the rat brain. J. Neurochem.52: 483-491.

10. Lapchak, P.A., Araujo, D.M., Quirion, R. and Collier, B. (1989) Binding sites for [3H]AF-DX 116 and effect of AF-DX 116 on endogenous acetylcholine release from rat brain slices. Brain Res. in press.

11. Lapchak, P.A., Araujo, D.M., Quirion, R. and Collier, B. (1989) Presynaptic cholinergic mechanisms in the rat cerebellum: evidence for nicotinic, but not muscarinic autoreceptors. J. Neurochem. in press.

12. Araujo, D.M., Lapchak, P.A., Regenold, W. and Quirion, R. (1989) Characterization of [3H]AF-DX 116 binding sites in rat brain: evidence for heterogeneity of muscarinic-M2 receptor sites. Synapse in press.

13. Flynn, D.D. and Mash, D.C. (1986) Characterization of L-[3H]nicotine binding in human cerebral cortex: comparison between Alzheimer's disease and the normal. J.Neurochem. 47: 1948-1954.

14. Whitehouse, P.J., Martino, A.M., Antuono, P.G., Lowenstein, P.R., Coyle, J.T., Price, D.L. and Kellar, K.J. (1986) Nicotinic acetylcholine binding sites in Alzheimer's disease. Brain Res. 371: 146-151.

15. Abood, L.G. and Grassi, S. (1986) [3H]Methylcarbamylcholine, a new radioligand for studying brain nicotinic receptors. Biochem. Pharmacol. 35: 4199-4202.

16. Boksa, P. and Quirion, R. (1987) [3H]N-Methylcarbamylcholine, a new radioligand specific for nicotinic acetylcholine receptors in brain. Eur. J. Pharmacol. 139: 323-333.

17. Araujo, D.M., Lapchak, P.A., Collier, B. and Quirion, R. (1988) Characterization of N-[3H]Methylcarbamylcholine binding sites and effect of N-Methylcarbamylcholine on acetylcholine release in rat brain. J. Neurochem. 51: 292-299.

18. Rowell, P.P. and Winkler, D.L. (1984) Nicotinic stimulation of [3H]acetylcholine release from mouse cerebral cortical synaptosomes. J. Neurochem. 43: 1593-1598.

19. Raiteri, M., Leardi, R. and Marchi, M. (1984) Heterogeneity of presynaptic muscarinic receptors regulating neurotransmitter release in the rat brain. J. Pharmacol. Exp. Ther. 228: 209-214.

20. Pohorecki, R., Head, R. and Domino, E.F. (1988) Effects of selected muscarinic cholinergic antagonists of [3H]acetylcholine release from rat hippocampal slices. J. Pharmacol. Exp. Ther. 244: 213-217.

21. Hadhazy, P. and Szerb, J.C. (1977) The effect of cholinergic drugs on [3H]acetylcholine release from slices of rat hippocampus, striatum and cortex. Brain Res. 123: 311-322.

22. Szerb, J.C., Hadhazy, P. and Dudar, J.D. (1977) Release of [3H]acetylcholine from rat hippocampal slices: effect of septal lesion and graded concentrations of muscarinic agonists and antagonists. Brain Res. 128: 285-291.

23. Marchi, M. and Raiteri, M. (1985) On the presence in the cerebral cortex of muscarinic receptor subtypes which differ in neuronal localization, function and pharmacological properties. J. Pharmacol. Exp. Ther. 235: 230-233.

24. Wang, J.X., Roeske, W.R., Gulya, K., Wang, W. and Yamamura, H.I. (1987) [3H]AF-DX 116 labels subsets of muscarinic cholinergic receptors in rat brain and heart. Life Sci. 41: 1751-1760.

25. Wang, J.X., Roeske, W.R., Wang, W. and Yamamura, H.I. (1988) Himbacine recognizes a high affinity subtype of M2 muscarinic cholinergic receptor in the rat cerebral cortex. Brain Res. 446: 155-158.

26. Hammer, R., Giraldo, E., Schiavi, G.B., Monferini, E. and Ladinsky, H. (1986) Binding profiles of a novel cardioselective muscarine antagonist, AF-DX 116, to membranes of peripheral tissues and brain in the rat. Life Sci. 38: 1653-1662.

27. Warburton, D.M., Wesnes, K., Shergold, K. and James, M. (1986) Facilitation of learning and state dependency with nicotine. Psychopharmacology 89: 55-59.

28. Wesnes, K. and Warburton, D.M. (1983) Smoking, nicotine, and human performance. Pharmacol. Ther. 21: 189-208.

29. Wesnes, K. and Revell, A. (1984) The separate and combined effects of scopolamine and nicotine on human information processing. Psychopharmacology 84: 5-11.

30. Goldberg, S.R. and Henningfield, J.E. (1988) Reinforcing effects of nicotine in humans and experimental animals responding under intermittent schedules of iv drug injection. Pharmacology Biochemistry and Behavior 30: 227-234.

31. Revell, A.D. (1988) Smoking and performance: a puff-by-puff analysis. Psychopharmacology 96: 563-565.

32. Sunderland, T., Tariot, P.N. and Newhouse, P.A. (1988) Differential responsivity of mood, behavior, and cognition to cholinergic agents in elderly neuropsychiatric populations. Brain Res. Rev. 13: 371-389.

33. Newhouse, P.A., Sunderland, T., Tariot, P.N., Blumhardt, C.L., Weingartner, H., Mellow, A. and Murphy, D.L. (1988) Intravenous nicotine in Alzheimer's disease: pilot study. Psychopharmacology 95: 171-175.

34. Benwell, M.E.M., Balfour, D.J.K. and Anderson, J.M. (1988) Evidence that tobacco smoking increases the density of (-)-[3H]nicotine binding sites in human brain. J. Neurochem. 50: 1243-1247.

35. Whitehouse, P.J. (1988) Intraventricular bethanechol in Alzheimer's disease. Neurology 38: 307-308.

36. Tariot, P.N., Cohen, R.M., Welkowitz, J.A., Sunderland, T., Newhouse, P.A., Murphy, D.L. and Weingartner, H. (1988) Multiple dose arecoline infusions on Alzheimer's disease. Arch. Gen. Psychiatry 45: 901-905.

POTENTIAL PHARMACOLOGICAL USE OF NEUROTROPHIC FACTORS

IN THE TREATMENT OF NEURODEGENERATIVE DISEASES

Franz Hefti

Andrus Gerontology Center and Department of
Biological Sciences
University of Southern California
Los Angeles, CA 90089

INTRODUCTION

   There is growing evidence that development, maintenance
of function, and regeneration of neurons are influenced by
trophic hormones or neurotrophic factors. These
neurotrophic factors stimulate mechanisms necessary for
survival, neurite growth and functions related to
transmitter production and release. Nerve growth factor
(NGF) is the first and best characterized neurotrophic
factor and serves as a paradigm for more recently discovered
molecules. NGF trophically acts on peripheral sympathetic
and sensory neurons, and cholinergic neurons in the brain.
Other neurotrophic molecules characterized so far influence
various other neuronal populations. Brain-derived
neurotrophic factor is a protein purified from pig brain
which supports the survival of chick sensory neurons and rat
retinal ganglion cells. Glia- derived nexin produced by
glial cells and inducing neurite growth of neuroblastoma
cells was found to be an inhibitor of cell- derived
proteases. This finding is in line with other evidence for
a role of proteases and protease inhibitors in neurite
growth and regeneration. Several laboratories have reported
partial or complete purification of neurotrophic factors for
spinal cord motoneurons. Besides these neurotrophic factors
which were found by means of purification and a neuronal
cell assay system, there is a number of earlier
characterized growth factors or hormones which also affect
neurons and, therefore, are often considered neurotrophic
factors. Among these are fibroblast growth factors which
stimulate the proliferation of non-neuronal cells but also
promote survival of rat brain neurons in vitro. Receptors
for insulin and insulin-like growth factors I and II occur
in the brain and these hormones promote growth of various
neuronal populations in culture. Neurotrophic actions have
been described for epidermal growth factor and transforming
growth factor alpha. Besides the neurotrophic factors
described so far, which are soluble proteins, there are
membrane-bound molecules promoting adhesion of neurons and
neurite extension. Various aspects of the field of

neurotrophic factors have been subject of recent reviews (1, 2, 3, 4, 5, 6, 7, 8, 9).

The discovery of neurotrophic factors has prompted considerations that such factors may play a role in neurodegenative diseases. Appel (10) formulated a general hypothesis stating that the lack of neurotrophic factors is responsible for the degeneration of selective neuronal populations as it occurs in Parkinson's disease, Alzheimer's disease, and in amyotrophic lateral sclerosis, and, furthermore, that application of the corresponding neurotrophic factor might prevent the neuronal degeneration. Since NGF is a trophic factor for the population of basal forebrain cholinergic neurons which degenerates in Alzheimer's disease, it has been speculated that NGF may be useful in the treatment of this disease (11, 12 13).

Neurotrophic factors may become useful as replacement therapy if lack of endogenous molecules plays a crucial role in the pathogenesis of a disease. Other deficits in neurotrophic factor-related mechanisms may be overcome by exogenously administered molecules. Furthermore, even in absence of a direct involvement of a neurotrophic factor in a pathological process, elevating the quantity of this factor above endogenous levels is likely to induce hypertrophy of responsive cells. Such hypertrophy is manifested by increased expression of structural proteins and molecules responsible for transmitter synthesis and release. Structural changes will improve the resistance of neurons to insults; hypertrophy of transmitter-related mechanisms will facilitate the neurons' ability to influence postsynaptic cells. This general concept is supported by studies on the interaction between NGF and basal cholinergic neurons (7, 8, 14, 15).

Classical neuropharmacology which has grown to a major field during the past few decades attempts to influence mechanisms related to neuronal impulse flow and transmission at the synapse. Currently used drugs and available pharmacological tools do not affect the structural features of the central nervous system and there are no compounds able to promote regeneration, plasticity, and maintenance of structural integrity of selected neuronal systems. According to the concepts outlined above, the area of neurotrophic factors may lead to the development of a new, structurally oriented neuropharmacology. In particular, the available data suggest that neurotrophic factors may be useful in the treatment of neurodegenerative diseases which are associated with structural disintegration of selected neuronal systems or brain areas. The following sections discuss possible strategies for the development of pharmacological interference of brain function based on neurotrophic factors. A more detailed review of these concepts has been published elsewhere (15).

INTRACEREBRAL ADMINISTRATION OF NEUROTROPHIC FACTORS

To be able to reach neuronal populations in the brain, neurotrophic factors will have to be given intracerebrally, since these proteins do not cross the blood-brain barrier. In experimental animals, NGF has been injected through

chronically implanted cannulas or has been chronically
infused with the help of osmotic minipumps (16, 17, 18).
Both these procedures are inadequate for human use and other
approaches are necessary to find suitable ways of
neurotrophic factor administration to humans.

Neurotrophic factors purified from natural sources or
produced by recombinant techniques may be chronically
infused into the brain with the help of mechanical pump
devices. Subcutaneous pumps are available which deliver
proteins through a small tubing to the cerebral ventricles.
Pumps can be refilled through the skin and their delivery
rate can be set without surgical intervention. Subcutaneous
pump devices have been used for the administration of
cholinergic agonists to Alzheimer patients (19). Pumps and
the intraventricular delivery systems apparently are well
tolerated (19, 20). Stability of the neurotrophic factors
during storage in these pump devices may require special
preparations. NGF is a relatively stable and soluble
protein, whereas other known neurotrophic factors are
unstable in solution. In the case of basic fibroblast
growth factor, stability was improved by single amino acid
substitutions (21). Self-assembly may become a problem when
proteins are packed at high concentrations in pumps or
polymers. In the case of insulin this problem was solved by
substitution of single amino acids (22).

If intraventricular infusion of a neurotrophic factor
is proven to be clinically effective, it may become
worthwhile to test slow-releasing intracerebral implants.
Such implants contain the active protein embedded in a
biodegradable polymer matrix. Existing polymers provide
stable release rates over a period of several weeks (23).

DEVELOPMENT OF FRAGMENTS AND ANALOGS OF NEUROTROPHIC FACTORS

Rather than administering entire trophic factor
molecules, it may be possible to use modified molecules or
active fragments. So far, very little is known about this
approach. A trypsin fragment of NGF, claimed to be
effective several years ago, was later shown to be inactive
(24). The lack of demonstrated success, however, does not
prove that such an approach is not feasible. Fragments of
EGF, bFGF and IGF-I appear to retain activity (25, 26, 27,
28). Despite their advantages, active fragments of trophic
factors will still require intraventricular administration.
This problem may be overcome by non-peptide agonistic
molecules for neurotrophic factors which pass the
blood-brain barrier. While theoretically possible, this may
prove a very difficult task.

GRAFTING OF CELL PRODUCING NEUROTROPHIC FACTORS

Grafting of brain tissue replacing degenerated cells is
frequently proposed as a potential approach to treat brain
dysfunction. Such techniques are not limited to natural
cells but could include genetically modified cells as
proposed by Gage et al. (14). In the case of NGF, cells
expressing this protein have been implanted in the vicinity
of the cell bodies of cholinergic neurons, and shown to
provide chronic and stable supply of NGF protecting the

cholinergic neurons from lesion- induced degeneration (29). It seems possible to produce cells which do not proliferate after implantation and are well tolerated by the host. If expression of the desired neurotrophic factor is put under control of a promoter responding to drugs, it will be possible to regulate and terminate its production. However, engineered cells probably will release other proteins besides the desired neurotrophic factor and production of these molecules may be difficult to control.

PHARMACOLOGICAL MANIPULATION OF NEUROTROPHIC FACTOR SYNTHESIS

A feasible approach to influence neurotrophic actions may be to search for ways to manipulate specifically the synthesis of endogenous neurotrophic factors. At the present time, very little is known about the regulation of synthesis of NGF or other neurotrophic factors and the mechanisms controlling the selective expression of their genes are poorly understood. The gene promoter regions of NGF were recently isolated and cloned from rodent genomic libraries as a first step in the analysis of the transcriptional regulation of NGF expression (30).

Molecules eventually able to regulate NGF expression are retinoic acid and thyroid hormones. Retinoic acid has recently been reported to increase the number of receptors for NGF in neuroblastoma cells (31) and to elevate the levels of NGF and its mRNA in L cells (32). The same compound has previously been shown to induce neuron-like differentiation of embryonic carcinoma cells (33, 34). Morphological and biochemical differentiation of human neuroblastoma cells is also affected by retinoic acid (35, 36).

Thyroid hormones are essential for the normal development of the brain, and these hormones have been reported to influence axonal regeneration in adult animals. Several findings suggest a relationship between thyroid hormones and NGF at least in relation to cholinergic neurons of the basal forebrain. Thyroid deficiency is associated with a reduction of ChAT activity in the brain of experimental animals (37). Triiodothyronine (T3) has been found to increase ChAT activity in various cultures system with rat neurons (38, 39, 40). The effects of T3 and NGF were found to be additive in one study (39) and synergistic in another (38). Interestingly, thyroid hypofunction in humans is associated with dementia (41, 42). This observation, together with the cholinergic deficit in Alzheimer's disease, promoted us to hypothesize that thyroid hormones may be useful in attenuating the atrophy of cholinergic neurons. However, application of thyroid hormones to patients with normal thyroid function would result in a multitude of undesired effects given the fact that these hormones influence the function of most organs. This problem might be circumvented with thyroxine analogs selectively stimulating central cholinergic neurons. Our own studies with a limited number of such analogs suggested that the structural requirements of central and peripheral receptors are similar (39). However, more recent structural data on thyroid hormone receptors indicate the existence of tissue specific receptors (43) and novel analogs have been described which differentiate between receptors of various peripheral organs (4 4) .

Transection of the sciatic nerve and its NGF responsive sympathetic and sensory neurons results in a robust and prolonged elevation of the expression of NGF and NGF receptors in the distal part of the transected nerve (45, 46) suggesting an involvement of NGF in peripheral neuronal regeneration. These experimental lesions of peripheral neurons result in infiltration of macrophages which release interleukin-1 which then stimulates NGF synthesis (47). Although experimental lesions of central NGF responsive pathways do not result in comparable massive changes in NGF or NGF receptor synthesis, it is possible that interleukin-1 is involved in the regulation of central NGF synthesis which then could be controlled by manipulating levels of interleukin-1.

CONCLUSION

Neurotrophic factors are potent molecules involved in regulation of neuronal survival, growth, plasticity and maintenance of function. Such molecules or active fragments may be pharmacologically useful after intracerebral administration. Alternatively, it may be possible to manipulate mechanisms involved in the regulation of neurotrophic factors.

Acknowledgment. The author was supported by NIH grant N522933, NSF grant BN5-8708049, and by grants from the Alzheimer's Disease and Related Disorders Association, Chicago IL, and the National Parkinson Foundation, Miami FL.

REFERENCES

1. Barde, Y.A., Davies, A. M., Johnson, J.E., Lindsay, R. M. and Thoenen, H. (1987) Brain-derived neurotrophic factor. Prog. Brain Res . 71:185-189 .
2. Baskin, D.G., Wilcox, B.J., Figlewicz, D.P. and Dorsa, D.M. (1888) Insulin and insulin-like growth factors in the CNS. Trends in Neurosci. 11(3):368-389.
3. Jessell, T.M. (1988) Adhesion molecules and the hierarchy of neural development. Neuron 1:3-13.
4. Monard, D. (1987) Role of protease inhibition in cellular migration and neuritic growth. Biochem. Pharmacol. 36:1389-1392 .
5   Morrison, R.S. (1987) Fibroblast growth factors: potential neurotrophic agents in the central nervous system. J. Neurosci. Res. 17:99-101.
6. Thoenen, H. and Edgar, D. (1985) Neurotrophic factors. Science, 229:238-242.
7   Thoenen, H., Bandtlow, C. and Heumann, R. (1987) The physiological function of nerve growth factor in the central nervous system: comparison with the periphery. Rev. Physiol. Biochem. Pharmacol. 109:145-178.
8. Whittemore, S.R. and Seiger, A. (1987) The expression, localization and functional significance of beta-nerve growth factor in the central nervous system. Brain Res. Revs. 12:439-464.

9. Yankner, B.A. and Shooter, E.M. (1982) The biology and mechanism of action of nerve growth factor. Ann. Rev. Biochem. 51:845-868.

10. Appel, S.H. (1981) A unifying hypothesis for the cause of amyotrophic lateral sclerosis, Parkinsonism, and Alzheimer's disease. Ann. Neurol. 10:499-505.

11. Hefti, F. (1983) Alzheimer's disease caused by a lack of nerve growth factor? Ann. Neurol. 13:109-110.

12. Hefti, F. and Weiner, W.J. (1986) Nerve growth factor and Alzheimer's disease. Ann. Neurol. 20:275-281.

13. Phelps, C.H., Gage, F.H., Growdon, J.H., Hefti, F., Harbaugh, R., Johnston, M.V., Khachaturian, Z.S., Mobley W.C., Price D.L., Raskind M., Simpkins, J., Thal, L.J., and Woodcock, J. (1989) Potential use of nerve growth factor to treat Alzheimer's disease. Neurobiol. Aging 10:205-207.

14. Gage, F.H., Wolff, J.A., Rosenberg, M.B., Xu, L., Yee, J.E., Shults, C. and Friedmann, T. (1987) Grafting genetically modified cells to the brain: possibilities for the future. Neuroscience 23:795-807.

15. Hefti, F., Hartikka, J. and Knusel, B. (in press) Function of neurotrophic factors in the adult and aging brain and their possible use in the treatment of neurodegenerative diseases. Neurobiol. Aging.

16. Hefti, F. (1986) Nerve growth factor (NGF) promotes survival of septal cholinergic neurons after fimbrial transections. J. Neurosci. 6:2155-2162.

17. Kromer, L.F. (1987) Nerve growth factor treatment after brain injury prevents neuronal death. Science 235:214-216.

18. Williams, L.R., Varon, S., Peterson, G.M., Wictorin, K., Fischer, W., Bjorklund, A. and Gage, F.H. (1986) Continuous infusion of nerve growth factor prevents basal forebrain neuronal death after fimbria fornix transection. Proc. Natl. Acad. Sci. USA 83:9231-9235.

19. Harbaugh, R.E. (1987) Intracerebroventricular cholinergic drug administration in Alzheimer's disease: preliminary results of a double-blind study. J. Neural. Transm. [Suppl] 24:271-277.

20. DeYebenes, J.G., Fahn, S., Lovelle, S., Jackson-Lewis, V., Jorge, P., Mena, M.A., and Reiriz, J., (1987) Continuous intracerebroventricular infusion of dopamine and dopamine agonists through a totally implanted drug delivery system in animal models of Parkinson's disease. Movement Disorders 2:143-158.

21. Seno, M., Sasada, R., Iwane, M., Sudo, K., Kurokawa, T., Ito, K. and Igarashi, K. (1988) Stabilizing basic fibroblast growth factor using protein engineering. Biochem. Biophys. Res. Commun. 151:701-708.

22. Brange, J., Ribel, U., Hansen, J.F., Dodson, G., Hansen, M.T., Havelund, S., Melberg, S.G., et al. (1988) Monomeric insulins obtained by protein engineering and their medical implications. Nature 333:679-691.

23. Leong, K.W., Brott, B.C. and Langer, R. (1986) Bioerodible polyanhydrides as drug-carrier matrices. I. Characterization, degradation, and release characteristics. J. Biomed. Materials Res. 20:51-64.

24. Romani, S., Moroder, L., Gohring, W., Scharf, R.,
    Wunsch, E., Barde, Y.A. and Thoenen, H. (1987)
    Synthesis of the trypsin fragment 10-25/75-88 of mouse
    nerve growth factor. Int. J. Protein Res. 29:107-117.
25. Baird, A., Schubert, D., Ling, N. and Guillemin, R.
    (1988) Receptor- and heparin-binding domains of basic
    fibroblast growth factor. Proc. Natl. Acad. Sci. USA
    85:2324-2328.
26. Ballard, F.J., Francis, G.L., Ross, M., Bagley, C.J.,
    May, B. and Wallace J.C. (1987) Natural and synthetic
    forms of insulin-like growth factor-1 (IGF-1) and the
    potent derivative, destripeptide IGF-1: biological
    activities and receptor binding. Biochem. Biophys. Res.
    Commun. 149:398-404.
27. Klagsburn, M., Smith, S., Sullivan, R., Shing, Y.,
    Davidson, S., Smith, J.A. and Sasse, J. (1987) Multiple
    forms of basic fibroblast growth factor: amino-terminal
    cleavages by tumor cell- and brain- derived acid
    proteinases. Proc. Natl. Acad. Sci. USA 84:1839-1843.
28. Komiriya, A., Hortsch, M., Meyers, C., Smith, M.,
    Kanety, H. and Schlessinger, J. (1984) Biologically
    active synthetic fragments of epidermal growth factor:
    localization of a major receptor-binding region. Proc.
    Natl. Sci. USA 81:1351-1355.
29. Rosenberg, M.B., Friedmann, T., Robertson, R.C.,
    Tuszynski, M., Wolff, J.A., Breakefield, X.O. and Gage,
    F.H. (1988) Grafting genetically modified cells to
    damaged brain: restorative effects of NGF expression.
    Science 242:1575-1578.
30. Zheng, M. and Heinrich, G. (1988) Structural and
    functional analysis of the promoter region of the nerve
    growth factor gene. Mol. Brain Res. 3:133-140.
31. Haskell, B.E., Stach, R.W., Werrbach-Perez, K. and
    Perez- Polo J.R. (1987) Effect of retinoic acid on
    nerve growth factor receptors. Cell Tissue Res.
    247:67-73.
32. Wion, D., Houlgatte, R., Barbot, N., Barrand, P.,
    Dicou, E. and Brachet, P. (1987) Retinoic acid
    increases the expression of NGF gene in mouse L cells.
    Biochem. Biophys. Res. Comm. 149:510-514.
33. Jones-Villeneuve, E.M.V., McBurney, M.W., Rogers, K.A.
    and Kalnins, V.I. (1982) Retinoic acid induces
    embryonal carcinoma cells to differentiate into neurons
    and glial cells. J. Cell Biol. 94:253- 262.
34. Kuff., E.L. and Fewell, J.W. (1980) Induction of
    neural-like cells and acetylcholinesterase activity in
    cultures of F9 teratocarcinoma treated with retinoic
    acid and dibutyryl cyclic adenosine monophosphate.
    Develop Biol 77:103-115.
35. Sidell, N. (1982) Retinoic acid-induced growth
    inhibition and morphologic differentiation of human
    neuroblastoma cells in vitro. J. Nat. Cancer Inst.
    68:565-571.
36. Thiele, C.J., Reynolds, C.P. and Israel, M.A. (1985)
    Decreased expression of N-myc precedes retinoic-acid
    induced morphological differentiation of human
    neuroblastoma. Nature 313:404-406.
37. Kalaria, R.N. and Prince, A.K. (1985) The effects of
    neonatal thyroid deficiency on acetylcholine synthesis
    and glucose oxidation in rat corpus striatum. Dev.
    Brain Res. 20:271-279.

38. Hayashi, M. and Patel, A.J. (1987) An interaction between thyroid hormone and nerve growth factor in the regulation of choline acetyltransferase activity in neuronal cultures derived from the septal-diagonal band region of the rat. Dev. Brain Res. 36:109-120.

39. Hefti, F., Hartikka, J. and Bolger, M.B. (1986) Effect of thyroid hormone analogs on the activity of choline acetyltransferase in cultures of dissociated septal cells. Brain Res. 375:413-416.

40. Honegger, P. and Lenoir, D. (1980) Triiodothyronine enhancement of neuronal differentiation in aggregating fetal rat brain cells cultured in a chemically defined medium. Brain Res. 199:425-434.

41. Rosenthal, M.J. and Sanchez, C.J. (1985) Thyroid disease in the elderly - missed diagnosis or overdiagnosis. West. J. Med. 143:643-647.

42. Swanson, J.W., Kelly, J.L. and McConahey, W.M. (1981) Neurologic aspects of thyroid dysfunction. Mayo Clin. Proc. 56:504-512.

43. Nakai, A., Seino, S., Sakurai, A., Szilak, I., Bell, G.J. and DeGroot, L.J. (1988) Characterization of a thyroid hormone receptor expressed in human kidney and other tissues. Proc. Natl. Acad. Sci. USA 85:2781-2785.

44. Underwood, A.H., Emmett, J.C., Ellis, D., Flynn, S.B., Leeson, P.D., Benson, G.M., Novelli, R. et al. (1986) A thyromimetic that decreases plasma cholesterol levels without increasing cardiac activity. Nature 324:425-429.

45. Heumann, R., Korsching, S., Bandtlow, C. and Thoenen, H. (1987) Changes of NGF synthesis in non-neuronal cells in response to sciatic nerve transection. J. Cell Biol. 104:1623-1631.

46. Taniuchi, M., Clark, H.B. and Johnson, E.M. (1986) Induction of nerve growth factor receptor in Schwann cells after axotomy. Proc. Natl. Acad. Sci. USA 83:4094-4098.

47. Lindholm, D., Heumann, R., Meyer, M. and Thoenen, H. (1987) Interleukin-1 regulates synthesis of nerve growth factor in non- neuronal cells of rat sciatic nerve. Nature 230:658-661.

THE USE OF REAGGREGATING CELL CULTURES AND IMMORTALIZED CENTRAL NERVOUS SYSTEM CELLS TO STUDY CHOLINERGIC TROPHIC MECHANISMS

B. H. Wainer[1,2,4], H. J. Lee[1], J. D. Roback[2], and D. N. Hammond[3,4]

Departments of Pharmacological and Physiological Sciences[1], Pathology[2], Neurology[3], and Pediatrics[4], The University of Chicago, Chicago, Illinois

ABSTRACT

A salient feature of Alzheimer's and other neurodegenerative diseases is the selective vulnerability of particular neural pathways. Since the development and maintenance of neural connections is supported by neural trophic factors, trophic dysfunction represents one possible pathogenetic mechanism for such neurological and age-associated diseases. This laboratory has utilized primary reaggregating cell cultures and developed immortalized central nervous system cell lines to study the trophic interactions that establish and maintain the septohippocampal pathway, which plays an essential role in cognitive function and is prominently affected in Alzheimer's Disease. The results of the primary cell culture studies have demonstrated the importance of trophic signals elaborated by the hippocampus in mediating the development of septal cholinergic neurons. Nerve growth factor plays an important trophic role in this pathway, but it cannot account for all of the effects of authentic hippocampal target cells. The development of clonal cell lines of septal and hippocampal lineage offers the prospect of investigating both the response to and elaboration of neural trophic signals at a more precise level of resolution than can be achieved with primary cultures. In addition, one of the hippocampal-derived cell lines, HN10, expresses what appears to be a novel cholinergic trophic activity. These cell lines represent a potential source for isolation of such factors, and also a potential "delivery system" via neural grafting techniques. The technology and information that are generated from these investigations will serve as a strategy to study trophic interactions in other brain circuits in future years, and to investigate possible changes or dysfunctions that occur both in the aging brain and in age-associated brain diseases.

INTRODUCTION

Alzheimer's Disease (AD) and other neurodegenerative disorders share the pathogenetic feature of progressive deterioration and loss of specific neural pathways (1-3). In AD, this degeneration involves both cortico-cortical association pathways, elements of the entorhinal-hippocampal circuitry, and subcortical diffuse ascending systems such as the cholinergic basal forebrain cell groups (Figure 1). All of these pathways are synaptically linked and contribute to cognitive function. A major therapeutic strategy has focused on enhancing cholinergic transmission either by providing precursors of acetylcholine, or attempting to prolong degradation with anticholinesterases (4,5). This strategy has not produced dramatic results clinically (5,6), and it does not take into account the degeneration that occurs in numerous noncholinergic pathways in AD. One possible pathogenetic mechanism to explain the pattern of neuronal degeneration observed is a dysfunction of essential trophic interactions that maintain the viability of particular neural circuits (2,6-8). This latter possibility has recently received substantial attention with the observation that nerve growth factor (NGF) is expressed in the central nervous system (CNS) and is likely to function as an important trophic factor for central cholinergic neurons that degenerate in AD (6,8-10). It is also likely that other growth factors, previously isolated in the periphery, are active in the brain and that additional substances are yet to be identified (11). This theoretical construct raises the possibility of a new era in therapeutic management that would consist of the delivery of growth factors to the nervous system in order to repair or prevent the degeneration of neural pathways (12). A recent report by Gage and his co-workers (13) has demonstrated the efficacy of grafting genetically modified fibroblasts that express NGF into the brains of lesioned rats and preventing septal cholinergic neuronal degeneration. The purpose of the present review is to discuss work carried out in this laboratory to: i) Investigate trophic interactions that establish and maintain one of the pathways at risk in AD, the septohippocampal projection; and ii). To present a CNS cell immortalization strategy that we have employed to identify novel neural trophic factors. For a discussion of other approaches to study neural trophic interactions with respect to NGF and other growth factors, the reader is referred to other chapters in this monograph and recent reviews (6,8-11).

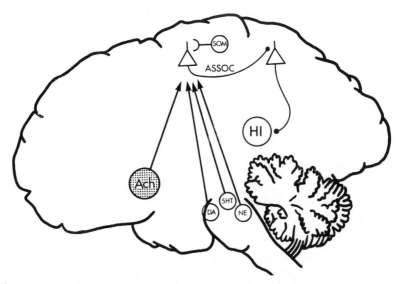

Figure 1. Schematic diagram illustrating some of the major neural connections that are at risk in Alzheimer's Disease. Assoc, cortico-cortico association pathways; HI, hippocampal circuitry, including entorhinal cortical inputs (i.e. perforant pathway); SOM, cortical somatostatin-containing neurons; Ach, the magnocellular basal forebrain cholinergic projections to cortex (including septohippocampal); Other diffuse ascending projections at risk include: DA, Dopaminergic; 5HT, Serotoninergic; NE, Noradrenergic. Diagram modified from (2).

CHOLINERGIC TROPHIC INTERACTIONS

This laboratory has studied the detailed anatomical principles of organization of central cholinergic pathways (14-17). The septohippocampal pathway contains a significant cholinergic component (i.e. part of the cholinergic basal forebrain system) (15,17,18), plays an important role in memory (19,20), and is severely affected in AD (1,3). Although this pathway is not the only locus of vulnerability in AD (1,3), it serves as a useful model system to examine the factors that establish and sustain neural connectivity. Information that is obtained from a careful study of this system may be directly applied as a therapeutic strategy in AD, and may serve as a rationale for the study and approach to both the repair and prevention of degeneration in other pathways which are at risk.

More recently, we have employed reaggregating cell culture techniques to examine the mechanisms that instruct developing septal cholinergic neurons to establish and maintain stable synaptic contacts with hippocampal target cells (Figure 2) (21,22). In this system, the brain areas of interest (hippocampus and/or septum) are dissected from mouse embryos, "dissociated" into a single cell suspension, and cultured under conditions which promote the reassociation, or "reaggregation", of these single cells into spheres, or "reaggregates" of approximately 200 μm in diameter (Figure 2). Within these reaggregates, cells are surrounded by, and may interact with, neighboring cells in three-dimensions (23). This situation closely approximates the environment *in vivo*. In fact, this environment is essential for some physiological interactions involved in the development of neural systems. Glutamine synthetase, an enzyme found in the Mueller glia of the retina, is induced by hydrocortisone if the intact retina is grown in explant culture (24), or if the dissociated retina is grown in reaggregating culture (25). However, if the dissociated cells are plated in monolayer culture, where the cell-cell interactions are more restricted, there is no steroidal induction (25). Work by Heller and colleagues (26) has demonstrated an increased survival of the developing dopaminergic neurons of the substantia nigra when they are coaggregated with a normal target area, the corpus striatum, but not with a non-target area, the tectum. No such survival effects are observed in monolayer cultures (27).

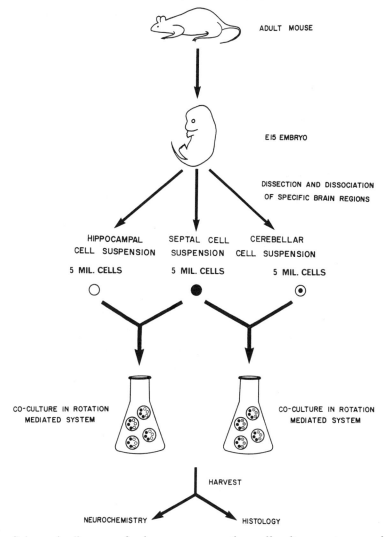

Figure 2. Schematic diagram of primary reaggregating cell culture system employed to study cholinergic trophic interactions in the developing septohippocampal pathway (21, 22, 34). See text for details.

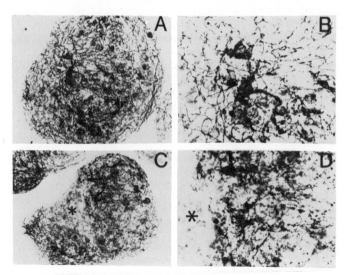

Figure 3. Photomicrographs of sections of a Septal-Hippocampal (S-H) coaggregate [(A) and (B)] and a Septal-Cerebellar (S-Cb) coaggregate [(C) and (D)] with AChE staining, counter-stained with thionine. Arrows in (A) and (B): AChE-positive neuron with proximal neurites. Note swollen AChE-positive fibers in the S-Cb coaggregate are often broken (D) compared to those in the S-H coaggregate which are well-defined and of fine caliber with extensive arborizations and varicosities (B). In addition, there is amorphous AChE reaction product in the S-Cb coaggregate. The asterisks in (C) and (D) mark cells from which AChE-positive fibers are excluded. This area is occupied by cerebellar cells (Fig 4). Scale bars = 30 μm. From Hsiang et al. (21).

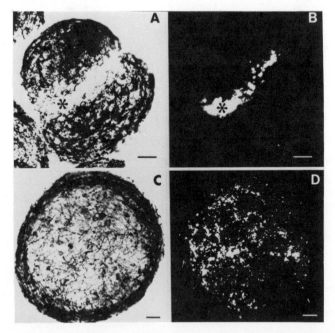

Figure 4. Sections of S-H and S-Cb coaggregates in which the hippocampal and cerebellar cells were internally labeled with rhodamine-wheatgerm agglutinin prior to culture. Photo-micrograph of S-Cb coaggregate (A) with AChE staining shows a band of cells (asterisk) from which AChE fibers are excluded. (B) Matching photo of rhodamine histofluoresence shows that this area is occupied by cerebellar non-target cells. (C) Photomicrograph of a S-H coaggregate with AChE staining showing the fine, varicose AChE-positive fibers. (D) Matching photo of rhodamine histofluoresence shows the rhodamine-labeled hippocampal cells and AChE-positive fibers are co-extensive. Scale bars = 30 μm. From Hsiang et al. (21).

Initially, we studied the effects of hippocampal target cells on the development of septal cholinergic neurons in reaggregate co-cultures (S-H coaggregates) derived from embryonic day 15 (E15) mouse brains (Figure 2) (21). As a control, nontarget cells from the cerebellum were coaggregated with the septal cells (S-Cb coaggregates). The results demonstrated a significant increase in the numbers of cholinergic cells in S-H coaggregates (relative to S-Cb), and proliferation of numerous fibers with axon-like morphologies (Figures 3 & 4). In septal-cerebellar coaggregates, the cells and fibers appeared to be degenerating by light microscopic observation and cholinergic fibers were excluded from regions of the coaggregates occupied by the nontarget cerebellar cells (Figures 3 & 4). In a follow-up ultrastructural study, it was determined that cholinergic axons form synaptic contact with hippocampal target cells in this culture system (Figure 5) (22). In contrast, in the presence of nontarget cerebellar cells, the cholinergic neurons develop initially, but subsequently undergo a process of cell degeneration and death. These results demonstrate that hippocampal cells elaborate trophic signals that are essential for the development, survival, and synaptogenic potential of septal cholinergic neurons.

One obvious putative trophic signal is NGF, which is present in the brain (9,10), is retrogradely transported by basal forebrain cholinergic neurons (28), and prevents retrograde degeneration of septal cholinergic neurons following axotomy (29-31). We have begun to study the expression of NGF in the *in vitro* reaggregate system and also its effects on early cholinergic development (32-34). It was previously proposed that NGF might be released from either peripheral or central target structures to serve as a neurite-guidance as well as survival factor during development (35,36). This hypothesis does not appear to be supported by the recent work of Davies et al. (37) who demonstrated that NGF synthesis in the mouse whisker pad is initiated precisely at the time of arrival of sensory innervation; sensory neurons, moreover, do not begin to express the NGF receptor until their axons arrive at their peripheral targets. Although these latter findings suggest that ingrowing axons might be involved in the induction of NGF expression, studies in denervated limb buds (38) and in heart (39) suggest that NGF expression appears at the appropriate developmental stage regardless of whether or not innervation occurs. In yet other studies, it has been shown that interleukin-1ß can upregulate NGF expression in adult sciatic nerve explants (40). This observation raises an additional possibility that lymphokines and perhaps other humoral factors might be implicated in the developmental regulation of NGF expression. To date, most of the studies of NGF expression in the CNS have been descriptive. In the developing rat hippocampus, NGF mRNA and protein are present at very low levels at birth (approximately 10% and 25% of adult levels respectively), then increase and peak by postnatal day 21 (approximately 350% and 120% of adult levels respectively), and finally decline to a plateau that is maintained throughout adulthood (41). The developmental peak occurs during the most active period of synaptogenesis in the hippocampus, especially with respect to septal afferent inputs.

In initial studies, we determined the capacity of the developing mouse hippocampus grown in reaggregating culture to synthesize NGF mRNA and protein in a developmentally-regulated manner (32,33). We utilized hippocampi from E15 mouse embryos, a developmental stage at which the hippocampus has not yet received afferent fibers from the septum (42), and is thus "naive" with respect to septal influences. Hippocampal cells were then grown in reaggregate culture for up to 28 days. During this period, flasks were harvested at specific time points for the determination of NGF mRNA and protein, using a Northern blot assay (43) and a 2-site enzyme-linked solid phase immunoassay (ELISA) (44). Previously published studies on NGF mRNA and protein expression in the developing hippocampus *in vivo* were performed in rats (41). We have repeated the *in vivo* developmental time course in the mouse in order to obtain a baseline for comparison to *in vitro* measurements (Figure 6), and the mouse results are in good agreement with previous rat studies. The hippocampal reaggregates synthesize significant levels of NGF protein in culture (Figure 6A). At the developmental stage at which the reaggregate cultures were initiated, E15, NGF protein is barely detectable; over the next 21 days, there is a significant increase in NGF protein expression in the reaggregates which closely parallels that seen *in vivo* (Figure 6B) (32). Because the septal afferents retrogradely transport NGF protein from the hippocampus, we considered the possibility that the levels of NGF protein *in vivo* may represent an underestimation of the actual synthetic rate. Similarly, the hippocampal reaggregates, devoid of normal septal innervation, may sequester NGF protein, resulting in an overestimation of the synthetic rate.

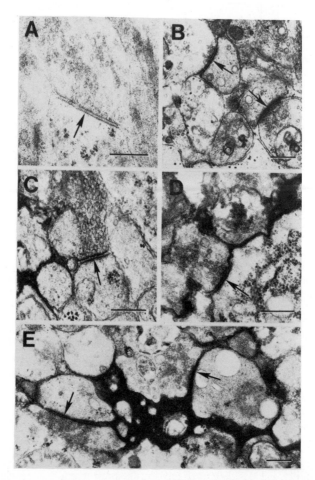

Figure 5. High-power electron micrographs of synapses (arrows) in septal-hippocampal (S-H) and septal-cerebellar (S-Cb) coaggregates. A: an unlabeled synapse in a 21-day-old S-H coaggregate is shown for comparison. Note that there is no AChE reaction product at the synaptic junction (in contrast to B-E). B: AChE-labeled axodendritic synapses within the hippocampal cell (target) area of a 15-day-old S-H coaggregate. Note that both pre- and postsynaptic membranes stain discretely and completely at the area of synaptic contact (arrows). C: AChE-labeled axodendritic synapse in the target area of a 21-day-old S-H coaggregate. D: AChE-labeled axosomatic synapse in the hippocampal area of a 21-day-old S-H coaggregate. This type of synapse is uncommon in the S-H coaggregates. E: AChE-labeled synapse in a 21-day-old S-Cb coaggregate. There are only occasional labeled synapses observed in S-Cb coaggregates, and they are not found in the cerebellar cell areas. Bars = 0.25 μm. From Hsiang et al. (22).

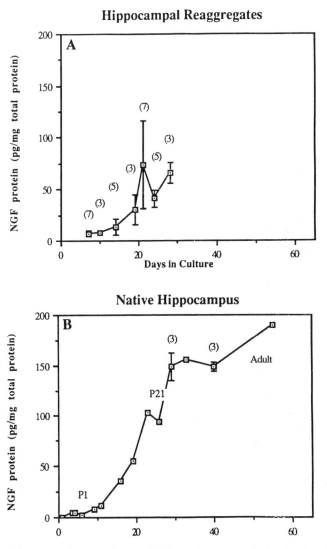

Figure 6. Preliminary studies on the synthesis of NGF protein in the developing mouse hippocampus *in vitro* (**A**) and *in vivo* (**B**). Hippocampal samples were harvested from reaggregate culture (**A**) or removed from the developing brain (**B**) at the indicated time points. NGF protein was quantitated using a 2-site enzyme-linked immunosorbent assay (ELISA) (44), and values were normalized for total protein in the samples. **A** and **B** have been positioned in register for comparison, with day 15 of gestation (E15) at the origin on the x-axes; developmental ages have been indicated on **B**. The early profile of NGF protein expression in hippocampal reaggregates closely parallels that seen in the hippocampus *in vivo*. Numbers above the curves represent the number of reaggregate flasks or tissue samples assayed; a triplicate determination was performed on each sample from Roback et al. (32).

In order to compare more closely developmental induction of NGF expression in the two systems, we employed Northern blot analyses of NGF mRNA (Figure 7) (33). Hippocampal reaggregates synthesize NGF mRNA which co-migrates electrophoretically with that seen in the Northern blot standard, which is derived from adult mouse hippocampus and cortex. At E15, there is no detectable expression of NGF mRNA in the hippocampus (Figure 7C). The expression then rises significantly *in vivo* (Figure 7C). In the developing rat hippocampus, NGF mRNA expression peaks between postnatal days 19 and 21. We have not yet examined this time point in the mouse hippocampus *in vivo*; however, if the situation is analogous, we would expect to see a signal at postnatal day 21 which is significantly greater than that seen in the adult hippocampus. Hippocampal reaggregates at 7 and 21 days in culture display a modest developmental induction in NGF mRNA expression (Figure 7B) when compared with the nearly undetectable levels seen at the time of dissection, E15 (Figure 7C). However, there is no increase in the mRNA levels between days 7 and 21 in culture, and these observations contrast with the developmental increases observed *in vivo* (Figure 8).

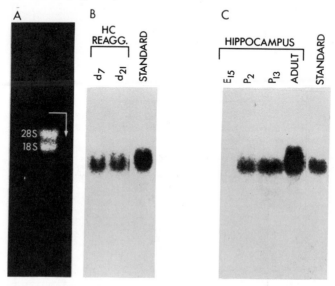

Figure 7. Preliminary Northern blot analyses of NGF mRNA expression in hippocampal reaggregates (**B**) and native hippocampus (**C**). Total RNA was extracted (70) from samples of selected developmental ages and 25 µg from each sample was size fractionated on a 1.2% agarose gel; a tissue standard (total RNA, extracted from hippocampus and neocortex of 50 adult mice, pooled and divided into 25 µg aliquots which were stored at -37°C until use) was co-electrophoresed on each gel to enable comparison between blots. RNA was transferred to GeneScreen and hybridized with a ^{32}P-labelled DNA probe made from the 0.9 kb *Pst I* fragment of the NGF cDNA (43). **A.** Ethidium bromide staining of total RNA. 5 µg of total reaggregate RNA, prepared as above, was electrophoresed on a 1.2% agarose minigel, and stained with ethidium bromide (71). The figure is a 100% enlargement of a polaroid 47 instant print, accounting for the grainy appearance. The tail of the arrow indicates the position of the well; 28S and 18S rRNA bands are indicated. **B.** Representative autoradiogram of NGF mRNA in hippocampal reaggregates grown in culture for 7 and 21 days. **C.** Autoradiogram depicting developmental induction in hippocampal NGF mRNA synthesis *in vivo* between E15 and adulthood. Note that the autoradiogram **B** was from a longer exposure than C (by comparison of the respective tissue standards). Hippocampal aggregates synthesize NGF mRNA, but do not display the full developmental induction in NGF mRNA expression observed *in vivo*. From Roback et al. (33).

These preliminary results suggest that the "naive" hippocampus retains the ability to synthesize NGF mRNA and protein when removed from the brain at E15 and grown in reaggregate culture. The fact that the dissection is performed prior to interactions between septal and hippocampal neurons indicates that these interactions are not necessary for the synthesis of NGF mRNA and protein by the hippocampus. However, the full developmental induction seen *in vivo* is not recapitulated in the hippocampal reaggregates. Because previous work in our laboratory has shown normal neuronal morphology (including axons, dendrites, and synapses) in reaggregates between 7 and 21 days in culture (21), we do not believe that the relatively low NGF mRNA expression observed at 21 days can be simply attributed to degenerative changes in the cultures. To rule out this possibility, however, it will be important to reprobe the membranes for other mRNA species, such as cytoskeletal proteins, in order to assess general neuronal maturation. Taken together, the available data suggest that the developmental induction in hippocampal NGF expression may be a multi-step process. The cells within the reaggregates may have been exposed to certain "early" developmental cues, leading to a modest induction in NGF mRNA between E15 and day 7 in culture; however, they may not have encountered all of the appropriate developmental signals necessary to recapitulate the pattern of NGF induction observed *in vivo*. One obvious signal may come from septal inputs and this possibility is currently being evaluated in S-H coaggregates, but it is also possible that other, perhaps humoral, signals are involved.

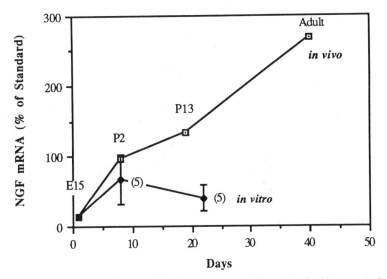

Figure 8. Preliminary studies on the time course of NGF mRNA expression in the developing hippocampus *in vitro* and *in vivo*. NGF mRNA expression was quantitated from autoradiograms (including those shown in Appendix 2) using a scanning laser densitometer (LKB Ultroscan XL). Values were normalized to the standards on each blot. Note that at the developmental stage at which reaggreagate cultures are initiated (E15), NGF mRNA expression is at approximately the lower limit of sensitivity of the techniques. NGF mRNA synthesis *in vitro* and *in vivo* increases over the next 7 days, but then plateaus in the reaggregates. Numbers on the *in vitro* curve represent the number of reaggregate flasks assayed. From Roback et. al. (33).

We have also investigated the actions of both "exogenous" and "endogenous" NGF as a putative cholinergic trophic factor in the reaggregate culture system (34). In the presence of exogenous NGF, septal reaggregates demonstrated increased levels of ChAT activity (Figure 9), increased numbers of cholinergic cells, and an increased density of fibers (Figure 10). However, when anti-NGF was added to S-H coaggregates in order to neutralize the putative actions of "endogenous" NGF, there was only a partial decrement in the levels of cholinergic markers observed. In contrast to other studies demonstrating destruction of sympathetic and sensory neurons following anti-NGF treatment *in vivo* (45,46), this *in vitro* procedure produced no qualitative changes in cholinergic cells or fibers at the light microscopic level, or synapse formation at the ultrastructural level (Figure11) (34).

Although data analysis is still in progress, follow-up ultrastructural studies of healthy versus degenerating cholinergic neurons in reaggregate cultures, grown either in the presence or absence of NGF, have demonstrated a modest enhancement of cell survival with a more dramatic enhancement of the histochemical marker employed to identify the cells (47,48). Our conclusion from these studies is that NGF is likely to act in concert with an unknown number of additional target cell-associated cues to mediate cholinergic neuronal development, synaptogenesis and maintenance in the septohippocampal pathway. These conclusions are supported by observations of other groups: Crutcher and Collins (49) and Heacock et al. (50) have demonstrated a non-NGF activity for cholinergic ciliary ganglion neurons, while Appel and coworkers (51,52) and Wise and colleagues (53) provided evidence for non-NGF molecule(s) influencing basal forebrain cholinergic cells.

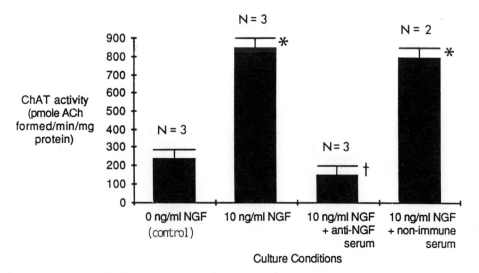

Figure 9. Effects of NGF and Anti-NGF antiserum on ChAT activity within septal reaggregates. Cultures were grown for 17 days in the following conditions: Culture medium only; 10 ng/ml NGF added to the medium beginning at day 6 of culture; 10 ng/ml NGF plus Anti-NGF antiserum (1 : 200 dilution) added; or 10 ng/ml NGF plus non-immune serum (1 : 200 dilution) added. Values represent the mean ± S.E.M. Assays were performed in triplicate from each flask. N indicates the number of flasks. *Differs from the control at p< 0.001 (one-tailed t test). †No significant difference from the control group (Student's t test). Data presentation modified from Hsiang et al. (34).

CNS CLONAL CELL LINES

The challenge of identifying novel trophic factors is complex because of the cellular heterogeneity of the brain and the likelihood that such factors are expressed in extremely minute quantities. Although a trophic "activity" may be detected in a crude brain extract or through the use of primary cell cultures, purification and characterization of the bioactive molecule(s) are still quite formidable. The utilization of clonal cell lines provides an alternative approach that can circumvent the problems cited above (54). In fact, the original identification of NGF was achieved by virtue of its expression in a rat sarcoma cell line (55). Relatively little work has been carried out with respect to the establishment of permanent cell lines from specific brain regions that elaborate trophic signals which are likely to participate in the establishment and maintenance of the synaptic circuitry of those regions. Two general

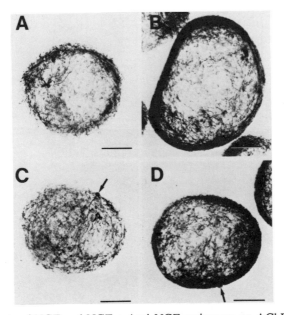

Figure 10. Effects of NGF and NGF + Anti-NGF antiserum on AChE-staining in 17-day old septal reaggregate cultures. NGF and antiserum treatments were initiated at day 6 of culture. A: Septal reaggregate grown in a culture medium without NGF. B: Septal reaggregate cultured in the presence of 10 ng/ml NGF. The AChE histochemistry reveals dense, heavily-stained AChE fibers which are most prominent at the periphery of the reaggregate section. C: Septal reaggregate cultured in the presence of 10 ng/ml NGF and Anti-NGF antiserum (1:200 dilution). AChE histochemistry reveals a fiber density similar to A, indicating that the effect of NGF on fiber staining intensity is antagonized. Arrow indicates a cell situated at the edge of the reaggregate section which has prominent proximal fibers. D: Septal reaggregate cultured in the presence of 10 ng/ml NGF and non-immune serum (1:200 dilution). AChE histochemistry demonstrates that the fiber density is the same as that of the NGF-treated in B, confirming the specificity of the NGF effect on fiber staining intensity. A cell body (arrow) situated at the edge of the reaggregate section is obscured by the dense plexus of heavily-stained fibers. Scale bars = 100 µm. From Hsiang et al. (34).

strategies are available for engineering such cell lines. The first approach is the use of retroviral vectors or other oncogenes to transform primary brain cells (56,57). This approach has been recently exploited to generate cell lines that recapitulate neuronal developmental stages. For example, a temperature sensitive mutant of the SV-40 virus has been employed to immortalize embryonic rat brain cells (57,58). Several cell lines were generated that expressed varying degrees of neuronal or glial differentiation and which could be induced either to divide at the permissive temperature, 33°C, or to "differentiate" at the nonpermissive temperature, 37-39°C. A hippocampal cell line generated through this

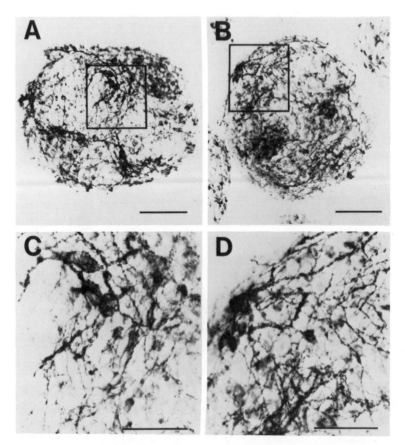

Figure 11. Effect of anti-NGF antiserum on septal-hippocampal (S-H) coaggregates: Photomicrographs of sections of 21-day old AChE-stained S-H coaggregates cultured in media alone, media containing non-immune serum, or media containing Anti-NGF antiserum beginning at day 2 in culture. A: S-H coaggregate grown in culture medium alone. AChE histochemistry reveals a typical target cell-induced pattern of fibers and cells similar to that described in previous studies (21). The boxed area is shown at higher magnification in C. B: S-H coaggregate cultured in the presence of non-immune serum (1: 200 dilution). AChE histochemistry reveals a pattern of cells and fibers similar to those in A. The boxed area is shown at higher magnification in D. C: Higher-power photomicrograph of boxed area of AChE-positive cells and fibers in A. These fine caliber fibers are well-defined with extensive arborizations and varicosities. D: Higher-power photomicrograph of boxed area of AChE-positive cells and fibers in B. The appearance of these cells and fibers does not differ from those shown in C. E: S-H coaggregate

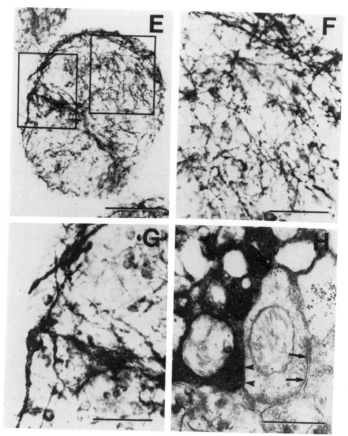

Figure 11 (Cont.) cultured in the presence of Anti-NGF antiserum (1:200 dilution). AChE histochemistry reveals fibers and cells similar to those in A. The boxed areas are showed at higher magnification in F and G. F & G: Higher-power photomicrographs of boxed areas of AChE-positive cells (G) and fibers (F) in E. The appearance of these cells and fibers are similar to those shown in A and B suggesting that NGF antibodies do not inhibit cholinergic fiber proliferation in S-H coaggregates. H: High-power electron micrograph showing AChE-labeled synapse (arrowheads) and unlabeled synapse (arrows) in a 21-day old S-H coaggregate which was cultured in the presence of Anti-NGF antiserum beginning on the second day of culture. The identification of labeled synapses in this case suggests that anti-NGF does not inhibit the process of synaptogenesis between septal cholinergic terminals and hippocampal target cells. Scale Bars: A, B, E = 200 μm; C, D, F, G = 50 μm; H = 0.5 μm. From Hsiang et al. (34).

approach, HT4, exhibits an immature neuronal phenotype and also expresses NGF mRNA and protein. This cell line has been examined in other laboratories including ours (unpublished observations). A preliminary report by Whittemore and co-workers (59) has demonstrated that the HT4 cells can be grafted into the adult rat brain and the cells do not appear to proliferate. In addition, when the recipient rats receive lesions of the septohippocampal pathway, the grafted cells partially prevent retrograde degeneration of septal cholinergic neurons possibly through the elaboration of NGF. While this approach is attractive, there are also some disadvantages. Retroviral transduction is only effective with cells that retain the capacity to replicate DNA and therefore divide. In addition, once a cell is "immortalized", it tends to remain locked within a particular developmental window. This phenomenon has been exploited by immunologists to study the stages of lymphocyte differentiation (60,61). Therefore, while viral gene transduction might yield cell lines to study the early stages of neuronal development, it is less likely to provide cell lines that express the phenotypic repertoire of mature neurons which are almost invariably post-mitotic.

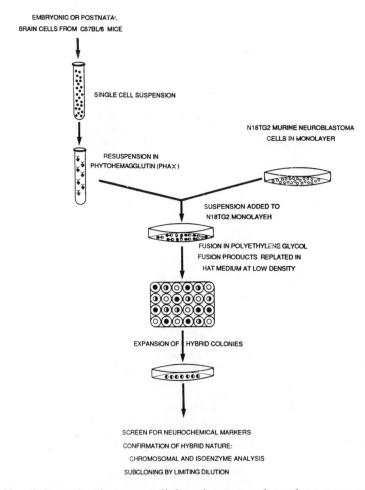

Figure 12. Schematic diagram outlining the protocol used to generate septum x neuroblastoma or hippocampus x neuroblastoma hybrid cell lines from C57BL/6 mice and the N18TG2 neuroblastoma (62). To facilitate adherence of primary cells to neuroblastoma cells, the primary cells are incubated with phytohemagglutinin (PHA) prior to fusion. Somatic cell fusion is mediated by polyethylene glycol. The fusion products are grown in hypoxanthine, aminopterin, and thymidine (HAT) media to select for hybrid cells. N18TG2 cell are deficient in hypoxanthine phosphoribosyltransferase and cannot survive in HAT media.

A second cell immortalization approach, one utilized by this laboratory, employs somatic cell fusion techniques (Figure 12) (62). This is precisely the approach that has been used to generate monoclonal antibody-producing hybridomas (63). The fusion technique allows one to "immortalize" cell populations that are postmitotic and therefore more likely to

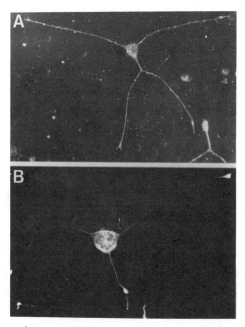

Figure 13. Septum x neuroblastoma cells in culture. **A.** Phase contrast photomicrograph of a septum x neuroblastoma cell line (SN 55) grown in serum-free medium for 3 days. Note the elaboration of very long, thin neurites. Magnification = 450x. **B.** Indirect immunofluorescence staining of a postnatal day 21 septum x neuroblastoma cell line (SN 48.B12.2.C6) with anti-neurofilament monoclonal antibodies. Cells were grown on untreated tissue culture plastic with 10% fetal calf serum in DMEM and then fixed with 2% formaldehyde in methanol. The cells were incubated with a primary antibody solution containing monoclonal antibodies to the low, middle, and high molecular weight neurofilaments proteins. Immunoreactivity was visualized with a fluorescein-conjugated secondary antibody. Magnification = 800x. From Lee et al. (64).

express highly differentiated neuronal phenotypes (64,65). Once neural cell lines are established, the probability of identifying a cell line which expresses interesting trophic activities is increased because of their clonal nature. Finally, the likelihood of successfully purifying and characterizing the molecules responsible for a "trophic activity" is enhanced since the cell lines represent an infinite source of starting material.

Using somatic cell fusion, we generated hybrid cell lines from both the septal and hippocampal regions of fetal mouse brains (Figure 12) (62,65). Embryonic septal or hippocampal cells were somatically fused to N18TG2 neuroblastoma cells via polyethylene glycol. The neuroblastoma, N18TG2, is deficient in hypoxanthine phosphoribosyl transferase (HPRT) and can be selectively eliminated in media containing hypoxanthine, aminopterin, and thymidine (HAT). The hybrid nature of the cell lines was further documented by chromosome and isozyme analyses. Subsequently, young adult septal and hippocampal cells were immortalized by this technique (64,66). However, a buoyant density centrifugation cell isolation procedure was devised in order to maintain viability of the primary cells at the time of dissection. To date, 56 septal (SN, septum x neuroblastoma) and 45 hippocampal (HN, hippocampus x neuroblastoma) cell lines have been generated from embryonic days 14, 15, and 18 and postnatal day 21 tissues.

Many septal cell lines exhibit phenotypes typical of differentiated neurons (62,64). Their somata and processes are highly refractile when viewed by phase contrast microscopy. The cell lines further differentiate when cultured in serum-free medium and extend long, thin processes (Figure 13A) (64,67). The neuronal origin of these cell lines is supported by the presence of immunoreactivity for neurofilament proteins (Figure 13B & 14) (62,64,67). In postnatal lines, an array of neurofilaments characteristic of a mature neuron is observed; no other cell-specific intermediate filaments are detected (Figure 14) (67). Taking into account the late age of the primary tissues used in the fusion, these findings suggest that such cell lines were derived from postmitotic neurons.

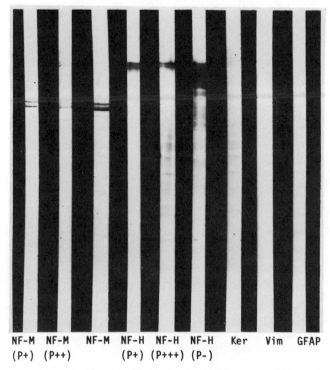

NF-M   NF-M   NF-M   NF-H   NF-H   NF-H   Ker   Vim   GFAP
(P+)   (P++)   (P+)   (P+++)   (P-)

Figure 14. Immunoblots for intermediate filaments expressed by a postnatal day 21 septum x neuroblastoma cell line (SN 48.B12.2.C6). Crude cell lysate preparations of the cell line were separated by SDS-Disc PAGE and transferred onto nitrocelluose. Each immunoblot was probed with a different antibody to visualize intermediate filament proteins: *Lane 1*, the middle molecular weight neurofilament protein (NF-M) in its weakly phosphorylated state (P+); *Lane 2*, NF-M in its moderately phosphorylated state (P++) ; *Lane 3*, NF-M in all its phosphorylation states; *Lane 4*, the high molecular weight neurofilament protein (NF-H) in its P+ state; *Lane 5*, NF-H in its highly phosphorylated state (P+++); *Lane 7*, NF-H in all its phosphorylation states. Note the broad range of electrophoretic mobility due to variable phosphorylation; *Lane 7*, cytokeratins 8, 18, and 19 (Ker); *Lane 8*, vimentin (Vim); and *Lane 9*, glial fibrillary acidic protein (GFAP). Not included: immunoblot for the low molecular weight neurofilament protein which is also positive. From Lee et al. (67).

The septal lines express neurochemical markers typical of septal cholinergic neurons (62,64). Significant levels of ChAT activity are radiochemically detected in a number of septal lines (Figure 15). In general, postnatal cell lines exhibit higher levels of ChAT activity than embryonic lines (64). Further evaluation of several lines has revealed that they are positive for ChAT immunocytochemistry and acetylcholinesterase (AChE) histochemistry (62). Since administration of exogenous NGF supports the development of septal cholinergic neurons *in vitro*, septal cell lines expressing a particularly differentiated phenotype were evaluated for their capacity to respond to NGF. When septal lines are grown on tissue culture plastic in the presence of 10% fetal calf serum, the addition of NGF does not increase ChAT activity or qualitatively change process formation. It may be that these particular septal lines constitutively express maximal ChAT activity in the presence of serum, and that any effect of exogenous NGF is not detectable. Alternatively, these SN lines may not express the NGF receptor (NGFR). We have examined three cholinergic septal lines for NGFR message expression by Northern blot analysis, and found that all three indeed express NGFR mRNA (unpublished observations). Future studies will therefore concentrate on the responsiveness of septal cell lines to NGF under serum-free culture conditions and in the presence of differentiating reagents.

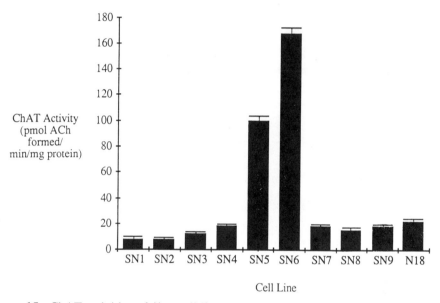

Figure 15. ChAT activities of nine cell lines generated by fusion of septal and N18TG2 cells, and of N18TG2 (N18) cells, as measured in picomoles of acetylcholine formed per minute per milligram of protein. The values shown are means ± SEM (n=3). SN5 and SN 6 demonstrate ChAT activities clearly greater than N18TG2. From Hammond et al. (62).

The hippocampal lines were screened for their capacity to express NGF (65,66). Several embryonic cell lines express high levels of NGF mRNA as detected by Northern blot analysis with a cDNA probe to the rat NGF message (Figure 16). Most of these lines also synthesize high levels of NGF protein as detected by a 2-site ELISA specific for ß-NGF (Figure 16). However, some lines display relatively high levels of NGF mRNA but no detectable NGF protein. This may indicate defects in translation or abnormal processing of the precursor protein to mature NGF. Postnatal lines contain up to 30,000 fg NGF/mg total protein (66). The N18TG2 neuroblastoma expresses neither NGF protein nor mRNA.

The production by these hippocampal cell lines of a central cholinergic trophic factor known to be produced in normal hippocampus, suggested that the cell lines may be capable of the synthesis of non-NGF trophic factors. We thus developed a monolayer bioassay to screen hippocampal cell lines for the expression of substances which affect cholinergic neurons (68). In this assay system, the primary septal cells are dissociated, suspended in a defined serum-free medium (N2), and plated at low density in monolayer in poly-lysine coated microtiter wells. After the cells have adhered, cell line extracts, membrane preparations, or conditioned media are added to the cultures. At the completion of the experiment, the microtiter plates are assayed for ChAT activity, and we have adapted the assay to be performed in the same wells in which the cells are grown. Studies employing this bioassay system indicate that it is sensitive to effects of NGF in a dose-dependent fashion, with ChAT increasing 2 to 4 fold depending on the concentration of NGF added (Figure 17).

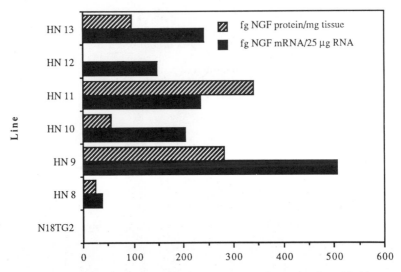

Figure 16. NGF protein and mRNA content of embryonic day 18 hippocampus x neuroblastoma (HN) cell lines. HN cell lines were grown in 10% fetal calf serum in DMEM, harvested, and assayed. NGF protein was measured by a 2-site ELISA specific for ß-NGF. NGF mRNA was quantitated by Northern blot analysis. The DNA probe was prepared from the 0.9 kb *Pst* I fragment of the NGF cDNA comprising a portion of the coding sequence as well as part of the 5' untranslated region. From Hammond et al. (65).

We have screened conditioned media from 22 HN cell lines, as well as N18TG2 cells, for effects on septal cell ChAT activity, using this bioassay system. Most of the lines have little effect (less than 75% increase in ChAT). However, one line, HN10, promotes a 4-fold increase in ChAT activity (Figure 17) (68). Polyacrylamide gel electrophoretic analysis of the serum-free conditioned media from HN10 demonstrates that HN10 secretes a unique spectrum of proteins, some of which are distinct from those secreted by the N18TG2 neuroblastoma cells (unpublished observations). We have found more recently that the HN10 bioactivity can be salt-extracted from a membrane preparation, with an approximately 6-fold increase in specific activity compared to conditioned medium (Figure 18) (69).

We have recently begun to address the question of whether the HN10 effect might be due to known polypeptide growth factors, such as NGF. We have directly quantitated NGF in the HN10 conditioned medium-treated wells by the 2-site ELISA, and find that the final concentration of NGF is over 10,000-fold less than the concentration of exogenous, purified NGF required to achieve the same effect on ChAT activity (68,69). Furthermore, the addition of the anti-NGF monoclonal antibody, 23C4, to primary septal cells blocks the effect of exogenous NGF, but not the effect of the HN10 membrane extract, providing further evidence that the HN10 activity is not mediated by NGF (Figure 19). When purified EGF or bFGF, two other polypeptides proposed as trophic molecules for neural cells, are added to basal forebrain cultures at 1 nM final concentration, ChAT activity increases by 50% and 60%, respectively, significantly less than the effect of HN10 conditioned medium (Figure 17). Taken together, then, these studies indicate that an HN10 membrane-associated factor(s) promotes the ChAT activity of central cholinergic cells in culture, and, furthermore, suggest that activity is not mediated by NGF, EGF, or bFGF.

Since hippocampal neurons express NGF and receive cholinergic innervation, hippocampal cell lines that produced NGF were additionally screened for muscarinic receptors. A radioligand binding assay for M_1-type receptors was employed utilizing N-methyl scopolamine and pirenzepine as ligands. HN 33 expressed 8 femtomoles of M_1-type receptors per million cells; 5 times as many as N18TG2 neuroblastoma cells and comparable to the number found on NGF-activated PC 12 cells (unpublished observations). RNA extracts from these cell lines are presently being probed for the presence of specific muscarinic receptor subtype mRNA species.

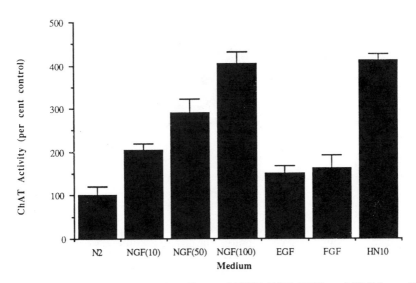

Figure 17. Preliminary studies on the effects of NGF, EGF, FGF, and HN10 conditioned media on septal cell ChAT activity. Embryonic septal cells were cultured using the microtiter bioassay culture system in serum-free N2 medium alone (N2), and in N2 with NGF at 10 ng/ml (NGF(10)), at 50 ng/ml (NGF(50)), or at 100 ng/ml (NGF(100)). Cells were also cultured in N2 medium with EGF at 1 nM (EGF), N2 with basic FGF at 1 nM (FGF), or with HN10 conditioned medium (CM) at a final protein concentration of 100 µg/ml (HN10). In this microtiter bioassay system, NGF treatment increases ChAT activity of septal cells in a dose-dependent fashion. At 1 nM concentrations, EGF and FGF increase ChAT activity over control N2 wells by approximately 50% and 60%, respectively. HN10 conditioned medium increases septal cell ChAT activity to approximately 410% of the control value. This increase is greater than that seen with 22 other cell lines tested (range 0 to 75% increase), or with EGF or FGF at 1 nM concentrations. Direct quantitation of NGF in the HN10 CM by ELISA (performed before the CM was added to the wells) indicates that the final concentration of HN10-derived NGF in the wells would be less than 1 pg/ml (over 10,000-fold less than the 100 ng/ml of purified, exogenous NGF required to stimulate approximately the same increase in ChAT). Values shown are means + SEM (n=3). These data suggest that the HN10 effect is not mediated by NGF, EGF, or FGF. From Hammond et al. (68).

In general, the cells lines produced via the cell fusion technique express higher levels of NGF and a more complete repertoire of neuronal cytoskeletal elements than retrovirally transduced embryonic cells (e.g. HT4). The disadvantage to the conventional fusion approach is that the growth characteristics of the hybrid cell lines are more difficult to control. This drawback probably relates to the overtly malignant nature of the neuroblastoma cell line that was employed as the fusion partner. If the hybrid cells are grafted into a mouse brain, they form tumor masses within a relatively short period of time; however, this effect can be prevented by prior treatment with antimitotic agents (unpublished observations). Studies are presently underway to evaluate whether or not grafted cell lines continue to express NGF or other trophic activities that may prevent cholinergic neuronal degeneration following axotomy.

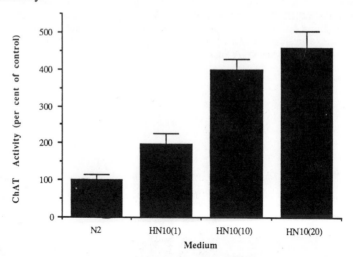

Figure 18. Preliminary studies on the effect of HN10 membrane extract on septal cell ChAT activity. Embryonic septal cells were cultured using the microtiter bioassay culture system in serum-free N2 medium alone (N2), and in N2 with an extract of an HN10 membrane preparation at final protein concentrations of 1, 10, and 20 μg/ml. The membranes were prepared and extracted as described in the Experimental Design and Methods section. Treatment with the membrane extract increases septal ChAT activity in a dose-dependent fashion. Additionally, the HN10 membrane extract displays an approximately 6-fold increase in specific activity compared to HN10 conditioned medium Values shown are means + SEM (n=3). From Hammond et al. (69).

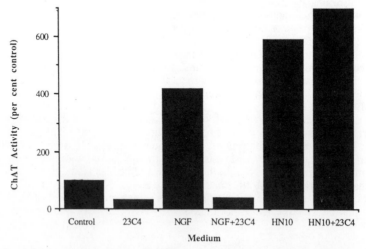

Figure 19. Preliminary studies on the effect of Anti-NGF monoclonal antibody 23C4 on the actions of NGF and HN10 membrane extract on septal cell ChAT activity. Embryonic septal cells were cultured using the microtiter bioassay culture system in serum-free N2 medium alone (N2), and in N2 with anti-NGF antibody 23C4, N2 with NGF, N2 with NGF plus 23C4, N2 with HN10 membrane extract, and N2 with HN10 membrane extract plus 23C4. The addition of anti-NGF antibody 23C4 blocks the effect of exogenous NGF on septal cell ChAT activity, but does not decrease the effect of HN10 membrane extract on septal cell ChAT activity. These data provide further evidence that the HN10 membrane extract activity is not mediated by NGF. From Hammond et al. (69).

CONCLUSIONS AND FUTURE DIRECTIONS

The results of the studies described above strongly suggest that the trophic interactions that influence both the development and maintenance of cholinergic basal forebrain neurons are likely to be mediated by more than one macromolecule such as NGF. The strategy outlined for the generation of region-specific clonal cell lines represents a powerful approach for elucidating the molecular basis of such interactions. This research will add to our knowledge of target hippocampal influences on basal forebrain neurons, and as such contribute to our understanding of basic mechanisms that sustain neural connections. In addition, similar strategies can be applied to study the trophic mechanisms sustaining neural connections in other pathways at risk in AD and in other neurodegenerative diseases. Ultimately, this research may lead to meaningful and potentially useful therapeutic approaches in AD, involving trophic factor therapy or neural grafting strategies. Cell lines expressing appropriate trophic factors may provide a ready source of this material. Importantly, such a therapeutic approach would promote the survival and normal function of neurons, rather than simply ameliorate symptoms as is the case with approaches which substitute exogenous compounds for a deficient neurotransmitter. Beneficial effects of trophic factor therapy on cell survival and function may occur even if factor deficit is not the primary cause of disease.

ACKNOWLEDGEMENTS

This research is supported by PHS RO1 NS25787, The Alzheimer's Disease and Related Disorders Association, The Illinois Department of Public Health, The Brain Research Foundation of The University of Chicago (BHW); PHS 5 KO8 NS01244, The French Foundation (DNH); and PHS 5 T32 HD070009 (HJL & JDR). The authors express gratitude for the excellent technical support of Ms. S.D. Nelson, Ms. L. Sherman, Mr. S.D. Price, and Mr. E. Anton.

REFERENCES

1. Price, D.L. (1986) New perspectives on Alzheimer's disease. Annu.Rev.Neurosci. 9:489-512.

2. Saper, C.B., Wainer, B.H. and German, D.C. (1987) Axonal and transneuronal transport in the transmission of neurological disease: potential role in system degenerations, including Alzheimer's disease. Neuroscience 23:389-398.

3. Saper, C.B. (1988) Chemical neuroanatomy of Alzheimer's disease. In: Handbook of Psychopharmacology Volume 20 (eds:Iversen, L.L., Iversen, S.D. and Snyder, S.H.),Plenum, New York, pp. 131-156.

4. Summers, W.K., Majovski, L.V., Marsh, G.M., Tachiki, K. and Kling, A. (1986) Oral tetrahydroaminoacridine in long-term treatment of senile dementia, Alzheimer type. NEJM 315:1241-1245.

5. Becker, R.E. and Giacobini, E. (1988) Mechanisms of cholinesterase inhibition in senile dementia of the Alzheimer type: Clinical, pharmacological, and therapeutic aspects. Drug Dev. Res. 12:163-195.

6. Hefti, F. and Weiner, W.J. (1986) Nerve growth factor and Alzheimer's Disease. Ann. Neurol. 20:275-281.

7. Appel, S.H. (1981) A unifying hypothesis for the cause of amyotrophic lateral sclerosis, Parkinsonism, and Alzheimer disease. Ann. Neurol. 10:499-505.

8. Hefti, F., Hartikka, J. and Knusel, B. (1989) Function of neurotrophic factors in the adult and aging brain and their possible use in the treatment of neurodegenerative diseases. Neurobiol. Aging (In Press)

9. Thoenen, H., Bandtlow, C. and Heumann, R. (1987) The physiological function of nerve growth factor in the central nervous system: comparison with the periphery. Rev. Physiol. Biochem. Pharmacol. 109:146-178.

10. Whittemore, S.R. and Seiger, A. (1987) The expression, localization and functional significance of ß-nerve growth factor in the central nervous system. Brain Res. Rev. 12:439-464.

11. Walicke, P.A. (1989) Novel neurotrophic factors, receptors, and oncogenes. Ann. Rev. Neurosci. 12:103-126.

12. Phelps, C.H., Gage, F.H., Growdon, J.H., Hefti, F., Harbaugh, R., Johnston, M.V., Khachaturian, Z.S., Mobley, W.C., Price, D.L., Raskind, M., Simpkins, J., Thal, L.J. and Woodcock, J. (1989) Potential use of nerve growth factor to treat Alzheimer's Disease. Neurobiol. Aging 10:205-207.

13. Rosenberg, M.B., Friedmann, T., Robertson, R.C., Tuszynski, M., Wolff, J.A., Breakefield, X.O. and Gage, F.H. (1988) Grafting genetically modified cells to the damaged brain restorative effects of ngf expression. Science 242:1575-1578.

14. Wainer, B.H., Levey, A.I., Mufson, E.J. and Mesulam, M.-M. (1984) Cholinergic systems in mammalian brain identified with antibodies against choline acetyltransferase. Neurochem. Int. 6:163-182.

15. Rye, D.B., Wainer, B.H., Mesulam, M.-M., Mufson, E.J. and Saper, C.B. (1984) Cortical projections arising from the basal forebrain: a study of cholinergic and noncholinergic components employing combined retrograde tracing and immunohistochemical localization of choline acetyltransferase. Neuroscience 13:627-643.

16. Rye, D.B., Saper, C.B., Lee, H.J. and Wainer, B.H. (1987) Pedunculopontine tegmental nucleus of the rat: cytoarchitecture, cytochemistry, and some extrapyramidal connections of the mesopontine tegmentum. J Comp.Neurol. 259:483-528.

17. Wainer, B.H. and Mesulam, M.-M. (1989) Ascending cholinergic pathways in the rat brain. In: Brain Cholinergic Systems (eds:Steriade, M. and Biesold, D.),Oxford University Press, New York, in press.

18. Wainer, B.H., Levey, A.I., Rye, D.B., Mesulam, M.-M. and Mufson, E.J. (1985) Cholinergic and non-cholinergic septohippocampal pathways. Neurosci.Lett. 54:45-52.

19. Meck, W.H., Church, R.M., Wenk, G.L. and Olton, D.S. (1987) Nucleus basalis magnocellularis and medial septal area lesions differentially impair temporal memory. J Neurosci. 7:3505-3511.

20. Zola Morgan, S., Squire, L.R. and Amaral, D.G. (1986) Human amnesia and the medial temporal region: enduring memory impairment following a bilateral lesion limited to field CA1 of the hippocampus. J Neurosci. 6:2950-2967.

21. Hsiang, J., Wainer, B.H., Shalaby, I.A., Hoffmann, P.C., Heller, A. and Heller, B.R. (1987) Neurotrophic effects of hippocampal target cells on developing septal cholinergic neurons in culture. Neuroscience 21:333-343.

22. Hsiang, J., Price, S.D., Heller, A., Hoffmann, P.C. and Wainer, B.H. (1988) Ultrastructural evidence for hippocampal target cell-mediated trophic effects on septal cholinergic neurons in reaggregating cell cultures. Neuroscience 26:417-431.

23. Garber, B.B. and Moscona, A.A. (1972) Reconstruction of brain tissue from cell suspensions. I. Aggregation of patterns of cells dissociated from different regions of the developing brain. Dev. Biol. 27:217-234.

24. Piddington, R. and Moscona, A.A. (1967) Precocious induction of retinal glutamine synthetase by hydrocortisone in the embryo and in culture. Age-dependent differences in tissue response. Biochim. Biophys. Acta 141:429-432.

25. Morris, J.E. and Moscona, A.A. (1970) Induction of glutamine synthetase in embryonic retina: Its dependence on cell interactions. Science 167:1736-1738.

26. Hoffmann, P.C., Hemmendinger, L.M., Kotake, C. and Heller, A. (1983) Enhanced dopamine cell survival in reaggregates containing telencephalic target cells. Brain Res. 274:275-281.

27. Prochiantz, A., diPorzio, U., Kato, A., Berger, B. and Glowinski, J. (1979) In vitro maturation of mesencephalic dopaminergic neurons from mouse embryos is enhanced in the presence of their striatal target cells. Proc. Natl. Acad. Sci. USA 76:5387-5391.

28. Seiler, M. and Schwab, M.E. (1984) Specific retrograde transport of nerve growth factor (NGF) from neocortex to nucleus basalis in the rat. Brain Res. 300:33-39.

29. Kromer, L.F. (1987) Nerve growth factor treatment after brain injury prevents neuronal death. Science 235:214-216.

30. Gage, F.H., Armstrong, M., Williams, L.R. and Varon, S. (1988) Morphological response of axotomized septal neurons to nerve growth factor. J Comp.Neurol. 269:147-155.

31. Montero, C.N. and Hefti, F. (1988) Rescue of lesioned septal cholinergic neurons by nerve growth factor: Specificity and requirement for chronic treatment. J. Neurosci. 8:2986-2999.

32. Roback, J.D., Wainer, B.H. and Large, T.H. (1988) The expression of nerve growth factor protein in the developing hippocampus in reaggregate culture. Soc. Neurosci. Abs. 14:303.

33. Roback, J.D., Large, T.H., Otten, U. and Wainer, B.H. (1989) Studies on the expression of NGF mRNA and protein in the developing hippocampus in vitro. Soc. Neurosci. Abs. in press.

34. Hsiang, J., Heller, A., Hoffmann, P.C., Mobley, W.C. and Wainer, B.H. (1989) The effects of nerve growth factor on the development of septal cholinergic neurons in reaggregate cell cultures. Neuroscience 29:209-223.

35. Gundersen, R.W. and Barrett, J.N. (1979) Neuronal chemotaxis: Chick dorsal-root axons turn toward high concentrations of nerve growth factor. Science 206:1079-1080.

36. Menesini-Chen, M.G., Chen, J.S. and Levi-Montalcini, R. (1978) Sympathetic nerve fibers ingrowth in the central nervous system of neonatal rodent upon intracerebral NGF injections. Arch. Ital. Biol. 116:53-84.

37. Davies, A.M., Bandtlow, C., Heumann, R., Korsching, S., Rohrer, H. and Thoenen, H. (1987) Timing and site of nerve growth factor synthesis in developing skin in relation to innervation and expression of the receptor. Nature 326:353-358.

38. Rohrer, H., Heumann, R. and Thoenen, H. (1988) The synthesis of nerve growth factor (NGF) in developing skin is independent of innervation. Dev. Biol. 128:240-244.

39. Clegg, D.O., Large, T.H., Bodary, S.C. and Reichardt, L.F. (1989) Regulation of nerve growth factor mRNA levels in developing rat heart is not altered by sympathectomy. Dev. Biol.

40. Lindholm, D., Heumann, R., Meyer, M. and Thoenen, H. (1987) Interleukin-1 regulates synthesis of nerve growth factor in non-neuronal cells of rat sciatic nerve. Nature 330:658-659.

41. Large, T.H., Bodary, S.C., Clegg, D.O., Weskamp, G., Otten, U. and Reichardt, L.F. (1986) Nerve growth factor gene expression in the developing rat brain. Science 234:352-355.

42. Bayer, S.A. (1980) The development of the hippocampal circuitry in the rat. II. Morphogenesis during embryonic and early postnatal life. J. Comp. Neurol. 190:89-106.

43. Shelton, D.L. and Reichardt, L.F. (1984) Expression of the ß-nerve growth factor gene correlates with the density of sympathetic innervation in effector organs. Proc. Natl. Acad. Sci. USA 81:7951-7955.

44. Weskamp, G. and Otten, U. (1987) An enzyme-linked immunoassay for nerve growth factor (NGF): A tool for studying regulatory mechanisms involved in NGF production in brain and peripheral tissues. J. Neurochem. 48:1779-1786.

45. Levi-Montalcini, R. and Booker, B. (1960) Destruction of the sympathetic ganglia in mammals by an antiserum to a nerve-growth protein. Proc. Natl. Acad. Sci. USA 46:384-391.

46. Johnson, E.M.Jr., Gorin, P.D., Brandeis, L.D. and Pearson, J. (1980) Dorsal root ganglion neurons are destroyed by in utero exposure to maternal antibody to nerve growth factor. Science 210:916-918.

47. Wainer, B.H., Price, S.D., Nelson, S.G. and Mobley, W.C. (1988) Does nerve growth factor (NGF) enhance survival of developing central cholinergic neurons? Soc. Neurosci. Abs. 14:366.

48. Wainer, B.H., Price, S.D., Nelson, S.G. and Mobley, W.C. (1989) Ultrastructural evidence for nerve growth factor-mediated enhanced survival of developing central cholinergic neurons in reaggregate cell culture. Soc. Neurosci. Abs. in press.

49. Crutcher, K.A. and Collins, F. (1982) In vitro evidence for two distinct hippocampal growth factors: Basis of neuronal plasticity? Science 217:67-68.

50. Heacock, A.M., Schonfeld, A.R. and Katzman, R. (1986) Hippocampal neurotrophic factor: Characterization and response to denervation. Brain Res. 363:299-306.

51. Ojika, K. and Appel, S.H. (1984) Neurotrophic effects of hippocampal extracts on medial septal nucleus in vitro. Proc. Natl. Acad. Sci. USA 81:2567-2571.

52. Bostwick, J.R., Appel, S.H. and Perez-Polo, J.R. (1987) Distinct influences of nerve growth factor and a central cholinergic trophic factor on medial septal explants. Brain Res. 422:92-98.

53. Emerit, M.B., Segovia, J., Alho, H., Mastrangelo, M.J. and Wise, B.C. (1989) Hippocampal membranes contain a neurotrophic activity that stimulates cholinergic properties of fetal rat septal neurons cultered under serum-free conditions. J. Neurochem. 52:952-961.

54. Banker, G. and Goslin, K. (1988) Developments in neuronal cell culture. Nature. 336:185-186.

55. Levi-Montalcini, R. (1987) The nerve growth factor 35 years later. Science 237:1154-1162.

56. Cepko, C. (1988) Immortalization of neural cells via oncogene transduction. Trends Neurosci. 11:6-8.

57. Cepko, C.L. (1989) Immortalization of neural cells via retroviral-mediated oncogene transduction. Ann. Rev. Neurosci. 12:47-65.

58. Frederiksen, K., Jat, P.S., Valtz, N., Levy, D. and McKay, R. (1988) Immortalization of precursor cells from the mammalian cns. Neuron 1:439-448.

59. Whittemore, S.R., Holets, V.R., Gonzalez-Carvajal, M. and Levy, D. (1988) Transplantation of a hippocampally-derived immortal, temperature-sensitive, neuronal cell line into adult rat CNS. Soc. Neurosci. Abs. 14:586.

60. Paige, C.J. and Wu, G.E. (1989) The B cell repertoire. FASEB J. 3:1818-1824.

61. Alt, F., Blackwell, K. and Yancopoulos, G.D. (1987) Development of the primary antibody repertoire. Science 238:1079-1087.

62. Hammond, D.N., Wainer, B.H., Tonsgard, J.H. and Heller, A. (1986) Neuronal properties of clonal hybrid cell lines derived from central cholinergic neurons. Science 234:1237-1240.

63. Kohler, G. and Milstein, C. (1975) Continuous cultures of fused cells secreting antibody of defined specifity. Nature 256:495-497.

64. Lee, H.J., Hammond, D.N. and Wainer, B.H. (1987) Generation of permanent cell lines derived from postnatal septal and hippocampal regions. Soc. Neurosci. Abs. 13:701.

65. Hammond, D.N., Wainer, B.H., Heller, A., Large, T.H. and Reichardt, L.F. (1987) Clonal hybrid cell lines derived from primary hippocampal cells express nerve growth factor (NGF) mRNA and protein. Neuroscience Suppl. 22:S278.(Abstract)

66. Lee, H.J., Hammond, D.N., Large, T.H. and Wainer, B.H. (1988) Expression of NGF by permanent cells lines derived from postnatal hippocampus. Soc. Neurosci. Abs. 14:365.

67. Lee, H.J., Elliot, G.J., Hammond, D.N., Lee, V.M.-Y. and Wainer, B.H. (1989) Expression of the mature array of neurofilament protein isoforms by a clonal cell line from the CNS. Soc. Neurosci. Abs. in press.

68. Hammond, D.N., Lee, H.J., Wainer, B.H. and Heller, A. (1988) Medium conditioned by a hippocampal cell line increase choline acetyltransferase activity of septal cells in serum-free culture. Soc. Neurosci. Abs. 14:366.

69. Hammond, D.N., Lee, H.J. and Wainer, B.H. (1989) A membrane-associated factor influences central cholinergic neuron development. Ann. Neurol. in press.

70. Chomczynski, P. (1987) Single-step method of RNA isolation by acid guanidinium thiocyanate-phenol-chloroform extraction. Analytical Biochemistry 162:156-159.

71. Maniatis, T., Fritsch, E.F. and Sambrook, J. (1987)Molecular Cloning - a Laboratory Manual. Cold Spring Harbor Laboratory, Cold Spring Harbor,

APPROACHES TO GENE THERAPY IN THE CNS: INTRACEREBRAL GRAFTING OF FIBROBLASTS GENETICALLY MODIFIED TO SECRETE NERVE GROWTH FACTOR

Michael B. Rosenberg[1], Mark H. Tuszynski,[2] Kazunari Yoshida,[2] Theodore Friedmann[1] and Fred H. Gage[2]

Departments of [1]Pediatrics and [2]Neurosciences
University of California at San Diego
La Jolla, CA 92093

INTRODUCTION

Considerable effort in recent years has been applied towards the development of methods for the genetic modification of mammalian cells to correct disease phenotypes *in vivo*, an approach that has been named gene therapy (1). In an ideal gene therapy system, the new genetic information would be applied directly to the affected tissue . This direct approach has not yet been attempted, because the current methods of gene transfer are limited to replicating cells. Because of this and other technical limitations, approaches to gene therapy in animal models of human disease have relied on removing mitotic cells from the target tissue, genetically modifying them in culture, and then returning the cells to the animal. Most of these studies have used genetic transducing vectors derived from murine retroviruses to introduce foreign genes (transgenes) into target cells, because retrovirus vectors offer several advantages over other current methods of gene transfer (2): 1) infection by retrovirus vectors is extremely efficient for a broad range of cell types and species, with up to 100% of the target cells expressing the transgene; 2) the viral genomes have a relatively large capacity for foreign DNA; and 3) infection generally causes little or no genetic or metabolic damage to recipient cells. Other methods of gene transfer, which utilize biochemical or physical means to introduce transgenes into cells, suffer from serious limitations in comparison. The first methods developed involve incubating cells with DNA complexed with DEAE-dextran (3) or calcium phosphate (4). More recent methods use direct microinjection (5), electric fields (electroporation) (6), liposomes (lipofection) (7), and tungsten microprojectiles (8).

Because of their accessibility and the presence of suitable replicating cell populations, the bone marrow (9-11) and skin (12-15) have been studied most extensively for gene therapy applications, and more recently, the liver has been actively investigated (16,17). Because of its relative inaccessibility and the lack of neuronal stem cell populations in adults, another potentially very important target organ, the brain, has not been pursued in gene therapy models. This is not meant to imply that neurons will always be the target cells for CNS gene therapy. There are certainly cases in which other cell types must be treated, such as oligodendrocytes in the demyelinating diseases. Neurons, however, will certainly be the target cells in the vast majority of disorders, and methods developed to treat neurons should be applicable to other cell types. The remainder of this chapter, therefore, will concentrate on neuronal therapy.

APPROACHES TO CNS THERAPY

Several approaches, both genetic and non-genetic, are theoretically available to restore missing functions to neurons (Fig. 1). The most direct approach would entail introducing the transgene directly into neurons using an appropriate vector (Fig. 1A). As discussed above, there are presently no available methods for gene transfer into post-mitotic cells. Suitable vectors may soon be developed, however. Herpes simplex virus (HSV) normally infects post-mitotic sensory neurons, in which it is capable of establishing a life-long latent, non-destructive infection. Several groups are developing vectors based on HSV (18,19), and such vectors may prove valuable for introducing transgenes into neurons and other post-mitotic cells, both *in vitro* and *in vivo*.

If effective treatment of a specific disease requires that the transgene be expressed in the target cell itself, direct vector application will be the only possible approach. In many disorders, however, it will not be necessary to treat neurons directly but instead it will be possible to allow the target cells to take up exogenously applied factors. For example, minipumps (20-23) and implanted solid polymers (24) have been investigated for delivery of substances to the CNS (Fig. 1B). Another approach that has received considerable attention is the grafting of donor cells or tissues that produce the needed substance, which can then enter the target cells by direct transfer through tight junctions or diffusion across the membrane (Fig. 1C) or by secretion and re-uptake via specific receptors or transport systems (Fig. 1D). This

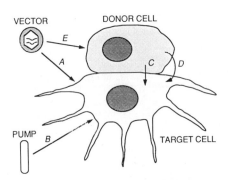

Figure 1. Theoretical approaches to CNS therapy (see text for description).

method has been widely applied to provide dopamine in Parkinson's disease patients and animal models, using both neural and non-neural tissue, i.e., fetal substantia nigra and adult adrenal gland (25-27). For this approach to be useful in treating a particular CNS disorder, several criteria must be met. A suitable donor tissue must be available that produces sufficient quantities of the desired factor, and this tissue must survive and continue to function when grafted to the brain. Ideally, the donor tissue should come from the patient himself, as the use of autologous grafts will avoid problems of histocompatibility. However, for most disorders there will not be a suitable non-neural tissue, eliminating the possibility of autografts. The use of fetal tissue poses serious ethical problems in addition to immunological problems.

As an alternative approach, we have been developing a model in which cells are genetically modified in culture to express the required function and then grafted to the brain (Fig. 1E) (28,29). This approach combines neural grafting with methods previously used for gene therapy models in bone marrow and skin. An advantage to this approach is donor cells need not be CNS-derived, nor do they have to express the desired function naturally. Instead, they may be selected based solely on their ability to be grown and manipulated in vitro and to survive as grafts. In addition, by using cells derived from the patient, many immunological problems may be circumvented. Although they are not necessarily the most well suited cells for intracerebral grafting, skin fibroblasts have several advantageous features: 1) they are easily obtained and grown from small biopsies with little discomfort to the patient; 2) they can be genetically manipulated in culture by a number of methods, including retrovirus vectors; and 3) they can survive as intracerebral grafts in rats. Therefore, we have developed a model for CNS gene therapy (Fig. 2) in which the patient would have a skin biopsy taken, cultured primary fibroblasts from the biopsy would be infected with a retrovirus vector (or treated by another suitable method) to express the desired transgene, and the cells would be grown to the necessary quantity and then stereotactically grafted into the patient's brain.

While our ultimate goal is to use autologous primary fibroblasts for grafting, many preliminary studies are facilitated by using established fibroblast cell lines instead, as they are even easier to manipulate in culture and allow one to select clonal lines that express the transgene at desired levels. For these reasons, we have compared the abilities of primary fibroblasts cultures and cell lines to survive as intracerebral grafts, and we have determined that both can survive for at least 2 months (28).

Although gene therapy has traditionally been thought of in terms of treating inherited diseases by replacing the dysfunctional gene, genetic strategies should also prove useful for treating other conditions in which a required function is lacking due to injury or cell death. In fact our most useful models for testing the feasibility of grafting genetically modified cells to the CNS have used mechanically or chemically induced lesions (see below). Thus, it is useful to expand the definition of gene therapy to include genetic treatment of any disorder, whether or not it is inherited.

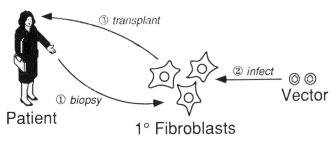

Figure 2. Proposed model for grafting genetically modified fibroblasts to treat disorders of the CNS.

INTRACEREBRAL GRAFTING OF GENETICALLY MODIFIED FIBROBLASTS

To test the therapeutic potential of this approach, we have chosen a well characterized rat model that provides the opportunity to observe a functional effect. Following transection of the fimbria-fornix, the pathway connecting cholinergic neurons of the basal forebrain to their target in the hippocampus, many of the cholinergic neurons undergo retrograde degeneration, exhibit a decrease in the activities of many enzymes and, in some cases, die (30,31). This degenerative response is attributed to the loss of trophic support from ß-nerve growth factor (NGF), which is normally transported retrogradely in the intact brain from the hippocampus to the septal cholinergic cell bodies (32-36). The importance of NGF in this response to damage is supported by experiments demonstrating that cholinergic neurons in the medial septum can be protected from retrograde degeneration by chronic infusion of exogenous NGF (20,22,23,37). We have used this model, which is also considered a model for the cholinergic degeneration seen in Alzheimer's disease, to determine whether grafted, genetically modified fibroblasts can produce a biological response (29).

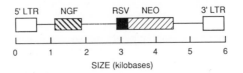

Figure 3. Retrovirus vector expressing NGF cDNA. LTR, long
terminal repeat; RSV, Rous sarcoma virus promoter; NEO, neomycin-
resistance gene.

A retroviral vector (Fig. 3) was constructed from Moloney murine leukemia virus (38) to
contain the 777 base pair HgaI-PstI fragment of mouse NGF cDNA (39,40) under control of
the promoter in the viral 5' long terminal repeat. This insert corresponds to the shorter NGF
transcript that predominates in mouse tissue receiving sympathetic innervation (41) and is
believed to encode the precursor to NGF that is secreted constitutively. The vector also
includes a dominant selectable marker encoding the neomycin-resistance function of trans-
poson Tn^5 (42) under control of an internal promoter from Rous sarcoma virus.
Transmissible ecotropic retrovirus was produced (29) and used to infect the established rat
fibroblast cell line Ratl (43). Individual neomycin-resistant colonies, selected in medium
containing the neomycin analog G418, were expanded and tested for NGF production and
secretion by two-site enzyme immunoassay. The highest producing clone, Ratl-N.8-8, contained 66 pg NGF per 10^5 cells and secreted NGF into the medium at a rate of 77 pg/hr per
10^5 cells. The secreted NGF was biologically active, as determined by its ability to induce
neurite outgrowth from PC12 rat pheochromocytoma cells (44,45). Uninfected Ratl cells, in
contrast, did not produce detectable levels of NGF.

Unilateral aspirative cavities were made through the cingulate cortex of Sprague-Dawley
rats, completely transecting the fimbria-fornix. Retrovirus-infected (NGF-secreting) and
control uninfected fibroblasts were suspended in PBS at 8 x 10^4 cells/µl, and 4 µl aliquots
were injected free-hand into the lesion cavity and lateral ventricle ipsilateral to the cavity.
Animals were sacrificed after 2 or 8 weeks and processed for immunohistochemistry.
Staining for fibronectin, a fibroblast-specific marker, revealed robust graft survival that was
comparable in both infected and control groups. Staining for choline acetyltransferase, to
evaluate the survival of cholinergic neurons, indicated a significantly greater number of remaining neurons on the lesioned side of the medial septum in animals that had received grafts
of infected cells than in animals that had received uninfected control grafts (Table 1). These
results are similar to our previous study with a different fibroblast cell line, 208F (29). It is
interesting to note that uninfected control grafts resulted in 60% survival of cholinergic
neurons, whereas previous studies have shown only a 40-50% survival in untreated control
animals (20,22,23,31,37). This suggests the possibility that the fibroblasts produce other as
yet unknown factors that can affect cholinergic survival. Basic fibroblast growth factor has
been shown to prevent the death of lesioned cholinergic neurons (46), and studies are in
progress to determine whether the fibroblasts secrete this or other agents believed to have
neurotrophic effects.

DISCUSSION

These and previous studies have demonstrated that genetically modified fibroblasts can
survive intracerebral grafting and continue to express transgenes for at least two months
(28,29). Furthermore, the grafts continue to produce and secrete sufficient NGF to have a
biological effect during this period. These results suggest that this system may prove feasible
for treating CNS disorders. There are several prerequisites for a neurological disease to be a
candidate for this approach: l) The pathogenesis of the disease must be sufficiently well
understood to allow identification of the relevant lacking function. 2) The relevant gene must
be available as a well characterized cDNA clone. 3) The affected region of the CNS must be
known and sufficiently localized to permit implantation into the appropriate area(s). 4)
Restoration of normal function must not, at present, require synaptic contact with target cells.

Table 1. Survival of cholinergic neurons in rats with unilateral fimbria-fomix lesions following fibroblast grafts.

| | Surviving ChAT$^+$ Neurons (% contralateral side) | |
Graft type	2 Weeks	8 Weeks
Rat1 control	62	60
Rat1-N.8-8	99	87

Instead, the donor cells must produce a factor that has a mechanism for release by the cells and uptake by neurons. In the example of NGF, these conditions are satisfied because the NGF precursor protein includes a putative signal sequence for secretion (41), and the secreted NGF binds to receptors on the target cholinergic neurons. In other cases, the needed factor may be packaged in specialized secretory vesicles or simply diffuse through the cell membrane. Alternatively, the donor cells can act as a toxin "sink" by expressing an enzyme that metabolizes a neurotoxin. This, of course, requires that the neurotoxin have a mechanism for leaving the neuron and entering the donor cell. S) Ideally, an animal model should be available.

With these issues in mind, we have been using this approach to deliver L-DOPA in a rat model of Parkinson's disease, and we have reported results comparable to those observed with adrenal medulla grafts (47). Other potentially applicable disorders include the various lysosomal storage diseases, in which a specific lysosomal enzyme is lacking, such as Krabbe's disease, i.e., galactosylceramidase deficiency. The twitcher mouse serves as an animal model for this disease, in which there is extensive CNS demyelination due to the buildup of the toxic substance psychosine in oligodendrocytes. When bone marrow from wild-type congenic mice is grafted into these animals, graft-derived macrophages infiltrate the CNS (48). The presence of these galactosylceramidase-positive cells serves to lower the CNS levels of psychosine significantly, resulting in decreased demyelination and prolonged survival. These results demonstrate that graft-derived cells can metabolize a toxic substance and ameliorate disease symptoms. It is likely that grafts of genetically modified fibroblasts may have similar effects in this and other lysosomal storage diseases. Although our studies have focused on the use of fibroblasts because of the features described earlier, other cell types should also prove useful for this approach and may be advantageous in specific situations. In particular, astrocytes may demonstrate longer-term survival and stability because of their CNS origin, although our preliminary studies have indicated survival comparable to that of primary skin fibroblasts. Endocrine cells may be valuable, too, because of their secretory capabilities. Pituitary-derived cells have been shown to express the retrovirus-transduced NGF cDNA and secrete NGF in response to a normal stimulator of pituitary secretion, corticotropin releasing factor (49). It should be stressed, however, that skin fibroblasts will be easier to obtain and culture than virtually all other cell types.

We conclude that the intracerebral grafting of genetically modified cells should eventually provide a means for CNS therapy. Together with traditional neuronal grafting and the upcoming vectors for direct genetic modification of neurons *in vivo*, this approach should permit the treatment of numerous CNS disorders that cannot be treated by standard drug therapies.

REFERENCES

1. Friedmann, T. and Roblin, R. (1972) Gene therapy for human genetic disease? Science 175: 949-955.
2. Miller, A.D., Jolly, D.J., Friedmann, T. and Verma, I.M. (1983) A transmissible retrovirus expressing human hypoxanthine phosphoribosyltransferase (HPRT): Gene transfer into cells obtained from humans deficient in HPRT. Proc. Natl. Acad. Sci. USA 80: 4709-4713.
3. McCutchan, J.H. and Pagano, J.S. (1968) Enhancement of the infectibility of simian virus 40 DNA with diethylaminoethyl dextran. J. Nat. Cancer. Inst. 41: 351-356.
4. Graham, F.L. and Van der Eb, A.J. (1973) A new technique for the assay of infectivity of human adenovirus 5 DNA. Virology 52: 456-467.
5. S. Capecchi, M. (1980) High efficiency transformation by direct microinjection of DNA into cultured mammalian cells. Cell 22: 479-488.

6. Shigekawa, K. and Dower, W.J. (1988) Electroporation of eukaryotes and prokaryotes: A general approach to the introduction of macromolecules into cells. BioTechniques 6: 742-

7. Felgner, P.L., Gadek, T.R., Holm, M., Roman, R., Chan, H.W., Wenz, M., Northrup, J.P., Ringold, G.M. and Danielsen, M. (1987) Lipofection: A highly efficient, lipid-mediated DNA-transfection procedure. Proc. Natl. Acad. Sci. USA 84: 7413-7417.

8. Klein, T.M., Wolf, E.D., Wu, R. and Sanford, J.C. (1987) High velocity micro-projectiles for delivering nucleic acids into living cells. Nature 327: 70-73.

9. Miller, A.D., Eckner, R.J., Jolly, D.J., Friedmann, T. and Verma, I.M. (1984) Expression of a retrovirus encoding human HPRT in mice. Science 225: 630-632.

10. Williams, D.A., Lemischka, I.R., Nathan, D.G. and Mulligan, R.C. (1984) Introduction of new genetic material into pluripotent haematopoietic stem cells of the mouse. Nature 310: 476-480.

11. Eglitis, M.A., Kantoff, P., Gilboa, E. and Anderson, W.F. (1985) Gene expression in mice after high efficiency retroviral-mediated gene transfer. Science 230: 1395-1398.

12. Selden, R.F., Skoskiewicz, M.J., Howie, K.B., Russell, P.S. and Goodman, H.M. (1987) Implantation of genetically engineered fibroblasts into mice: Implications for gene therapy. Science 236: 714-7 18.

13. St.Louis, D. and Verma, I.M. (1988) An alternative approach to somatic cell gene therapy. Proc. Natl. Acad. Sci. USA 85: 3150-3154.

14. Palmer, T.D., Thompson, A.R. and Miller, A.D. (1989) Production of human factor IX in animals by genetically modified skin fibroblasts: Potential therapy for hemophilia B. Blood 73: 438-445.

15. Morgan, J.R., Barrandon, Y., Green, H. and Mulligan, R.C. (1987) Expression of an exogenous growth hormone gene by transplantable human epidermal cells. Science 237: 1476-1479.

16. Wolff, J.A., Yee, J.-K., Skelly, H.F., Moores, J.C., Respess, J.G., Friedmann, T. and Leffert, H. (1987) Expression of retrovirally transduced genes in primary cultures of adult rat hepatocytes. Proc. Natl. Acad. Sci. USA 84: 3344-3348.

17. Ledley, F.D., Darlington, G.J., Hahn, T. and Woo, S.L.C. (1987) Retroviral gene transfer into primary hepatocytes: Implications for genetic therapy of liver-specific functions. Proc. Natl. Acad. Sci. USA 84: 5335-5339.

18. Palella, T.D., Silverman, L.J., Schroll, C.T., Homa, F.L., Levine, M. and Kelley, W.N. (1988) Herpes simplex virus-mediated human hypoxanthine-guanine phosphoribosyltransferase gene transfer into neuronal cells. Mol. Cell. Biol. 8: 457-460.

19. Geller, A.I. and Breakefield, X.O. (1988) A defective HSV-l vector expresses Escherichia coli ß-galactosidase in cultured peripheral neurons. Science 241: 1667-1669.

20. Williams, L.R., Varon, S., Peterson, G.M., Wictorin, K., Fischer, W., Bjorklund, A. and Gage, F.H. (1986) Continuous infusion of nerve growth factor prevents basal forebrain neuronal death after fimbria-fomix transection. Proc. Natl. Acad. Sci. USA 83: 7 9231-9235.

21. Fischer, W., Wictorin, K., Bjorklund, A., Williams, L.R., Varon, S. and Gage, F.H. (1987) Amelioration of cholinergic neuron atrophy and spatial memory impairment in aged rats by nerve growth factor. Nature 329: 65-68.

22. Hefti, F. (1986) Nerve growth factor (NGF) promotes survival of septal cholinergic neurons after fimbrial transection. J. Neurosci. 8: 2155-2162.

23. Kromer, L.F. (1987) Nerve growth factor treatment after brain injury prevents neuronal death. Science 235: 214-216.

24. Freese, A., Sabel, B.A., Saltzman, W.M., During, M.J. and Langer, R. (1989) Controlled release of dopamine from a polymeric brain implant: In vitro characterization. Exp. Neurol. 103: 234-238.

25. Dunnett, S.B., Bjorklund, A., Gage, F.H. and Stenevi, U. (1985) Transplantation of mesencephalic dopamine neurons to the striatum of adult rat. In: Neural grafting in the mammalian CNS (eds. Bjorklund, A. and Stenevi, U.) Elsevier, Amsterdam, pp. 451-469.

26. Becker, J.B. and Freed, W.J. (1988) Adrenal medulla grafts enhance functional activity of the striatal dopamine system following substantia nigra lesions. Brain Res. 462: 401-406.

27. Allen, G.S., Burns, R.S., Tulipan, N.B. and Parker, R.A. (1989) Adrenal medullary transplantation to the caudate nucleus in Parkinson's disease: Initial clinical results in 18 patients. Arch. Neurol. 46: 487-491.

28. Gage, F.H., Wolff, J.A., Rosenberg, M.B., Xu, L., Yee, J.-K., Shults, C. and Friedmann, T. (1987) Grafting genetically modified cells to the brain: Possibilities for the future. Neuroscience 23: 795-807.

29. Rosenberg, M.B., Friedmann, T., Robertson, R.C., Tuszynski, M., Wolff, J.A., Breakefield, X.O. and Gage, F.H. (1988) Grafting genetically modified cells to the damaged brain: Restorative effects of NGF expression. Science 242: 1575-1578.

30. Diatz, H.M. and Powell, T.P.S. (1954) Studies on the connexions of the fornix system. J. Neurol. Neurosurgery Psychiatry 17: 75-82.

31. Gage, F.H., Wictorin, K., Fischer, W., Williams, L.R., Varon, S. and Bjorklund, A. (1986) Retrograde cell changes in medial septum and diagonal band following fimbria-fornix transection: Quantitative temporal analysis. Neuroscience 19: 241-255.

32. Korsching, S. and Thoenen, H. (1983) Nerve growth factor in sympathetic ganglia and corresponding target organs of the rat: Correlation with density of sympathetic innervation. Proc. Natl. Acad. Sci. USA 80: 3513-3516.

33. Whittemore, S.R., Ebendal, T., Larkfors, L., Olson, L., Seiger, A., Stromberg, I. and Persson, H. (1986) Developmental and regional expression of ß-nerve growth factor messenger RNA and protein in the rat central nervous system. Proc. Natl. Acad. Sci. USA 83: 817-821.

34. Shelton, D.L. and Reichardt, L.F. (1986) Studies on the expression of the ß-nerve growth factor (NGF) gene in the central nervous system: Level and regional distribution of NGF mRNA suggest that NGF functions as trophic factor for several distinct populations of neurons. Proc. Natl. Acad. Sci. USA 83: 2714-2718.

35. . Seilor, M. and Schwab, M.E. (1984) Specific retrograde transport of nerve growth factor (NGF) from neocortex to nucleus basalis in the rat. Brain Res. 300: 33-39.

36. Gnahn, H., Hefti, F., Heumann, R., Schwab, M.E. and Thoenen, H. (1983) NGF-mediated increase in choline acetyltransferase (ChAT) in the neonatal rat forebrain: Evidence for a physiological role of NGF in the brain? Dev. Brain Res. 9: 45-52.

37. Gage, F.H., Armstrong, D.M., Williams, L.R. and Varon, S. (1988) Morphological response of axotomized septal neurons to nerve growth factor. J. Comp. Neurol. 269: 147-155.

38. Varmus, H. and Swanstrom, L. (1982) Replication of retroviruses. In: RNA Tumor Viruses (eds. Weiss, R., Teich, N., Varmus, H. and Coffin, J.) Cold Spring Harbor Press, Cold Spring Harbor, New York, pp. 233-249.

39. Scott, J., Selby, M., Urdea, M., Quiroga, M., Bell, G.I. and Rutter, W.J. (1983) Isolation and nucleotide sequence of a cDNA encoding the precursor of mouse nerve growth factor. Nature 302: 538-540.

40. Ullrich, A., Gray, A., Berman, C. and Dull, T.J. (1983) Human beta nerve growth factor gene sequence highly homologous to that of mouse. Nature 303: 821-825.

41. Edwards, R.H., Selby, M.J. and Rutter, W.J. (1986) Differential RNA splicing predicts two distinct nerve growth factor precursors. Nature 319: 784-787.

42. Southern, P.J. and Berg,P. (1982) Transformation of mammalian cells to antibiotic resistance with a bacterial gene under control of the SV40 early region promoter. J. Mol. Appl. Genet. 1: 327-341.

43. Mishra, N.K. and Ryan, W.L. (1973) Effect of 3-methylcholanthrene and dimethyl-nitrosamine on anchorage dependence of rat fibroblasts chronically infected with Rauscher leukemiavirus. Int. J. Cancer 11: 123-130.

44. Greene, L.A. and Tischler, A.S. (1976) Establishment of a noradrenergic clonal line of rat adrenal pheochromocytoma cells which respond to nerve growth factor. Proc. Natl. Acad. Sci. USA 73: 2424-2428.

45. Greene, L.A. (1977) A quantitative bioassay for nerve growth factor (NGF) activity employing a clonal pheochromocytoma cell line. Brain Res. 133: 350-353.

46. Anderson, K.J., Dam, D., Lee, S. and Cotman, C.W. (1988) Basic fibroblast growth factor prevents death of lesioned cholinergic neurons in vivo. Nature 332: 360-361.

47. Wolff, J.A., Xu, L., Friedmann, T., Rosenberg, M.B., Iuvone, M.P., O'Malley, K.L., Fisher, L.J., Shimohama, S. and Gage, F.H. (1988) Grafting of genetically engineered fibroblasts which produce L-DOPA in a rat model of Parkinson's. Soc. Neurosci. Abs. 14: 734.

48. Hoogerbrugge, P.M., Suzuki, K., Poorthuis, B.J.H.M., Kobayashi, T., Wagemaker, G. and van Bekkum, D.W. (1988) Donor-derived cells in the central nervous system of twitcher mice after bone marrow transplantation. Science 239: 1035-1038.

49. Wolf, D., Richter-Landsberg, C., Short, M.P., Cepko, C. and Breakefield, X.O. (1988) Retrovirus-mediated gene transfer of beta-nerve growth factor into mouse pituitary line AtT-20. Mol. Biol. Med. 5: 43-59.

EXOGENOUS NERVE GROWTH FACTOR STIMULATES CHOLINE ACETYLTRANSFERASE ACTIVITY IN BASAL FOREBRAIN OF AXOTOMIZED AND AGED RATS

Lawrence R. Williams[1], Karen S. Jodelis[1], Melody R. Donald[1], and Henry K. Yip[2]

[1]CNS Diseases Research, Unit 7251-209-5, The Upjohn Company, 301 Henrietta Street, Kalamazoo, MI 49001, and [2]Department of Anatomy, University of Utah, School of Medicine, Salt Lake City, Utah 84132

INTRODUCTION

Nerve growth factor (NGF) is physiologically critical for the survival and normal development of sympathetic and spinal sensory neurons, and for their maintenance in the adult (1,2). NGF has been found to have a similar role in the mammalian central nervous system (CNS) (3). NGF was first implicated in CNS function when Schwab et al. (4) found specific retrograde transport of exogenous NGF from cerebral and hippocampal cortices to neuronal cell bodies in the rat basal forebrain. NGF is now known to be present and produced in the CNS, and is in largest amount in the cortex and hippocampus, the target tissues for neurons in the basal forebrain (3).

The axonal projections from the medial septum and diagonal band of Broca (MS/DB) through the dorsal fornix and fimbria (F-F) to the hippocampus and the projections from the nucleus basalis of Meynert (NBM) to the cerebral cortices are systems used to examine the role of NGF in CNS neuronal function. The cholinergic components of these systems are particularly affected in Alzheimer's disease. Neurotrophic hypofunction is hypothesized to underlie such neurodegeneration (5-7). In several experimental paradigms, administration of mouse NGF (mNGF) either by repeated injection or continuous infusion is found to prevent the loss of cholinergic and non-cholinergic neurons (8-10) and to stimulate the expression of cholinergic phenotypes (11-18), particularly the activity of choline acetyltransferase (ChAT; acetyl-CoA: choline-O-acetyltransferase, EC 2.3.1.6), the enzyme that synthesizes the cholinergic transmitter, acetylcholine (ACh). In this report, we review recent data from our experiments examining the effects of mNGF on the basal forebrain following transection of the F-F. We also report the changes observed in the central cholinergic systems with age, and the stimulatory effect of exogenous mNGF on these systems.

MATERIALS AND METHODS

NGF Infusion Solution

Renin-free 2.5s mNGF was purchased from Bioproducts For Science
(Indianapolis, IN). The concentration of pure mNGF in a stock solution
of PBS was determined by molar extinction (1.64 O.D.280/mg/ml) and
aliquots of 1 mg/ml were stored at -70⁰C for later use. The concentration
and biological activity of the mNGF solutions were confirmed using the
morphological differentiation of PC12 cells in vitro (19). At the time of
animal surgery, working solutions were prepared by dilution of the
concentrate in Dubelco's PBS containing 0.1% rat serum albumin (Sigma),
i.e., the infusion vehicle. After filter sterilization, serial dilutions
were prepared where appropriate, and the sterile solutions were used to
prefill the infusion cannnlae and pumps. No loss of biological activity
was detected in sterile aliquots of stock solutions of mNGF at
concentrations ranging from 100 µg/ml to 1 µg/ml when stored _in vitro_ at
37⁰C for periods up to 1 month. Also, no loss in biological activity was
detected in 100 µg/ml mNGF solutions after 2 weeks infusion _in vivo_.
Control animals were infused with the vehicle, the albumin (1 mg/ml)
serving as a non-specific protein.

Infusion Cannula

NGF does not cross the blood-brain-barrier; treatment of the central
nervous system requires NGF infusion directly into the brain. Williams et
al. (20), described the methods for construction and stereotaxic
implantation of infusion cannula device. For the present experiments, the
cannula device was made from 30 gauge stainless steel tubing with an
intraparenchymal length of 4.5 mm. The device was used to infuse control
and experimental solutions always into the right lateral ventricle. Both
the cannula and an Alzet osmotic pump (Model 2002, 0.5 µl/hr for 14 days,
Alza Corp., Palo Alto, CA) were filled with the infusate prior to
implantation. At the end of the experiments, i.e., up to 2 weeks after
pump implantation and continuous infusion, the cannula device and pump
were removed from the animal and the device was checked for continued
patency. _All_ devices used in these experiments were patent at the end of
the experiment.

F-F Transection and mNGF Treatment of Young Adult Rats

Female albino rats of the Sprague-Dawley strain, 200 - 250 g in
weight, were used for F-F transection experiments. Details of the
Microsurgical procedures have been described for the selective unilateral
aspirative transections of the dorsal septo-hippocampal pathways (9,21).
Anesthesia for surgery and sacrifice was induced by intramuscular
injection with a mixture (4 ml/kg) of ketamine (25 mq/ml), rompun (1.3
mg/ml) and acepromazine (0.25 mg/ml). Most animals received complete
unilateral aspirative transections of the right supracallosal striae,
dorsal fornix and fimbria, i.e., all the dorsal pathways on the right
side _(F-F Aspiration)_. Other animals received a _sham_ aspiration where the
parietal and cingulate cortices, as well as the supracallosal striae and
corpus callosum were aspirated exposing the F-F, but leaving the F-F
undamaged. _Normal_, sham, and F-F Aspirated animals received a cannula
implantation and were infused with mNGF 1.2 µg/day for 2 weeks. Other
groups of F-F aspirated animals were infused with serial dilutions of
mNGF to establish a dose response.

mNGF Treatment of Aged Rats

The effect of mNGF in aged rats was examined in Fisher 344 male rats obtained from the National Institute of Aging colony at Harlan/Sprague-Dawley (Indianapolis, IN). Normal uninjured animals 4 months and 2 years old received a cannula implantation and were treated for two weeks with vehicle or mNGF at 1.2 μg/day.

Quantitation of NGF Receptor Density

NGF receptor density was quantitated using the 192-IgG monoclonal antibody to the receptor (22) as described by Yip (23). Animals were anesthetized and perfused intracandially with 200 - 300 ml of oxygenated Krebs-Ringer at 4^0C, until the effluent was clear of blood. The brains were quickly removed and frozen in liquid nitrogen vapor. Tissues were mounted onto cryostat chucks, and 16 μm serial sections were cut at -15^0C and thaw mounted onto gelatin/chrome alum-coated slides. Slide mounted sections were pre-incubated in incubation buffer (100 mM sodium phosphate pH 7.0, 120 mM sodium chloride, 0.1 mM bacitracin, 0.02% bovine serum albumin, containing 0.1% polyethylenimine) for 15 min. at $22-25^0$C. Brain sections were incubated in buffer containing 5 nM ^{125}I-192-IgG for 60 min. at $22-25^0$C. Non-specific binding was determined by inclusion of 1 μM of non-labeled 192-IgG. Slides were washed in 4^0C buffer, rinsed quickly in cold distilled water, dried under a stream of cold dry air, and then placed in slide boxes containing desiccant overnight at 4^0C. Brain sections were exposed for 3 days against LKB UltroFilm at room temperature to generate autoradiograms.

Autoradiograms were quantified using a microcomputer-assisted densitometer (Stahl Research Laboratories, Inc) at an anatomical resolution of 100 μM. The optic density readings were converted into the amount of radioligand bound/mg protein using 16 μm thick ^{125}I-labeled brain mesh standards. Five - eight densitametric readings were taken for each structure on a single brain section. NGF receptor density in fmol receptor per mg protein is expressed as the average from 3-4 animals (13).

Brain Micro-dissections

All tissue samples were taken from the right side of the brain ipilateral to the implanted cannula and/or F-F aspiration. Immediately after dissection, all samples were frozen on dry ice. The most extensive dissections were done in the experiments with the Fisher male rats. Under deep anesthesia the control and experimental animals were perfused through the heart with oxygenated Krebs-Ringer, 40C, until the effluent was cleared of blood (24). The cannula device was removed from the skull, the animal decapitated, and the brain was quickly removed for micro-dissection. A coronal brain matrix (Harvard Apparatus, South Natick, MA) was used to facilitate reproducible dissections. Frontal cortex was obtained from a coronal slice of the brain cut at the caudal end of the lateral olfactory tract. Under the dissecting microscope, a razor blade was used to hemiseat the slice, and the olfactory tract and tubercle were dissected away from the piece of frontal cortex. Next, a 4 mm coronal slice was cut using the caudal edge of the optic chiasm as a landmark. From the right hemisection of this slice, the MS/DB was dissected as previously described (21). The striatum was removed from this same slice. In the next 3 mm coronal slice, the NBM was micro-dissected as described by Cuello and Carson (24). From the remaining brain, a piece of parietal cortex (approximately 2 mm^2) overlying the septal pole of the hippocampus was removed, the whole hippocampus was dissected, and a 2 mm^2 piece of temporal cortex and entorhinal cortex overlying the temporal pole of the hippocampus was taken as the final piece of the dissection.

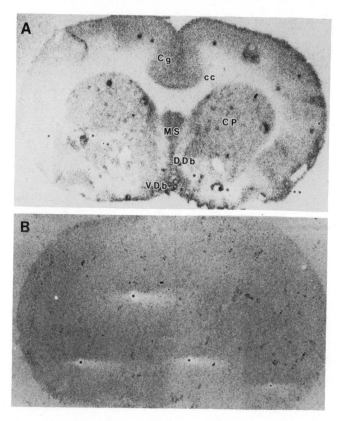

Fig. 1. Bright Field Photographic images of Autoradiagrams Generated by 5 nM ^{125}I-192-IgG exposed to Ultrofilm for 3 days. Serial sections were incubated in the absence (A, specific binding) or presence(B, non-specific binding) of 1 µm nonlabled ^{125}I-192-IgG. cc-corpus callosum; Cg - cingulate cortex; CP - striatum; DDb-dorsal diagonal band of Broca; MS - medial septal nucleus; VDb-ventral diagonal band of Broca.

Sprague-Dawley rats with F-F transections were not perfused prior to decapitation and brain micro-dissection. MS/DB and striatum were dissected as described (21).

Assay for Choline Acetyltransferase Enzymatic Activity

Each tissue-piece was sonicated at 20 watts in 1 ml of double distilled water on ice. The samples were diluted to contain approximately 0.5 mg/ml of protein, and 5 µl of this solution (in triplicate) was placed into a siliconized scintillation vial on ice. ChAt activity was determined by the micromethod of Fonnum (21). Protein concentration of the samples was estimated by the method of Lowry as modified by Fryer et al.(25), using BSA as the standard protein. Inclusion of Triton X-100 in the sonication solution was found to interfere with the Lowry protein determinations. The detectable amount of ChAT activity in the MS/DB sonicates was not affected by omission of the detergent from the solution. The ChAt reaction was linear over the range of protein used in these experiments and up to 15 min of incubation. The average ChAt enzyme activity is expressed as pmol acetylcholine synthesized per μg protein per min. Statistical significance was determined using the Kruskal-Wallis one-way analysis of variance and the Mann-Whitney U test.

RESULTS

NGF Administration Stimulates Receptor Binding After F-F Transection

In the normal young adult Sprague-Dawley female rat, there are high levels of specific ^{125}-192-IgG binding in the superficial layers of cerebral cortex, striatum, and MS/DB (Fig. 1). In the normal MS/DB, the average receptor density is equal to 30 fmol/mg protein (n=4). At two weeks after F-F transection, there is a significant 26% reduction of ^{125}I- 192-IgG binding to the NGF receptor in the right MS/DB iipsilateral

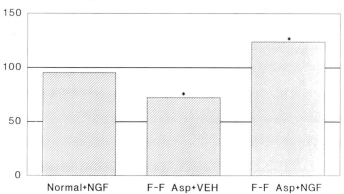

Fig. 2. NGF Receptor Density Following F-F Transection and mNGF Infusion. The density of 125I-192-IgG binding in the MS/DB of experimental animals is expressed as the percent of the specific binding in normal, untreated animals, i.e., 30 fmol/mg protein. n=4 in each group, *p<.05.

to the axotomy as compared to normal rats (Fig. 2). Infusion of mNGF at a dose of 1.2 μg/day (a pump concentration of 100 μg/ml) for 2 weeks, has no effect on the NGF receptor density of normal basal forebrain neurons. However, mNGF treatment of F-F transected animals results in a 134% increase in NGF receptor density on the side of transection compared to the same side of normal forebrain (13).

NGF Administration Stimulates ChAT Activity After F-F Transection

The average specific activity of ChAT in micro-dissections of the normal MS/DB is 2.3 pmol ACh/μg protein/min (n=4). Infusion of mNGF at a dose of 1.2 μg/day for 2 weeks has no effect on the ChAT activity in the

MS/DB of normal animals (Fig. 3). There is no detectable loss of ChAT activity in the right MS/DB of untreated or vehicle-treated animals 2 wks after aspirative transection of the right F-F (21). However, a substantial increase in ChAT activity is found in animals that received a F-F aspirative transection and were infused with mNGF. A 200% increase in ChAT specific activity is observed in the right transected MS/DB, as compared to untreated normal animals. The ChAT activity in MS/DB of axotomized, mNGF-treated animals is statistically greater than that in normal animals treated with mNGF, sham-operated animals treated with mNGF, and transected animals infused with vehicle (p = .001).

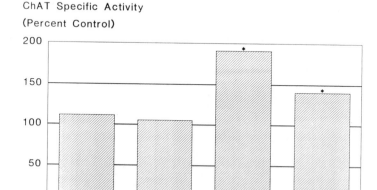

Fig. 3. Axotomy-Dependent Stimulation of ChAT Activity in Female Sprague-Dawley Rats. ChAT specific activity in the experimental groups is expressed as the percent of that measured in micro-dissections of the MS/DB and striatum in normal, untreated animals, i.e., 2.32, and 2.41 pmol ACh/μg protein/min, respectively, n=4 in each group. * p<.05.

NGF treatment also stimulates ChAT activity in dissections of the striatum of Sprague-Dawley rats. ChAT activity in normal untreated striatum is 2.4 pmol ACh/μg protein/min. In both normal and F-F transected animals, there is a 140% statistically significant stimulation of ChAT activity after mNGF infusion for 2 weeks compared to untreated animals (Fig. 3).

Stimulation of ChAT Activity is Dose Dependent

Animals received a right F-F aspiration and were infused for 2 weeks with serial dilutions of mNGF (Fig. 4). The $E.D._{50}$ of mNGF on the stimulation of ChAT activity in the MS/DB ipsilateral to the transection was obtained using an infusate mNGF concentration of 10 μg/ml, a dose to the rat brain equivalent to 120 ng/day.

Changes in ChAT Activity in the Aged Brain

The specific activity of ChAT varied amongst the various brain regions micro-dissected for analysis. In 4 month old untreated Control animals, the average specific activities in distilled water sonicates of micro-dissected brain regions are as follows (n=6): striatum - 3.2; MS/DB - 2.1; hippocampus - 1.6; frontal cortex - 1.2; temporal cortex - 1.1; parietal cortex - 0 . 7; and NBM - 0 . 7 . The effects of age on the ChAT activity of these brain regions is illustrated in Figures 5 and 6. The

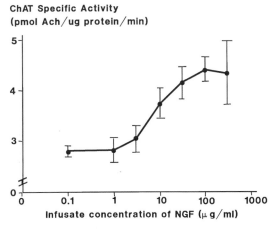

Fig. 4. mNGF Stimulation of ChAT Activity is Dose-Dependent. The dose response is illustrated for the mNGF effect after F-F transection. A pump concentration of 10 μg/ml delivers 120 ng of mNGF per day to the rat brain, n=4 for each concentration.

most consistent age-related losses of ChAT activity are in the MS/DB, hippocampus, and striatum (Fig. 5). All three areas have significant, 20 - 30% losses in enzyme activity compared to 4 month old untreated animals. A significant 15% loss of enzyme activity is also observed in the frontal and temporal cortices of this sample of 2 year old animals. No change is observed in the parietal cortex or in the NBM.

mNGF Stimulates Chat Activity in Aged Fisher 344 Rats

Infusion of mNGF into young adult Fisher 344 male rats has a significant effect on the ChAT activity in the MS/DB; enzyme activity is stimulated 120% above control values. However, the effect on the MS/DB in 2 year old animals is even larger. Treatment of 2 year old rats with mNGF stimulates ChAT activity 170% compared to control, levels that are significantly larger than those in the 4 month NGF-treated animals (p<.002). NGF treatment also stimulates ChAT activity in the hippocampus, frontal cortex, and temporal cortex of 2 year old animals compared to untreated and vehicle-treated 2 year old rats. Although there is an above average stimulation of ChAT activity by mNGF in the NBM of both 4 month and 2 year old rats, the differences from control values are not significant due to the large variability of these samples. As in the young adult Sprague-Dawley female rats, mNGF treatment stimulates ChAT activity in the striatum of 4 month old Fisher male rats as well as the 2 year old rats.

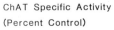

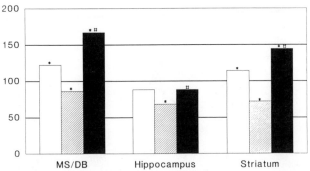

Fig. 5. Age-Related Stimulation of ChAT Activity by mNGF. Enzyme activity is expressed as the percent of activity in 4 month old untreated animals (pmol ACh/μg protein/min): MS/DB = 2.4; Hippocampus = 1.6; Striatum = 3.2. Open bars - 4 Month Old + mNGF; Hatched bars - 2 Year Old + Vehicle; Black bars - 2 Year Old + mNGF, n=6 in each group. *p<.05 compared to 4 Month Old Untreated animals. #p<.05 compared to 2 Year Old + Vehicle.

DISCUSSION

Axotomy-dependent Stimulation of ChAT in the MS/DB of Sprague-Dawley Rats

Developmental studies of the rat basal forebrain and striatum identified the sensitivity of the cholinergic neurons within these brain regions to the administration of exogenous mNGF (14-18). ChAT enzyme activity is stimulated up to 10-fold in normal embryonic and neonatal MS/DB upon treatment with exogenous mNGF. However, in older animals, the cholinergic neurons of the MS/DB appear to became less sensitive to exogenous mNGF, and in the adult rat, mNGF has considerably less effect on the ChAT activity in the normal MS/DB (18). In our experiments using normal female Sprague-Dawley rats, continuous infusion of mNGF at

1.2 µg/day has no effect on the ChAT activity in the MS/DB. However, identical treatment of Fisher 344 male rats results in a small but significant 120% stimulation of ChAT activity. This different sensitivity to exogenous mNGF in normal young adults may be related to the sex (26,27) or the species of the animal (28).

Transection of the F-F in adult female Sprague-Dawley rats triggers a sensitivity of the cholinergic neurons in the MS/DB to administration of exogenous mNGF. Continuous infusion of mNGF for 2 weeks after complete unilateral F-F aspiration stimulates ChAT specific activity in the MS/DB ipsilateral to the transection to a level that is 200% higher than that

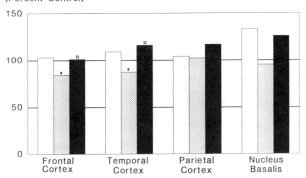

Fig. 6. Effects of mNGF on the Nucleus Basalis Projection System. Enzyme activity is expressed as the percent of activity in 4 month old untreated animals. Open bars - 4 Month Old + mNGF; Hatched bars - 2 Year Old + Vehicle; Black bars - 2 Year Old + mNGF, n=6 in each group. *p<.05 compared to 4 Month Old Untreated animals. #p<.05 compared to 2 Year Old + Vehicle.

measured in normal adult animals. The stimulation of enzyme activity is axotomy-dependent as administration of mNGF has no effect in sham operated animals with an intact F-F. The stimulation is also dose dependent. The E.D.50 was obtained at a pump concentration of 10 µg/ml, or 120 ng/day.

The mechanism(s) is unknown regulating this axotomy-induced sensitization to exogenous NGF. At 2 weeks after a F-F transection, there is a 26% decrease in receptor density on the side of aspiration (13). This agrees with the reported loss of NGF receptor using traditional immunohistochemical methodology (29). After mNGF administration, the loss of receptor density is not only prevented (12), but there is a supranormal, 130% increase of ^{125}I-192-IgG binding. These data indicate that the response of the transected neurons to exogenous mNGF is mediated by a feed-forward stimulation of cell surface NGF receptor expression. Increased NGF receptor expression could provide a mechanism for the increase in ChAT activity in the transected MS/DB after mNGF treatment.

Changes in ChAT Activity and NGF Sensitivity in Aged Fisher 344 Rats

Septo-Hippocampal System. There is a significant 40% loss of NGF mRNA and protein in the hippocampus of two year old Fisher male rats (28). This correlates with the 20-30% loss of ChAT activity in micro-dissections of the cholinergic cell bodies of the MS/DB and in their terminals within the hippocampus as observed in the present study, and the morphological atrophy of the MS/DB cholinergic neurons reported by others in aged Fisher rats (30). This age-related cholinergic dystrophy (see also 31-33) in the MS/DB may underlie the age-related sensitization of these neurons to exogenous mNGF. Treatment of two year old animals with mNGF for two weeks results in a 160% stimulation of MS/DB ChAT activity compared to 4 month untreated rats. Although mNGF treatment of 4 month Fisher males does result in a 120% stimulation of ChAT activity, the 2 year old rat apparently is even more sensitive; the effect of exogenous mNGF treatment in 2 year old rats is significantly greater than in 4 month old animals.

The stimulation of ChAT activity in the cell bodies of 2 year old rats is also reflected in the elevated enzyme activity detected in the hippocampus of the mNGF-treated aged rats. In this series of experiments, no stimulation of ChAT enzyme activity was detected in the hippocampus of 4 month old animals.

NEM - Cortex System. In the Fisher rat, the NBM system responds to age very differently than the MS/DB system. There is no detectable loss of NGF protein in the frontal cortex of aged Fisher rats (28), and there is no detectable loss of ChAT activity in the aged NBM. These neurons are reported to atrophy in both Fisher (30) and Sprague-Dawley (33) rats, and in the samples of frontal and temporal cortices analyzed in these experiments, there is a significant decrease in ChAT activity, indicating the possibility of NBM terminal degeneration in these areas.

The cholinergic neurons of the NBM show a range of responses to exogenous mNGF. In both 4 month and 2 year old Fisher male rats, some micro-dissections possessed higher ChAT levels than most of the samples from NGF-treated animals. Thus, there is a trend for stimulated ChAT activity in the NBM in both young and old animals, but the stimulation is not statistically significant in either case. Morphologic data indicate that NGF treatment reverses age-related neuronal atrophy in the NBM (33). Interestingly, in the samples of the two year old rats examined in these experiments, the ChAT activity in the terminal regions of the NBM, i.e., the frontal and temporal cortices, are stimulated by the mNGF treatment.

The NBM and the MS/DB have been hypothesized to represent similar populations of neurons (34). However, in the rat, the two groups of neurons can be distinguished by their expression of the neuropeptide, galanin. Galanin co-localizes with cholinergic neurons in rat MS/DB, but not rat NBM (35,36). Differential expression of galanin or other peptides may be related to the apparent differences in the aging response of the neurons in these nuclei.

Striatum. The sensitivity to exogenous mNGF of the cholinergic interneurons within the striatum persists throughout life. In neonatal (12), young adult Sprague-Dawley female, young adult Fisher 344 male, and 2 year old Fisher 344 male rats, administration of mNGF to the CNS results in a significant 115% - 140% stimulation of ChAT activity in the striatum compared to untreated controls.

Mature striatal interneurons are hypothesized to exist with less-than-maximal support from endogenous NGF (37). Such optimal or less-than-optimal conditions may maintain the sensitivity of these neurons to exogenous mNGF. The striatal cholinergic neurons atrophy with age (33), and exhibit a substantial age-related loss of ChAT enzyme activity in both Sprague-Dawley (32) and Fisher rats. This age-related dystrophy may underlie the apparent increased sensitivity of aged striatum to exogenous mNGF; treatment of 2 year old rats results in a 140% stimulation in ChAT activity, a level that is significantly larger than that in 4 month old mNGF-treated Fisher rats.

SUMMARY

Our results indicate that in the rat, there is a differential regulation of the cholinergic phenotypes expressed by the interneurons of the striatum, the projection neurons of the MS/DB to the hippocampus, and the projection neurons of the NBM to the cerebral cortex. these three cholinergic neuronal groups respond differently to the aging process, and express different sensitivities to exogenous mNGF. There is no detectable loss of ChAT enzyme activity with age in the NBM projection system, whereas both the striatal interneurons and the projection neurons in the MS/DB exhibit substantial losses of enzyme activity with age. The age-related dystrophy of these latter cholinergic systems may be mediated by the decreased levels of endogenous NGF (28), and underlie the behavioral impairments observed in aged animals (32,33).

Neurons of the young adult MS/DB are little affected by exogenous NGF. However, both axotomy and age appear to activate NGF-mediated mechanisms regulating cholinergic metabolism. NGF treatment of these sensitized neurons triggers a feed forward expression of NGF receptor and results in a supranormal stimulation of ChAT activity. Of interest is the similarity of age-dependent sensitization to that of the trauma of axotomy. It is also possible that the response of a given neuron to age is not only mediated by endogenous levels of trophic factor (6), but also by the influence of co-existing peptides such as galanin (38).

ACKNOWLEDGEMENTS

We extend our large gratitude to Dr. Stephen Buxser and Mr. Douglas Decker, Cell Biology Unit, The Upjohn Company, Kalamazoo, MI, for providing the well characterized nerve growth factor used in this study, and for monitoring NGF biologic activity during the course of the experiments.

REFERENCES

1. Levi-Montalcini, R., and Angeletti, P.U. (1968) Nerve growth factor. Physiol. Rev. 48:534-569.
2. Thoenen, H., Bandtlaw, C., and Heumann, R. (1987) m e physiological function of nerve growth factor in the central nervous system: Comparison with the periphery. Rev. Physiol Biochem. Pharmacol. 109:146-178.
3. Whittemore, S.R., and Seiger, A. (1987) The expression, localization and functional significance of ß-nerve growth factor in the central nervous system. Brain Research Rev. 12:439-464.
4. Schwab, M.E., Otten, U., Agid, Y., and Thoenen, H. (1979) Nerve growth factor (NGF) in rat CNS: Absence of specific retrograde axonal transport and tyrosine hydroxylase induction in locus coeruleus and substantia nigra. Brain Research 168:473-483.
5. Stewart, S.S., and Appel, S.H. (1988) Trophic factors in neurologic disease. Ann. Rev. Med. 39:193-201. 12

6. Varon, S., Manthorpe, M., and Williams, L.R. (1984) Neuronotrophic and neurite promoting factors and their clinical potentials. _Dev. Neurosci._ 62:73-100.

7. Hefti, F., and Weiner, W.J. (1986) Nerve growth factor and Alzheimer's disease. _Ann. Neurol_. 20:275-281.

8. Hefti, F. (1986) Nerve growth factor promotes survival of septal cholinergic neurons after fimbrial transections. _J. Neurosci_. 6:2155-2162.

9. Williams, L.R., Varon, S., Peterson, G.M., Wictorin, K., Fischer, W., Ejorklund, A. and Gage, F.H. (1986) Continuous infusion of Nerve Growth Factor prevents basal forebrain neuronal death after fimbria-fornix transection. _Proc. Nat. Acad. Sci_. (USA) 83:9231- 9235.

10. Kromer, L.F. (1987) Nerve growth factor treatment after brain injury prevents neuronal death. _Science_ 235:214-235.

11. Hefti, F., Dravid, A., and Hartikka, J. (1984) Chronic intraventricular injections of nerve growth factor elevate hippocampus choline acetyltransferase activity in adult rats with partial septo-hippocampal lesions. _Brain_ 293:305-311.

12. Montero, C.N., and Hefti, F. (1988) Rescue of lesioned septal cholinergic neurons by nerve growth factor: specificity and requirement for chronic treatment. _J. Neurosci_. 8:2986-2999.

13. Yip, H., and Williams, L.R. (1988) Plasticity of NGF receptors in the rat basal forebrain following axotomy and exogenous N. _Soc. Neurosci_ . Abstr. 14: 256 .

14. Mobley W.C., Rutkowski, J.L., Tennekoonn, G.I., Buchhanan, K., and Jonston, M.V. (1985) Choline acetyltransferase in striatum of neonatal rats increased by nerve growth factor. _Science_ 229:284-287.

15. Hefti, F., Hartikka, J., Eckenstein, F., Gnahn, H., Heuman, R., and Schwab, M. (1985) Nerve growth factor increases choline acetyltransferase but not survival or fiber outgrowth of cultured fetal septal cholinergic neurons. _Neuroscience_ 14:55-68.

16. Gnahn, H., Hefti, F., Heumann, R., Sc3hwab, M.E., and Thoenen, H. (1983) NGF-mediated increase of choline acetyltransferase (ChAT) in the neonatal rat forebrain: evidence for a physiological role of NGF in the brain? _Dev. Brain Research_ 9:45-52.

17. Mobley W.C., Rutkowski, J.L., Tennekoon, G.I., Gemski, J., Buchanan, K., and Johnston, M.V. (1986) Nerve growth factor increases choline aoetyltransferase activity in developing basal forebrain neurons. _Mol. Brain Research_ 1:53-62.

18. Johnston, M.V., Rutkawski, J.L., Wainer, B.H., Long, J.B., and Mobley, W.C. (1987) NGF effects on developing forebrain cholinergic neurons are regionally specific. _Neurochem. Res_. 12:985-994.

19. Buxser, S.E., Watson, L., and Johnson, G.L. (1983) A comparison of binding properties and structure of NGF receptor on PC12 pheochromocytoma and A875 melanoma cells. _J. Cellular Biochem_. 22:219-233.

20. Williams, L.R., Vahlsing, H.L., LindamoDd, T., Gage, F.H., Varon, S. and Manthorpe, M. (1987) A small gauge cannala device for continuous infusion of exogenous agents into the brain. _Exp. Neurol_. 95:743- 754.

21. Williams, L.R., Jodelis, K.S. and Donald, M.R. (1989) Axotomy-dependent stimulation of choline acetyltransferasle by exogenous mouse nerve growth factor in rat basal forebrain. _Brain Res_. in press.

22. Chandler, C.E., Parsons, L.M., Hosang, M., and Shooter, E.M. (1984) A monoclonal antibody modulates the interaction of nerve growth factor with PC12 cells. _J. Biol. Chem_. 259:6882-6889.

23. Yip, H.K. (1989) The localization of NGF receptors in the central nervous system of the rat-an _in vitro_ autoradiographic study with a monoclonal antibody against the NGF receptor. _J. Neurosci_. in press.

24. Cuello, A.C., and Carson, S. (1983) Microdissections of fresh rat brain tissue slices. In Methods in the Neurosciences, Vol. 2: Brain Dissection Techniques. (ed: Cuello, A.C.) John Wiley amd Sons, Chinchester, pp. 37-125.

25. Fryer, H.J.L., Davis, G.E., Manthorpe, M., and Varon, S. (1986) Lowry protein assay using an automatic microtiter plate spectrophotometer. Anal. Biochem. 153:262-266.

26. Loy, R., and Milner, T.A. (1983) Neonatal steroid treatment alters axonal sprouting in adult hippocampus: Sexually dimorphic development of target neruons. In: Nervous System Regeneration, (eds: Haber, B., Perez-Polo, R., Hashim, G.A., and Stella, A.M.G.), A.R. Liss, NY pp. 417-423.

27. Harrell, L.E., and Parsons, D.S. (1988) Role of gender in the behavioral effects of peripheral sympathetic in growth. Exp. Neurol. 99: 315-325 .

28. Larkfors, L., Ebendal, T., Whittemore, S.R., Perrsson, H., Hoffer, B., and Olson, L. (1988) Developmental appearance of nerve growth factor in the rat brain: significant deficits in the aged forebrain. Prog. Brain Res. 78:27-31.

29. Springer, J.E., Koh, S., Tayrien, M.W., and Loy, R. (1987) Basal forebrain magnocellular neurons stain for nerve grawth factor receptor: Correlation with cholinergic cell bodies and effects of axotomy. J. Neurosci. Research 17: 111-118.

30. Armstrong, D.M., Buzsaki, G., Chen, K., Ruiz, R., Sheffield, R., and Gage, F.H. (1987) Cholinergic neurotransmission in the aged rat: A behavioral, electrophysiological, and anatcmical study. Soc. Neurosci. Abstr. 13: 434 .

31. Decker, M.W. (1987) The effects of aginq on hippocampal and cortical projections of the forebrain cholinergic system. Brain Res. Rev. 12: 423-438 .

32. Strong, R., Hicks, P., Hsu, L., Bartus, R.T. and Enna, S.J. (1980) Age-related alterations in the rodent brain cholinergic system and beavior. Neurobiol. Aging 1:59-63.

33. Fischer, W., Wictorin, K., Bjorklund, A., Williams, L.R., Varon, S., and Gage, F.H. (1987) Intracerebral infusion of Nerve Growth Factor ameliorates cholinergic neuron atrophy and spatial memory impairments in aged rats. Nature 329: 65-68.

34. Schwaber, J.S., Rogers, W.T., Satoh, K., and Fibiger, H.C. (1987) Distribution and organization of cholinertic neurons in the rat forebrain demonstrated by computer-aided data acquisition and three-dimensional reconstruction. J. Comp. Neurol. 263:309-325.

35. Melander, T., Staines, W.A., Hokfelt, T., Rokaeus, A., Eckenstein, F., Salvaterra, P.M., and Wainer, B.H. (1985) Galanin-like immunoreactivity in cholinergic neurons of the septum-basal forebrain complex projecting to the hippocampus of the rat. Brain Res. 360:130-138.

36. Wenk, G.L., and Rokaeus, A. (1988) Basal forebrain lesions differentially alter galanin levels and acetylcholinergic receptors in the hippocampus and neocortex. Brain Res. 460:17-21.

37. Hagg, T., Hagg, F. Vahlsing, H.L., Manthorpe, M. and Varon, S. (1989) Nerve growoth factor effects on cholinergic neurons of neostriatum and nucleus accumbels in the adult rat. Neurosci. in press.

38. Chan-Palay, V. (1988) Galanin hyperinnervates surviving neurons ofthe human basal nucleus of Meynert in dementias of Alzheimer's and Parkinson's disease: A hypothesis for the role of galanin inaocentuating cholinergic dysfunction in dementia. J. Comp. Neurol.273: 453-557 .

NEURONOTROPHIC FACTORS, GANGLIOSIDES AND THEIR INTERACTION: IMPLICATIONS

IN THE REGULATION OF NERVOUS SYSTEM PLASTICITY

Stephen D. Skaper, Alberta Leon and Gino Toffano

Fidia Research Laboratories
Via Ponte della Fabbrica 3/A
35031 - Abano Terme, Italy

INTRODUCTION

The phenomenon of neuroplasticity can be discussed, in very broad terms, as the ability of a nerve cell to modify its behaviors under the influence of extrinsic factors. Like any living system, the nervous system represents a dynamic organization, whose various elements are in a continual state of change due to interactions not only with one another, but also with their extraneural environment. Neurons are exposed to such influences from cells with which they are in direct contact, and from humoral sources; this vast array of external influences constitutes the microenvironment of these cells. Agents affecting neuronal behaviors represent a diverse and crucial element in determining how nerve cells will respond to cues from this microenvironment. Our ability to alter the response(s) of neuronal cells to these extrinsic signals can constitute a powerful tool for modulating the neuroplastic behaviors of the former – an important consideration for promoting regeneration and/or repair processes in the brain. Such is the topic of the present article.

NEURONOTROPHIC FACTORS: NERVE GROWTH FACTOR

Peripheral Nerve System

One very important class of extrinsic agents directed to neurons are neuronotrophic factors. The current state of knowledge of trophic factors has come, in large part, from the discovery of Nerve Growth Factor (NGF) (1,2). This protein is required for the development and maintenance of function of sympathetic neurons and the majority of neural crest-derived sensory neurons, in terms of both survival (3,4) and neurite elongation and neurotransmitter enzyme induction (5,6). Selective responsiveness to NGF is linked to expression of specific cell surface receptors. NGF binds to its receptor, which is internalized as a receptor/NGF complex and transported in a retrograde fashion to the cell body where physiologic actions are mediated (7,8). NGF mRNA is present in peripheral tissues of various mammalian species, where a good correlation exists between the amounts of NGF mRNA and the density of sympathetic innervation (9,10).

In addition to its well-established role in the development of peripheral sympathetic and sensory neurons, a number of recent studies support a role for NGF also in the development of basal forebrain cholinergic neurons. NGF is selectively taken up by cholinergic nerve terminals in the neocortex and hippocampus, and retrogradely transported to these forebrain magnocellular cholinergic neurons (11). Exogenous NGF increases choline acetyltransferase (ChAT) activity (12) and survival and neurite outgrowth (13) of cultured fetal septal neurons, and also ChAT activity in the basal forebrain of neonatal rats in vivo (14,15). NGF and its mRNA in the developing rat brain parallel the growth of cholinergic neurons (16,17). Intraventricular administration of NGF leads to up-regulation of NGF receptor mRNA expression and receptor immunoreactivity (18), while antibodies to NGF given by the same route reduce ChAT activity (19).

The role of NGF goes beyond that of development, affecting the function of these neurons in the adult brain. Hippocampal and cortical target areas of basal forebrain cholinergic neurons express high levels of NGF and NGF mRNA (16,17,20). NGF receptors have been visualized in adult rat (21), primate (22) and human (23) brain. The mRNA encoding the NGF receptor has been detected in rat (24) and human (25) basal forebrain. Exogenously administered NGF is able to affect developed forebrain cholinergic neurons trophically after axonal injury. Fimbrial lesions, which interrupt the septohippocampal cholinegric pathway, lead to a retrograde degeneration of cholinergic neurons in the septum. Intraventricular application of NGF has been found to prevent this lesion-induced degeneration (26-28). Important also is the observation that NGF infusion is able to elevate ChAT activity in hippocampus and septum of non-lesioned adult rats (29).

In addition to the basal forebrain cholinergic neurons, other CNS populations may be affected by NGF. For example, transection of the optic nerve in the adult rat leads to degeneration of retinal ganglion cells. Application of NGF to the site of injury is reported to prevent this ganglion cell loss (30), or to reduce ganglion cell damage following ischemia (31).

OTHER NEURONOTROPHIC MOLECULES

A number of other macromolecules endowed with neuronotrophic activity have been identified and characterized since the discovery of NGF. These include the Ciliary Neuronotrophic Factors (CNTF) (32-34), Brain-Derived Neurotrophic Factor (35), fibroblast growth factors (36-40), and epidermal growth factor (41).

PHARMACOLOGICAL APPROACHES TO THE TREATMENT OF NEURAL INSULTS AND NEURODEGENERATIVE DISEASES

The capacity of a CNS neuron to undergo adaptive changes in response to microenvironmental cues - neuroplasticity - represents a finely tuned balance between promoting and inhibiting infuences. Disruption of this mechanism by axotomy or cutting off the blood supply are probably the two major causes of neuronal death in the CNS. Any considerations of intervention must take into account the order of biological events that follow a brain insult. Lesion or trauma will lead to an acute loss of neurons, accompanied by a delayed, secondary phase of neuronal death. The primary neuronal loss is likely an intractable occurrence, with nothing short of actual cell replacement having any chance of effecting amelioration (42,43). On the other hand, delayed (secondary) loss of neurons may be amenable to pharmacological treatment with subsequent neuronal survival providing for functional recovery.

Exogenous Trophic Factor Administration

Neuronotrophic factors similar, if not identical to those in development, may continue to function in the maintenance and repair capacities of adult neurons. Certain degenerative processes of the nervous system and/or the events that are associated with brain aging may actually result from defective or insufficient supplies of trophic factors. This concept has given rise to what has been termed the "trophic deficit hypothesis" (44,45). For example, the finding that exogenous NGF is able to reduce the loss of adult lesioned cholinergic neurons in the septum/diagonal band and nucleus basalis of the brain (26-28) has led to the speculation that availability of a trophic factor for these neurons (perhaps NGF) may control their survival and biological competence (44,45). In these terms, a trophic deficit may result in cholinergic cell deterioration as well as accompanying memory deficits - a situation known to occur in Alzheimer's disease (46).

The potential for application of trophic substances to therapy in the CNS is demonstrable in at least one case discussed above, in which cholinergic neurons in the medial septum can be protected from retrograde degeneration by chronic infusion of NGF (26-28). Another version of this therapeutic approach comes from experiments by Rosenberg et al. (47), who reported that cultured fibroblasts, genetically modified to produce and secrete NGF and then grafted to the cavity formed in creating a fimbria-fornix lesion, will prevent retrograde cholinergic degeneration and induce axonal sprouting.

One limitation to this strategy of exogenous trophic intervention derives from the apparent necessity of applying the desired material in close proximity to the lesion site. A way to circumvent this problem could lie in pharmacological treatment designed to enhance the action of endogenously occurring neuronotrophic activities. The following sections will discuss this idea in more detail.

Ganglioside Treatment and CNS Repair Processes

Agents involved in modulating neuronal behaviors, especially in reponse to neuronotrophic influences, have been seldom studied, with the possible exception of gangliosides. These molecules comprise a family of naturally occurring sialic acid-containing glycosphingolipids (48). Gangliosides are localized in the plasma membrane of vertebrate cells, with the highest concentrations in mammals being in the grey matter of the nervous system, in particular, in the region of synaptic terminals (49). Striking modifications of the ganglioside profile occur during development of the mammalian brain (50); changes also take place in aging (51) and in several neuropathological situation (52). The view that gangliosides, and in particular the monosialoganglioside GM1, play a distinctive role in the process of axonal growth is consistent with observations that anti-GM1 antibodies inhibit neurite regeneration in vitro (53), and axonal elongation in vivo (54), as well as produce long-lasting alterations in the maturation of CNS circuitry and behavioral processes when administered to developing animals (55).

Experiments with diverse neuronal cell types *in vitro* have provided clear evidence that exogenous gangliosides (mainly GMl) are able to enhance de novo neurite outgrowth or neurite regeneration in the presence of the appropriate trophic factor (56-59). The ability of GMl to potentiate neuronotrophic action is a broad one, in that GMl is also effective with NGF-unlike trophic activities (59,60). Exogenous GMl is observed to stimulate the biochemical development and survival of dopaminergic and GABAergic populations in cultured fetal mouse mesencephalic cells (61). In neuronal cells with neuronotrophic factor-linked survival or neurite outgrowth, ganglioside will improve the trophic action - but not substitute for it. These trophic-dependent ganglioside actions require the "correct" balance between stimulating and retarding influences (59,62). This principle is a key one, in that neuronal dysfunction and/or death resulting from pathological events or aging may also reflect an imbalance of environmental signals.

In addition to enhancing neuronal cell responsiveness to exogenous neuronotrophic factors *in vitro*, the potentiating action of GMl administration on postlesion recovery in the CNS is well-documented. GMl-induced improvement of biochemical, morphological and behavioral parameters after various types of brain lesion have been observed (63-65). Quite a large number of reports have described GMl ganglioside-stimulated recovery of lesioned nigral dopaminergic, serotonergic, and cholinergic neurons. GMl treatment has also been shown to facilitate behavioral recovery following brain damage (66,67).

The ability of GMl to act *in vivo* appears to be a function of the extent of the lesion applied (68,69), suggesting the need for a certain level ("set point") of trophic support. This idea is not inconsistent from the *in vitro* studies already discussed, where the facilitating action of GMl was found to depend on a particular balance between promoting and inhibiting factors acting together with NGF or other trophic influences. It is important to keep in mind the functional role that neuronotrophic factors may serve in the adult CNS. The above model thus implies that the effects of GMl *in vivo* are related to an enhancement of trophic activity which has increased as a result of lesion. In fact, neuronotrophic activities, including NGF, increase at the lesion site following brain damage (70, 71). Such trophic activities may be critical for the execution of repair processes, yet inadequate in titer or activity; however, together with ganglioside this set-point may be surpassed.

Some very recent findings provide *in vivo* support for the hypothesis of monosialoganglioside potentiation of neuronotrophic factor effects. In one study which used a peripheral nervous system model (72), GMl was shown to facilitate NGF effects following vinblastine-induced sympathectomy in newborn rats, as measured by NGF's ability to maintain noradrenergic innervation in the heart and spleen; GMl alone was inactive against vinblastine. In another case, both GMl and NGF prevented the biochemical and morphological changes accompanying lesions to rat basal forebrain cholinergic neurons: NGF and GMl acted synergistically to stimulate choline acetyltransferase activity in cultured septal neurons (73).

ALZHEIMER'S DISEASE AND BRAIN AGING: THERAPEUTIC PERSPECTIVES

Alzheimer's disease is a disease of unknown cause that is characterized by a progressive loss of memory and other cognitive functions, leading to eventual permanent disability, and death. Neuropathologically, senile plaques and neurofibrillary tangles evidence the main features of Alzheimer's disease (74).

tangles evidence the main features of Alzheimer's disease (74).

One of the most consistent findings in Alzheimer's brain is the degeneration of neurons forming the ascending cholinergic pathways of the basal forebrain (75). A good correlation between the observed reduction in ChAT activity and the severity of clinical dementia has been reported (76). This loss of cholinergic neurons has often been regarded as a major factor responsible for the memory loss in Alzheimer's disease.

Brain aging has also been hypothesized as reflecting a trophic deficit (44). Several similarities are evident between Alzheimer's disease and the apparent reduction in the regenerative capacity of neural systems with age. Most affected appear to be the cholinergic neurons of the nucleus basalis of Meynert and of the septum, the same areas as in Alzheimer's. Decreased levels of NGF and its mRNA have been described to occur in the hippocampus of the aged rat brain (77), with intraventricular infusion of NGF having been reported to improve the cognitive behavior of such age-impaired rats (78).

It has been suggested that the degeneration of cholinergic nerve cells is responsible, at least in part, for the symptoms of Alzheimer's disease. The recently described ability of NGF to prevent the degeneration of cholinergic neurons in adult rats with experimental lesions mimicking the cholinergic deficit in Alzheimer's disease (26-28) and to ameliorate cholinergic neuron atrophy in aged rats (78), may provide useful paradigms for examining the question of whether increasing the availability of NGF to cholinergic cells could promote their survival in clinical disease states (46). It is interesting that NGF seems to affect cholinergic neurons not only after axonal interruption (26-28), but also in other types of lesions. Intraventricular NGF administration attenuates the reduction of ChAT activity in the cortex induced by ibotenic acid-induced lesions in the nucleus basalis (79).

The prospects for an effective treatment of cholinergic dysfunction leave much work to be done. Clinical application of NGF presents certain logistical problems, in that NGF is a protein which must be administered directly into the brain, and that is available in only very limited amounts. This latter restriction may be overcome by the use of genetic engineering techinques to produce larger quantities of human NGF. The limitation of NGF administration could be approached by the use of drugs capable of potentiating the effects of endogenous NGF. As discussed in this article, monosialogangliosides would appear to be attractive pharmacological candidates for addressing this problem. Not only do gangliosides augment the effects in vivo of NGF on central cholinergic neurons (73), but they also are described to protect against brain damage induced by the excitotoxin ibotenic acid (80) - as does NGF (79). Given the lack of a viable therapy for Alzheimer's disease, further research related to gangliosides seems warranted.

REFERENCES

1. Levi-Montalcini, R. (1966) Nerve growth factor: its mode of action on sensory and sympathetic neurons. Harvey Lect. 60: 217-219.
2. Levi-Montalcini, R. (1987) The Nerve Growth Factor thirty five years later. Science 237: 1154-1162.
3. Gorin, P.D. and Johnson, E.M. (1979) Experimental autoimmune model of nerve growth factor deprivation: effects on developing peripheral sympathetic and sensory neurons. Proc. Natl. Acad. Sci. USA 76: 5383-5386.

4. Levi-Montalcini, R. and Angeletti, P.U. (1966) Immunosympathectomy. Pharmacol. Rev. 18: 619-628.
5. Levi-Montalcini, R. and Hamburger, V. (1951) Selective growth stimulating effects of mouse sarcoma on the sensory and sympathetic nervous system of the chick embryo. J. Exp. Zool. 116: 321-362.
6. Thoenen, H., Angeletti, P.U., Levi-Montalcini, R. and Kettler, R. (1971) Selective induction by nerve growth factor of tyrosine hydroxylase and dopamine-beta-hydroxylase in the rat superior ganglion. Proc. Natl. Acad. Sci. USA 68: 1598-1602.
7. Hendry, I.A., Stoeckel, K., Thoenen, H. and Iversen, L.L. (1974) The retrograde axonal transport of nerve growth factor. Brain Res. 68: 103-121.
8. Stoeckel, K., Schwab, M. and Thoenen, H. (1975) Specificity of retrograde transport of nerve growth factor (NGF) in sensory neurons: a biochemical and morphological study. Brain Res. 89: 1-14.
9. Heumann, R., Korsching, S., Scott, J. and Thoenen, H. (1984) Relationship between levels of nerve growth factor (NGF) and its messenger RNA in sympathetic ganglia and peripheral target tissues. EMBO J. 3: 3183-3189.
10. Shelton, D.L. and Reichardt, L.F. (1984) Expression of the beta nerve growth factor gene correlates with the sympathetic innervation in effector organs. Proc. Natl. Acad. Sci. USA 81: 7951-7955.
11. Seiler, M. and Schwab, M.E. (1984) Specific retrograde transport of nerve growth factor from neocortex to nucleus basalis in rat. Brain Res. 400: 33-39.
12. Hefti, F., Hartikka, J., Eckenstein, F., Gnahn, H., Heumann, R. and Schwab, M. (1985) Nerve growth factor (NGF) increases choline acetyltransferase but not survival or fiber outgrowth of cultured fetal septal cholinergic neurons. Neuroscience 14: 55-68.
13. Hartikka, J. and Hefti, F. (1988) Development of septal cholinergic neurons in culture: plating density and glial cells modulate effects of NGF on survival, fiber growth, and expression of transmitter-specific enzymes. J. Neurosci. 8: 2967-2985.
14. Gnahn, H., Hefti, F., Heumann, R., Schwab, M. and Thoenen, H. (1983) NGF-mediated increase of choline acetyltranferase (ChAT) in the neonatal forebrain: evidence for a physiological role of NGF in the brain? Dev. Brain Res. 9: 45-52.
15. Mobley, W.C., Rutkowski, J.L., Tennekoon, G.I., Gemski, J., Buchanan, K. and Johnston, M.V. (1986) Nerve growth factor increases choline acetyltransferase activity in developing basal forebrain neurons. Molec. Brain Res. 1: 53-62.
16. Auburger, G., Heumann, R., Hellweg, R., Korsching, S. and Thoenen, H. (1987) Developmental changes of nerve growth factor and its mRNA in the rat hippocampus: comparison with choline acetyltransferase. Dev. Biol. 120: 322-328.
17. Whittemore, S.R., Ebendal, T., Lärkfors, L., Olson, L. and Seiger, A. (1986) Developmental and regional expression of beta nerve growth factor messenger RNA and protein in the rat central nervous system. Proc. Natl. Acad. Sci. USA 83: 817-821.
18. Caviccioli, L., Flanigan, T.P., Vantini G., Fusco, M., Polato, P., Toffano, G., Walsh, F.S. and Leon A. (1989) NGF amplifies expression of NGF receptor messenger RNA in forebrain cholinergic neurons of rats. Eur. J. Neurosci., in press.
19. Vantini, G., Schiavo, N., Di Martino, A., Polato, P., Triban, C., Callegaro, L., Toffano, G. and Leon, A. (1989) Evidence for a physiological role of nerve growth factor in CNS of neonatal rats. Neuron, in press.
20. Shelton, D.L. and Reichardt, L.F. (1986) Studies on the expression of the beta nerve growth factor (NGF) gene in the central nervous system: level and regional distribution of NGF mRNA suggest that NGF

functions as a trophic factor for several distinct populations of neurons. Proc. Natl. Acad. Sci. USA 83: 2714-2718.

21. Yan, Q. and Johnson, E.M. Jr. (1988) An immunohistochemical study of nerve growth factor (NGF) receptor in developing rats. J. Neurosci. 8: 3481-3498.

22. Schatterman, G.C., Gibbs, L., Lanahan, A.A., Claude, P. and Bothwell, M. (1988) Expression of NGF receptor in the developing and adult primate central nervous system. J. Neurosci. 8: 860-873.

23. Hefti, F., Hartikka, J., Salvatierra, A., Wiener, W.J. and Mash, D.C. (1986) Localization of nerve factor receptors in cholinergic neurons of the human basal forebrain. Neurosci. Lett. 69: 37-41.

24. Buck, C.R., Martinez, H.J., Chao, M.V. and Black, I.B. (1988) Differential expression of the nerve growth factor receptor gene in multiple brain areas. Dev. Brain Res. 44: 259-268.

25. Goedert, M., Fine, A., Dawbarn, D., Wilcock, G.K. and Chao, M.V. (1989) Nerve growth factor receptor mRNA distribution in human brain: normal levels in basal forebrain in Alzheimer's disease. Molec. Brain Res. 5: 1-7.

26. Hefti F. (1986) Nerve growth factor (NGF) promotes survival of septal cholinergic neurons after fimbrial transection. J. Neurosci. 6: 2155-2162.

27. Williams, L.R., Varon, S., Peterson, G.M., Wictorin, K., Fischer, W., Björklund, A. and Gage, F.H. (1986) Continuous infusion of nerve growth factor prevents basal forebrain neuronal death after fimbria fornix transection. Proc. Natl. Acad. Sci. USA 83: 9231-9235.

28. Kromer, L.F. (1987) Nerve growth factor treatment after brain injury prevents neuronal death. Science 235: 214-216.

29. Fusco, M., Oderfeld-Nowak, B., Vantini, G., Schiavo N., Gradkowska, M., Zaremba, M. and Leon, A. (1989) NGF effects uninjured, adult rat septohippocampal cholinergic neurons. Neuroscience, in press.

30. Carmignoto, G., Maffei, L., Candeo, P., Canella, R. and Comelli, C. (1989) Effects of NGF on the survival of rat retinal ganglion cells following optic nerve section. J. Neurosci., 9: 1263-1272.

31 Siliprandi, R., Canella, R., Zanoni, R. and Carmignoto, G. (1989) Retinal ganglion cell vulnerability after ischemia in the cat. Effects of NGF. Soc. Neurosci. Abstr. 15: in press.

32. Barbin, G., Manthorpe, M. and Varon, S. (1984) Purification of the chick eye ciliary neuronotrophic factor (CNTF). J. Neurochem. 43: 1468-1478.

33. Manthorpe, M., Skaper, S.D., Williams, L.R. and Varon, S. (1986) Purification of adult rat sciatic nerve ciliary neuronotrophic factor. Brain Res. 367: 282-286.

34. Watters, D.J. and Hendry, I.A. (1987) Purification of a ciliary neurotrophic factor from bovine heart. J. Neurochem. 49: 705-713.

35. Barde, Y.-A., Edgar, D. and Thoenen, H. (1982) Purification of a new neurotrophic factor from brain. EMBO J. 1: 549-553.

36. Hatten, M.E., Lynch, M., Rydel, R.R., Sanchez, J., Joseph-Silverstein, J., Moscatelli, D. and Rifkin, D.B. (1988) In vitro neurite extension by granule neurons is dependent upon astroglial-derived fibroblast growth factor. Dev. Biol. 125: 280-289.

37. Ferrari, G., Minozzi, C.-M., Toffano G., Leon, A. and Skaper, S.D. (1989) Basic fibroblast growth factor promotes the survival and development of mesencephalic neurons in culture. Dev. Biol. 133: 140-147.

38. Walicke, P.A. (1988) Basic and acidic fibroblast growth factors have trophic effects on neurons from multiple CNS regions. J. Neurosci. 8: 2618-2627.

39. Walicke, P., Cowan, W.M., Ueno, N., Baird, A. and Guillemin, R. (1986) Fibroblast growth factor promotes survival of dissociated

hippocampal neurons and enhances neurite extension. <u>Proc. Natl. Acad. Sci. USA</u> 83: 3012-3016.

40. Unsicker, K., Reichert-Preibsch, H., Schmidt, R., Pettmann, B., Labourdette, G. and Sensenbrenner, M. (1987) Astroglial and fibroblast growth factors have neurotrophic functions for cultured peripheral and central nervous system neurons. <u>Proc. Natl. Acad. Sci. USA</u> 84: 5459-5463.

41. Morrison, R.S., Kornblum, H.I., Leslie, F.M. and Bradshaw, R.A. (1987) Trophic stimulation of cultured neurons from neonatal rat brain by epidermal growth factor. <u>Science</u> 238: 72-75.

42. Freed, W.J., Morihisa, J.M., Spoor, E., Hoffer, B.J., Olson, L., Seiger, A. and Wyatt, R.J. (1981) Transplanted adrenal chromaffin cells in rat brain reduce lesion induced rotational behavior. <u>Nature</u> 292: 351-352.

43. Gage, F.H. and Björklund, A. (1986) Cholinergic septal grafts into the hippocampal formation improve spatial learning and memory in aged rats by an atropine-sensitive mechanism. <u>J. Neurosci.</u> 6: 2837-2847.

44. Appel, S.H. (1981) A unifying hypothesis for the cause of amyotrophic lateral sclerosis, parkinsonism, and Alzheimer's disease. <u>Ann. Neurol.</u> 10: 599-605.

45. Varon, S., Manthorpe, M., Davis, G.E., Williams, L.R., and Skaper, S.D. (1988) Growth factors. In: <u>Functional Recovery in Neurological Disease</u> (ed: Waxman, S.G.), vol. 47, Raven Press, New York, NY, pp. 493-521.

46. Hefti, F., and Weiner, W.J. (1986) Nerve growth factor and Alzheimer's disease. <u>Ann. Neurol.</u> 20: 275-281.

47. Rosenberg, M.B., Friedmann, T., Robertson, R.C., Tuszynski, M., Wolff, J.A., Breakefield, X.O. and Gage, F.H. (1988) Grafting genetically modified cells to the damaged brain: restorative effects of NGF expression. <u>Science</u> 242: 1575-1578.

48. Svennerholm, L. (1984) Biological significance of gangliosides. In: <u>Cellular and Pathological Aspects of Glycoconjugate Metabolism</u> (eds: Dreyfus, H., Massarelli, R., Freysz, L. and Rebel, G.), vol. 126, INSERM, Paris, pp. 21-44.

49. Ledeen, R.W. (1983) Gangliosides. In: <u>Handbook of Neurochemistry</u> (ed: Lajtha, A.), vol. 3, Plenum Press, New York, NY, pp. 41-90.

50. Willinger, M. and Schachner, M. (1980) GM1 ganglioside as a marker for neuronal differentiation in mouse cerebellum. <u>Dev. Biol.</u> 74: 101-117.

51. Ando, S., Tanaka, Y. and Kon, K. (1986) Membrane aging of the brain synaptosomes with special reference to gangliosides. In: <u>Gangliosides and Neuronal Plasticity</u> (eds: Tettamanti, G., Ledeen, R.W., Sandhoff, K., Nagai, Y. and Toffano, G.), Fidia Research Series, vol. 6, Liviana Press, Padova, pp. 105-112.

52. Purpura, D.P. and Suzuki, K. (1976) Distortion of neuronal geometry and formation of aberrant synapses in neuronal storage diseases. <u>Brain Res.</u> 116: 1-21.

53. Spirman, N., Sela, B.A. and Schwartz, M. (1982) Anti-ganglioside antibodies inhibit neuritic outgrowth from regenerating goldfish retinal explants. <u>J. Neurochem.</u> 39: 847-877.

54. Sparrow, J.R., McGuinness, C., Schwartz, M. and Grafstein, B. (1984) Antibodies to ganglioside inhibit goldfish optic nerve regeneration in vivo. <u>J. Neurosci. Res.</u> 12: 233-243.

55. Kasarskis, E.J., Karpiak, S.E., Rapport, M.M., Yu, R.K. and Bass, N.H. (1981) Abnormal maturation of cerebral cortex and behavioral deficit in adult rats after neonatal administration of antibodies to ganglioside. <u>Dev. Brain Res.</u> 1: 25-35.

56. Ferrari, G., Fabris, M. and Gorio, A. (1983) Gangliosides enhance neurite outgrowth in PC12 cells. <u>Dev. Brain Res.</u> 8: 215-221.

57. Leon, A., Benvegnù, D., Dal Toso, R., Presti, D., Facci, L.,

Giorgi, O. and Toffano, G. (1984) Dorsal root ganglia and nerve growth factor: a model for understanding the mechanisms of GM1 effects on neuronal repair. J. Neurosci. Res. 12: 277-287.

58. Roisen, F.J., Bartfeld, H., Nagele, R. and Yorke, G. (1981) Ganglioside stimulation of axonal sprouting in vitro. Science 214: 577-578.

59. Skaper, S.D., Katoh-Semba, R. and Varon, S. (1985) GM1 ganglioside accelerates neurite outgrowth from primary peripheral and central neurons under selected culture conditions. Dev. Brain Res. 23: 19-26.

60. Spoerri, P.E. and Roisen, F.J. (1988) Ganglioside potentiation of NGF-independent agents on sensory ganglia. Neurosci. Lett. 90: 21-26.

61. Leon, A., Dal Toso, R., Presti, D., Benvegnù, D., Facci, L., Kirschner, G., Tettamanti, G. and Toffano, G. (1988) Development and survival of neurons in dissociated fetal mesencephalic serum-free cultures: II. Modulatory effects of gangliosides. J. Neurosci. 8: 746-753.

62. Skaper, S.D. and Varon, S. (1985) Ganglioside GM1 overcomes serum inhibition of neuritic outgrowth. Internatl. J. Dev. Neurosci. 3: 187-198.

63. Tettamanti, G., Ledeen, R.W., Sandhoff, K., Nagai, Y. and Toffano, G. (1986) Gangliosides and Neuronal Plasticity. Fidia Research Series, vol. 6, Liviana Press, Padova.

64. Mahadik, S.P. and Karpiak, S.K. (1988) Gangliosides in treatment of neural injury and disease. Drug Dev. Res. 15: 337-360.

65. Skaper, S.D., Leon, A. and Toffano G. (1989) Ganglioside function in the development and repair of the nervous system: from basic science to clinical application. Molec. Neurobiol., in press.

66. Sabel, B.A., Slavin, M.D. and Stein, D.G. (1984) GM1 ganglioside treatment facilitates behavioral recovery from bilateral brain damage. Science 225: 340-342.

67. Karpiak, S.E. (1983) Ganglioside treatment improves recovery of alteration behavior after unilateral entorhinal cortex lesion. Exp. Neurol. 81: 330-339.

68. Toffano, G., Agnati, L.F., Fuxe, K., Aldinio, C., Consolazione, A., Valenti, G. and Savoini, G. (1984) Effect of GM1 ganglioside treatment of the recovery of dopaminergic nigrostriatal neurons after different types of lesion. Acta Physiol. Scand. 122: 313-321.

69. Gradkowska, M., Skup, M., Kiedrowski, L., Calzolari, S. and Oderfeld-Nowak, B. (1986) The effect of GM1 ganglioside of cholinergic and serotoninergic systems in the rat hippocampus following partial denervation is dependent on the degree of fiber regeneration. Brain Res. 375: 417-422.

70. Gasser, U.E., Weskamp, G., Otten, U. and Dravid, A.R. (1986) Time course of elevation of nerve growth factor (NGF) content in the hippocampus and septum following lesions of the septohippocampal pathway in rats. Brain Res. 376: 351-356.

71. Nieto-Sampedro, M., Manthorpe, M., Barbin, G., Varon, S. and Cotman, C.W. (1983) Injury-induced neuronotrophic activity in adult rat brain. Correlation with survival of delayed implants in a wound cavity. J. Neurosci. 3: 2219-2229.

72. Vantini, G., Fusco, M., Bigon, E. and Leon, A. (1988) GM1 ganglioside potentiates the effect of nerve growth factor in preventing vinblastine-induced sympathectomy in newborn rats. Brain Res. 448: 252-258.

73. Cuello, A.C., Garofalo, L., Kenigsberg, R.L. and Maysinger, D. (1989) Gangliosides potentiate in vivo and in vitro effects of nerve growth factor on central cholinergic neurons. Proc. Natl. Acad. Sci. USA 86: 2056-2060.

74. Price, D.L. (1986) New Perspectives on Alzheimer's disease. Ann. Rev. Neurosci. 9: 489-512.

75. Whitehouse, P.J., Price, D.L., Struble, R .G., Clark, A.W., Coyle, J.T. and De Long, M.R. (1982) Alzheimer's disease and senile dementia: loss of neurons in the basal forebrain. Science 215: 1237-1239.

76. Perry, E.K., Tomlinson, B.E., Blessed, G., Bergmann, K., Gibson, P.H. and Perry, R.H. (1978) Correlation of cholinergic abnormalities with senile plaques and mental test scores in senile dementia. Brit. Med. J. II: 1457-1459.

77. Lärkfors, L., Ebendal, T., Whittemore, S.R., Persson, H., Hoffer, B.J. and Olson, L. (1987) Decreased level of nerve growth factor (NGF) and its messenger RNA in the aged rat brain. Mol. Brain Res. 3: 55-60.

78. Fischer, W., Wictorin, K., Björklund, A., Williams, L.R., Varon, S. and Gage, F.H. (1987) Amelioration of cholinergic neuron atrophy and spatial memory impairment in aged rats by nerve growth factor. Nature 329: 65-68.

79. Haroutunian, V., Kanof, P.D. and Davis, K.L. (1986) Partial reversal of lesion-induced deficits in cortical cholinergic markers by nerve growth factor. Brain Res. 386: 397-399.

80. Mahadik, S.P., Vilim, F., Korenowsky, A. and Karpiak, S.E. (1988) GM1 ganglioside protects nucleus basalis from excitotoxin damage: reduced cortical cholinergic losses and animal mortality. J. Neurosci. Res. 20: 479-483.

SUPPRESSION OF ACTIVE NEURONAL DEATH BY IMMUNE INTERFERON

Eugene M. Johnson, Jr., David P. Martin, Beth K. Levy and
Jason Y. Chang

Department of Pharmacology
Washington University Medical School
St. Louis, MO. 63110, USA

Neuronal cell death is an active process

The survival of neuronal cells depends on the presence of trophic factors. To date, nerve growth factor (NGF) is the only trophic factor which is chemically well characterized and of proven physiological significance (1). NGF is necessary for the survival and function of sympathetic and neural crest-derived sensory neurons. It is becoming clear that NGF is also important for the basal forebrain cholinergic neurons in CNS (2), a cell group involved in memory and which degenerates in Alzheimer's disease.

Since NGF is critical for the survival of a variety of neurons, one central question that needs to be addressed is the molecular mechanisms by which NGF keeps neurons alive. This survival-promoting effect may result from either one of the following mechanisms. First, NGF may nourish the neurons, exerting a positive effect on the general metabolism, thus keeping the neurons alive. Many of these general stimulatory effects (such as enzymatic synthesis of neurotransmitters, hypertrophy of the cells) require protein synthesis. In this case, neuronal survival is a direct result of the nourishing (or trophic) effects. Upon removal of NGF, the cells lose the positive stimulation, and die in a passive fashion. This has been the implicit view in the literature. Alternatively, NGF may have a "death¬suppressing" effect which is mechanistically separable from its trophic effects. The neurons may possess an endogenous "death program" which is suppressed by NGF. This "death program" will be initiated when the neuronal cells are deprived of NGF. In other words, instead of a passive process, this view sees that the death resulting from NGF deprivation is an active process.

There are some predictions can be made if either of these mechanisms mentioned above is true. If the death resulting from NGF deprivation is a passive process, one would expect inhibition of macromolecular synthesis (such as protein and RNA synthesis) will be detrimental to these neurons. As a result, addition of inhibitors of protein synthesis (such as cycloheximide) or RNA synthesis (such as actinomycin D) to cells deprived of NGF should hasten the dying process. On the other hand, if NGF deprivation initiates an active process which kills the neurons, one would expect protein and RNA synthesis inhibitors will interrupt the process and save these cells.

We designed experiments using sympathetic neurons in culture to address this question. Sympathetic neurons were obtained from embryonic rat superior cervical ganglia, and the culture was established in the presence of NGF for a week. Removal of NGF by anti-NGF antibodies at this time resulted in massive death of these cells in two days. To see the effects of protein and RNA synthesis inhibitors on the NGF-deprived neurons, anti-NGF antibodies were added to the culture with or without the presence of these inhibitors. Our results (Fig.1) (3) indicated that the presence of cycloheximide or actinomycin D prevented the death of the NGF¬deprived neurons. Looked at another way, inhibiting protein or RNA synthesis non-specifically mimicked the effect of NGF. These results support the notion that there is an intrinsic "death program" in these cells which can be activated by NGF deprivation. Upon removal of NGF, these cells initiate an active process which involves the synthesis of new RNA(s) and protein(s), or increased synthesis of pre¬existing molecules, that ultimately kill the cells. Cycloheximide and Actinomycin D may interrupt this "death program" by inhibiting the synthesis of some death-associated protein(s) or RNA(s), thus preventing these cells from dying. In addition to the sympathetic neurons described here, protein and RNA synthesis inhibitors have been shown to block the neuronal cell death in other systems. Very importantly, Oppenheim and Prevette (4) showed that these agents could block the naturally occurring cell death of sensory and motor neurons in the chicken embryo. These results indicate that the requirement of macromolecular synthesis is a general property of these "physiologically appropriate" cell deaths.

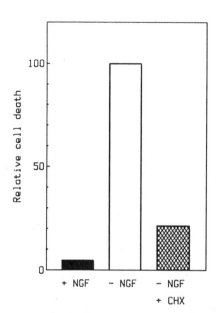

Fig.1. Inhibition of NGF deprivation-induced cell death by cycloheximide. Primary culture of sympathetic neurons was prepared from superior cervical ganglia of neonatal rats. The culture was established in the presence of NGF for 7 days. To initiate the experiment, anti-NGF antibodies were added to the culture with or without the presence of 1 ug/ml of cycloheximide. Neuronal cell death after NGF deprivation resulted in massive release of the intracellular enzyme, adenylate kinase, into the medium, which can be taken as a measure of cell death (3). The degree of cell death was assessed 2 days after the addition of anti-NGF antibodies. Results from this experiment indicate that the presence of cycloheximide significantly reduced the neuronal cell death resulted from NGF deprivation. Those cells saved by cycloheximide at the end of the experiment will go on to live indefinitely as the untreated cells if the drug is removed from the culture, and NGF is added at this time.

Suppression of inadvertently activated "proframmed cell death" by interferons

Since RNA synthesis inhibitors (such as actinomycin D) and protein synthesis inhibitors (such as cycloheximide) have been shown to prevent a number of "programmed cell death", one might ask if there is any physiologically important agents other than trophic factors which can serve to modify the death program. Interferon (IFN) should be a prime candidate for this purpose. IFN's are a family of proteins which have antiviral and anti-proliferative effects (5,6). There are two major types of IFN, namely type I and type II IFN. Type I IFN consists of IFN-a (produced by leukocytes) and IFN-ß (produced by fibroblasts), and they share the same receptor type. Type II IFN (IFN-γ), produced by activated T cells) has unique immunoregulatory activity in addition to the antiviral and anti proliferative effects, has its own receptor.

IFN is known to activate an enzyme, the 2',5'-oligoadenosine synthetase, thus stimulating the synthesis of 2',5'-oligoadenosine (2,5-A). 2,5-A is able to activate a RNAse, which degrades a certain mRNA's. It can also activate a protein kinase which can phosphorylate the "elongation factor 2" in protein synthesis pathway, and hence inhibit protein synthesis with some selectivity. IFN thus is an agent which possesses the ability to inhibit certain mRNA and protein syntheses. Recently, it was demonstrated that NGF could induce the 2,5-A synthetase activity in PC12 cells, a pheochromocytoma cell line commonly used as a model for neurons (7). Conceivable, NGF may be able to induce the production of 2,5-A, thus inhibiting the synthesis of some "death program" associated mRNA's and proteins.

If IFN indeed can inhibit the production of the death-associated mRNAs and proteins, then one should be able to remove NGF from an established neuronal culture, and halt or retard the progression of the death program by adding IFN to the culture. To test this possibility, we prepared sympathetic neuronal cultures from embryonic rat superior cervical ganglia as described above, removed NGF from the established culture by addition of anti-NGF antibodies, and added recombinant IFN-γ (Genentech, South San Francisco, CA.) into this NGF-deprived culture. The effects of IFN was assessed after two days, by which time those cells treated with anti-NGF antibodies only were dead. Our results (Fig.2) indicated that IFN-γ was able to suppress neuronal death resulting from NGF deprivation in a dose-dependent manner. The maximal protection could be seen at 5 units/ml, while the EC_{50} for this neuronal saving is approximately 1 unit/ml (1.3×10^{-11} M). It is worth mentioning that, by definition, 1 unit/ml is the EC_{50} of IFN in a standard antiviral assay. This suggests that the mechanism by which IFN-γ inhibits viral RNA and protein synthesis is related to its ability to prevent the putative "death-associated" RNA and protein from synthesis. Subsequent experiments indicated that IFN-α/ß (Lee Biochemicals, San Diego, CA.) also had the ability to protect the neurons deprived of NGF, with an EC_{50} of approximately 1,000 units/ml. IFN did not have the ability to replace NGF; this can be seen from the fact that the cells treated concurrently with anti-NGF antibodies and IFN had slightly atrophic cell bodies. This implies that IFN has the "death-suppressing" ability, but not the trophic functions associated with NGF.

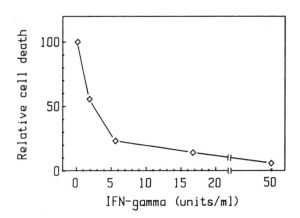

Fig.2. Inhibition of NGF deprivation¬induced cell death by recombinant murine IFN-γ. The experimental conditions were the same as those described in Fig.1 except that recombinant murine IFN-γ (Genentech, South San Francisco, CA.) was used in combination with anti-NGF antibodies. Results from this experiment indicate that IFN-γ was able to prevent neuronal cell death in a dose-dependent manner. The EC_{50} of this neuronal saving is approximately 1 unit/ml.

Further experiments indicated that upon short-term NGF deprivation, IFN could prevent a majority of cells from dying. IFN could retard the cell death during long-term NGF deprivation, but could not prevent the ultimate death. In order to examine the effects of IFN on cells deprived of NGF for a longer period of time, we performed the following experiment. Neuronal cells from an established culture were treated with antibodies against NGF for one, two, three, four or five days. At the end of this antibodies treatment, fresh medium containing regular concentration of NGF (50 ng/ml) was added to the culture. The cells were grown to the end of the experiment, and then quantified. As shown in Fig.3, the majority of neuronal cells were dead when they were deprived of NGF for two days without supplement of IFN. However, a significant number of neurons were still alive when they were treated with IFN during this period of NGF deprivation. When the condition of NGF deprivation was extended to day 5, most of the cells were dead whether or not IFN was present in the culture.

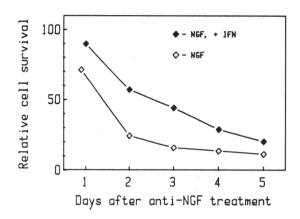

Fig.3. IFN-γ retards neuronal cell death upon long-term NGF deprivation. Anti-NGF antibodies were added to an established cell culture for 1, 2, 3, 4, or 5 days. The anti-NGF antibodies were then removed from the cultures, and the cells treated with complete medium containing regular concentration of NGF (50 ng/ml). These cells were grown to the 8th day after the initiation of the experiment, lysed with Triton X-100, and the total amount of adenylate kinase determined as a measure of cell remained in the culture. Results from this experiment indicate that the presence of IFN-γ in the culture significantly decreased the cell death induced by NGF deprivation.

The effects of IFN appear to be directly on the neuronal cells instead of indirectly mediated through non-neuronal cells. Since our experiments were performed in the presence of excess anti-NGF antibodies, it is not likely IFN induces NGF production, thereby supporting the neurons. Furthermore, our results (Chang, et al., in preparation) from receptor binding indicate these neurons have specific receptors for IFN-γ. Receptor autoradiography indicates the receptors are present both on the cell bodies and neurites. Experiments which crosslinked IFN-updside down lambda to its receptor revealed a major protein complex at the range of 100,000 daltons, which is consistent with reports from other cell types. These results strongly suggest that IFN-γ exerts its effects directly on the neuronal cells.

Programmed cell death

It is becoming clear that programmed cell death occurs in a number of systems. The common feature of this type of cell death is that it involves new protein and RNA synthesis, thus inhibitors of protein and RNA synthesis can prevent this type of cell death. Besides the neuronal cell death described above, examples of "programmed cell death" include glucocorticoids-induced cell death in thymocytes (8), interleukin-2 withdrawal induced lymphocyte death (9), castration induced cell death in prostate epithelium (10,11), and death of intersegmental muscles of the moth Manduca sexta due to withdrawal of ecdysteroid level (12). It is likely that these cells respond to an external signal (such as NGF withdrawal in sympathetic neurons, or a drop of androgen level resulting from castration) by initiating a "cascade" of death-associated RNA and protein synthesis, which leads to the production of the proximal "killer protein" that ultimately kills the cells. Actinomycin D and cycloheximide can non¬selectively mimic the effects of NGF by inhibiting this cascade from propagating, thus prevent the cells from dying. Consistent with this idea, Buttyan et al. (13) showed that there is a cascade of gene induction in rat ventral prostate gland upon castration induced cell death. Conceivably, loss of transcriptional control of the "death program" could play a role in neurodegenerative disease or in cellular attrition seen in aging.

Conclusion

We have presented data which argue that the neuronal cell death resulting from NGF deprivation is an active process. Neurons appear to posses an intrinsic "death program" which is constantly suppressed by NGF. NGF deprivation may initiate a cascade of new RNA and protein syntheses, which ultimately kill the cells. Inhibitors of RNA or protein synthesis can interrupt this cascade from propagating, thus preventing neuronal death. Sympathetic neurons have receptors for the IFN-γ, and IFN-γ can retard neuronal cell death upon NGF deprivation. It is possible that this is a self-defense mechanism during trauma. There are two events that may occur concurrently during external trauma which involves bleeding and extensive tissue damage, namely, inflammation in the local area, and neuronal damage in the affected tissue. During local inflammation, IFN is likely to be secreted by activated T cells, and serve its antiviral and immunoregulatory functions. In the meantime, neuronal damage, such as axotomy, may deprive the neurons from trophic factors, which may result in neuronal cell death within several days. The fact that IFN can retard neuronal cell death indicates that this agent, in addition to its other functions in immune system, may have a role in nervous system. This death-suppressing ability of IFN can give these neurons an extended time to search for other trophic support, thus minimizing the damage resulting from trauma. In this respect, it is relevant to note that IFN-γ can potentiate the production of interleukin-1 by monocytes (14,15), and interleukin-1 has the ability to stimulate NGF production from Schwann cells and fibroblasts (16). These results suggests that while IFN can directly prevent neurons from dying by acting on the receptors on neuronal cells, this agent can also indirectly stimulate non-neuronal cells to produce NGF, thus minimizing the extent of cell death during trauma. These ideas are summarized and presented in Fig.4.

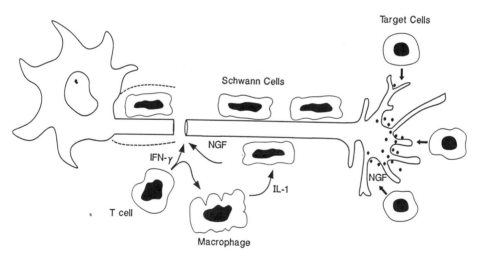

Fig.4 Hypothetical conditions describing possible roles of IFN-γ in neuronal injury. Under normal condition, NGF produced by target cells is taken up in the neuronal terminal and retrogradely transported to the cell body. Two events are envisioned after trauma which involves extensive tissue damage and blood shedding. First, axotomy may occur in the affected area, and the transport of NGF to the cell body will be interrupted. A "death program" may be initiated as a result of this NGF deprivation. Second, immune cells may migrate into this area and perform their various functions. In addition to the antiviral and immunoregulatory roles, the IFN-γ produced by T cells may also have a role in preventing neuronal cell death. The IF-γ may bind to the IFN-γ receptors on neuronal cells, and directly retard the progression of the "death program". Indirectly, IFN-γ may stimulate the macrophages to secret interleukin-1, which, in turn, will stimulate the Schwann cells (or fibroblasts) to secret NGF. A combination of these direct and indirect events may help the neurons survive trauma.

References

1. Thoenen, H., and Barde, Y. A., 1980, Physiology of nerve growth factor, <u>Physiol. Rev.</u>, 60:1284.
2. Mobley, W. C., Rutkowski, J. L., Tennekoon, G. I., Buchanan, K., and Johnston, M. V., 1985, Choline acetyltransferase activity in striatum of neonatal rats increased by nerve growth factor, <u>Science</u>, 229:284.
3. Martin, D. P., Schmidt, R. E., DiStefano, P. S., Lowry, O. H., Carter, J. G., and Johnson, E. M., Jr., 1988, Inhibitors of protein synthesis and RNA synthesis prevent neuronal death caused by nerve growth factor deprivation, <u>J.Cell Biol.</u>, 106:829.
4. Oppenheim, R. W., and Prevette, D. M., 1988, Reduction of naturally occurring neuronal death in vivo by the inhibition of protein and RNA synthesis, <u>Soc. Neurosci. Abstr.</u>, 14:368.
5. Mannering, G. J., and Deloria, L. B., 1986, The pharmacology and toxicology of the interferons: an overview, <u>Annu. Rev. Pharmacol. Toxicol.</u>, 26:455.
6. Pestka, S., Langer, J. A., Zoon, K. C., and Samuel, C. E., 1987, Interferons and their actions, <u>Annu. Rev. Biochem.</u>, 56:727.
7. Saarma, M., Toots, U., Raukas, E., Zhelkovsky, A., Pivazian, A., and Neuman, T., 1986, Nerve growth factor induces changes in (2'-5')oligo(A) synthetase and 2'-phosphodiesterase activities during differentiation of PC12 pheochromocytoma cells, <u>Exp. Cell. Res.</u>, 166:229.
8. Cohen, J. J., and Duke, R. C., 1984, Glucocorticoid activation of a calcium-dependent endonuclease in thymocyte nuclei leads to cell death, <u>J. Immunol.</u>, 132:38.
9. Duke, R. C., and Cohen, J. J., 1986, IL-2 addiction: Withdrawal of growth factor activates a suicide program in dependent T cells, <u>Lymphokine Res.</u>, 5:289.
10. Stanisic, T., Sodlowski, R., Lee, C. and Grayhack, J. T., 1978, Partial inhibition of castration-induced ventral prostate regression with actinomycin D and cycloheximide, <u>Invest. Urol.</u>, 16:15.
11. Kyprianou, N., English, H. F., and Isaacs, J. T., 1988, Activation of Ca^{+2}-Mg^{+2}-dependent endonuclease as an early event in castration-induced prostatic cell death, <u>Prostate</u>, 13:103.
12. Lockshin, R. A., 1969, Programmed cell death-- Activation of lysis by a mechanism involving the synthesis of protein, <u>J. Insect Physiol.</u>, 15:1505.
13. Buttyan, R., Zakeri, Z, Lockshin, R., and Wolgemuth, D., 1988, Cascade induction of c-fos, c-myc, and heat shock 70K transcripts during regression of the rat ventral prostate gland, <u>Mol. Endocrinol.</u>, 2:650.
14. Arenzana-Seisdedos, F., Virelizier, J. L., and Fiers, W., 1985, Interferons as macrophage-activating factors. III. Preferential effects of interferon-gamma on the interleukin-1 secretory potential of fresh or aged human monocytes, <u>J. Immunol.</u>, 134:2444.
15. Gerrard, T. L., Siegel, J. P., Dyer, D. R., and Zoon, K. C., 1987, Differential effects of interferon-a and interferon-gamma on interleukin-1 secretion by monocytes, <u>J. Immunol.</u>, 138:2535.
16. Lindholm, D., Heumann, R., Meyer, M., and Thoenen, H., 1987, Interleukin-1 regulates synthesis of nerve growth factor in non-neuronal cells of rat sciatic nerve, <u>Nature</u>, 330:658.

BASIC FIBROBLAST GROWTH FACTOR, AN EXAMPLE OF A

MULTIFUNCTIONAL TROPHIC FACTOR WITH NEUROTROPHIC ACTIVITY

Patricia Ann Walicke

Department of Neuroscience
University of California, San Diego
La Jolla, CA 92093

All neurons are believed to require trophic factors for support of their survival and process growth. Conversely, neuronal atrophy and death after CNS injury or during aging have been ascribed to deficiencies of trophic factors (1). For many years, the only known neurotrophic factor (NTF) was nerve growth factor (NGF). Studies with NGF have led to significant insights into neuronal cell biology and development, particularly in the peripheral nervous system. Models constructed from its actions on sympathetic and sensory neurons have been generalized to principles guiding the growth of all neurons. The recent recognition that NGF is a NTF for cholinergic septal and basal neurons has allowed seminal studies on the regulation of neuronal growth in the CNS and holds potential implications for the treatment of Alzheimer's disease. But it also must be remembered that NGF is not a universal NTF, and that its targets in the CNS are limited to only a few populations of neurons (2-4). Even many of the other neuronal populations affected in Alzheimer's disease, such as entorhinal cortical and hippocampal neurons, are not responsive to NGF. Therefore, many laboratories have searched for the novel NTFs hypothesized to exist for these other neurons, but the results have been frustrating. Only one other NTF closely resembling NGF in its chemistry and biological activity has been isolated, brain-derived neurotrophic factor (BDNF). But as with NGF, most of the known targets of BDNF are peripheral sensory neurons (2,5,6).

While progress has been discouragingly slow in purification of NTFs, discovery and isolation of trophic factors has proceeded rapidly in other sectors of medical biology. As the distribution of these factors was examined, it often became apparent that either the factor or its receptor was present in the CNS. In some cases, the association appeared to be specifically with neurons in the CNS. Among these factors are the fibroblast growth factors (FGF), insulin and the insulin-like growth factors (IGF), epidermal growth factor (EGF), transforming growth factor alpha (TGF-alpha), some types of transforming growth factor beta (TGF-beta), platelet derived growth factor (PDGF), interleukin 1 (IL-1), and the nexins (5). Although some of these peptides may act as neuromodulators in the CNS, it seems likely that growth regulation is one of their functions in brain as in other tissues.

These factors differ from NGF in several respects, perhaps the most obvious being that they are all multifunctional or pleiotropic. For example, basic fibroblast growth factor (bFGF) is known to affect fibroblasts, endothelial cells (including those from brain capillaries), vascular smooth muscle cells, skeletal myoblasts, astrocytes, immature oligodendroctyes, a variety of neurons, and pituitary lactotropes and thyrotropes (7-10). Most of the current theories and explanations of CNS development start with the assumption that NTFs are restricted in their actions to neurons (2, 6, 11) . Therefore the existence of a factor with the spectrum of activities attributed to bFGF appears surprising, if not improbable. Yet bFGF is abundant in the CNS, as are several of the other multifunctional factors mentioned above.

Attempting to understand the function of these pleiotropic factors in the brain poses a significant challenge and has already produced considerable controversy (6,11) . Perhaps they chiefly regulate infrastructure, modulating growth of blood vessels and connective tissue components which brain shares with other tissues. Perhaps their significant role is restricted to regulation of glial proliferation and differentiation. But since several of these factors address neurons, they may play a significant role as NTFs. If these factors are really NTFs, it would suggest that some major revisions may be required in our conceptualization of the control of neuronal and brain growth.

For example, if cortical neurons, astrocytes and endothelial cells all share a common trophic factor, it appears likely that there are multiple opportunities for coordinate or competitive interactions among these cell types. Traditionally, neuronal growth has been viewed in isolation from other cell types except for synaptic targets (2,6,11). Such a restricted viewpoint may be rather artificial, if not potentially misleading, since the brain is an organ which contains a variety of cell types. A major issue for future research will be elucidation of the mechanisms which restrict and regulate the actions of multifunctional factors. For example, bFGF injected into the cortex might principally cause blood vessel growth under some conditions or axonal growth under others. Likely overall response will in some way be determined by the underlying configuration and pattern of endogenous growth regulatory substances, which is being disrupted by the sudden interjection of a single trophic agent. This type of model is considerably more complex than the "magic bullet" NTF usually postulated in models derived purely from studies with NGF (6,11); however, it is entirely consistent with current thinking about peptide trophic factors in other sectors of medical biology (12).

This chapter will focus on one of the pleiotropic factors present in brain, bFGF, reviewing particularly the evidence supporting its identification as an NTF. This evidence includes:
1) Support of neuronal survival and growth in cultures lacking detectable glial cells (13-15);
2) Presence of bFGF receptors on hippocampal and other CNSneurons (9, 16);
3) Internalization and degradation of bFGF by hippocampalneurons *in vitro* (17);

4) Immunohistochemical evidence for bFGF in CNS neurons inintact brain tissue (18-21);
5) Availability of bFGF to neurons in their normal environment as suggested by the presence of bFGF (22) and its mRNA (23, 24) in brain tissue, and astrocytes *in vitro* (14,23,25);
6) Enhancement of neuronal survival *in vivo* after injury (26,27) by exogenously applied bFGF.

Although many questions remain about the role and function of brain bFGF, together these studies present a good argument that bFGF is an NTF. Speculations concerning its possible role in both normal and pathological brain tissue will be presented.

ACTIONS OF bFGF *IN VITRO*

In vitro, bFGF enhances the survival of at least some neurons from many regions of the CNS, including frontal, parietal, occipital, and entorhinal cortex, hippocampus, basal ganglion, septum and basal forebrain, anterior thalamus, brainstem, cerebellum and spinal cord (14,15,28-32). In many of these regions, it appears likely that only subpopulations of neurons may respond, but their phenotypes are not necessarily as yet well defined. More specific subpopulations of neurons which have been observed to respond to bFGF *in vitro* include hippocampal pyramidal neurons (28), septal and basal cholinergic neurons (32), dopaminergic mesencephalic neurons (31), cerebellar granule cells (14), and spinal cord motoneurons neurons (15) . At least some retinal ganglion cells respond to the closely related factor, acidic FGF (aFGF) (33). Many of these neurons can be maintained *in vitro* with bFGF for periods of one to several weeks (14,28,29). Neurons in the peripheral nervous system responding to bFGF include parasympathetic neurons (15,34) and sympathetic neurons during a brief developmental period preceding onset of NGF sensitivity (35) .

In addition to supporting survival, bFGF enhances growth of neurites from many of these types of neurons. The response can be observed within 24 hours of exposure, before any demonstrable change in neuronal survival in at least hippocampal and cortical cultures (28,30). After one or more weeks, neurons exposed to bFGF still display longer neurites (14, 29) . PC12 cells have also been demonstrated to extend neurites in response to bFGF, mimicking their response to NGF (3 4, 3 6, 3 7) . Neurite outgrowth has been reported on atypical substrates such as heparin, which may in part be related to the high affinity of heparin for members of thê FGF family (28, 38) . bFGF also appears to enhance production of the neurotransmitter appropriate to the phenotype of the responding neurons. It increases indices of cholinergic function in spinal cord motoneurons (15), cholinergic and GABAergic function in septal cultures (32), and catecholaminergic and GABAergic function in cultures of brainstem neurons (31). The neuronal responses of increased survival, process growth and transmitter production to bFGF are reminiscent of the responses of sympathetic neurons to NGF.

The minimal required concentration of bFGF for neuronal survival has been reported to be in the vicinity of about 1 to 100 pM (14,15,29,30). The variability likely reflects different potencies among preparations of bFGF as well as differences in the assay methods. Neurite outgrowth appears to require about 5-10 fold higher concentrations of bFGF (28). Even higher amounts of bFGF have been reported to decrease rather than enhance neuronal survival (14,29).

Since bFGF is a mitogen for astrocytes, the possibility that it acts indirectly through stimulating growth of glial cells was raised (11). It should be noted that all of the above studies used highly enriched populations of neurons in which glial contamination was less than 10% even in the presence of bFGF. Furthermore, bFGF has been demonstrated to support neuronal survival in glial-free cultures of hippocampal neurons (13), cerebellar granular cells (14) and parasympathetic neurons (15). Therefore, it appeared likely that bFGF acted directly on neurons.

In highly purified cultures of astrocytes, bFGF stimulates mitosis, induces morphological differentiation to a more fibrillar form, and augments GFAP synthesis (13,39,40). Reported effects on immature oligodendrocytes include stimulation of mitosis and induction of marker enzymes (9,41,42). With mesenchymal cells, bFGF is also not only a mitogen, but also regulates expression of differentiated characteristics (7,8,10,43).

CHARACTERIZATION OF NEURONAL RECEPTORS FOR bFGF

Radioreceptor binding assays have demonstrated the presence of two types of binding sites for bFGF on all cell types studied, including hippocampal neurons. The first is labile to high salt concentrations (2M NaCl) and to heparinase or hepartinase and is generally ascribed to glycosoaminoglycans (GAG). The second is stable to these treatments but labile to detergents and proteases and is generally thought to represent a membrane receptor (16,44,45). Scatchard analyses of [^{125}I]bFGF binding to cultures of hippocampal neurons indicate that the GAG sites have a Kd of around 1.0 nM and a density of about 1-2 x 10^5 sites/neuron. At a concentration of about 100 pM [^{125}I]bFGF, GAGs account for about 40-60% of total binding. The receptor site has an apparent Kd of about 150 pM and is present at a density of about 2-6 x 10^4/neuron (16). Comparison with previous binding studies performed on mesenchymal cells such as endothelial cells (44) reveal some potentially interesting differences. Specifically, neurons compared to mesenchymal cells have: 1) only 10-20% as many GAG sites; 2) a decrease in the relative role of GAGs from 90-99% of total binding to only 40-60%; 3) a receptor with roughly ten-fold lower affinity for bFGF; 4) a 5-10 fold higher density of receptor sites/cell. Preliminary studies indicate that binding characteristics of astrocytes more closely resemble those of mesenchymal cells than neurons (P. Walicke, in preparation).

Multiple mechanisms could be postulated to account for the somewhat different kinetics of neuronal and mesenchymal receptors. Perhaps the set of differences between neurons and mesenchymal cells are interdependent. For example, GAGs might provide a first stage of binding which increases the efficiency of later receptor binding. The higher density of receptor sites on neurons might contribute to the apparently lower Kd (46). Possibly all cells bear the same receptor molecules, but their affinity is regulated by processes such as phosphorylation. Or finally, the receptor molecules on neurons and mesenchymal cells may be somewhat different. Whatever the mechanism, these kinetic differences could affect the amount of bFGF which is bound by competing endothelial cells and neurons in brain tissue, and therefore the eventual biological effect observed.

Some attempts have been made to characterize the molecules responsible for both GAG and receptor binding. The active GAG appears to be heparan sulfate because: 1) only heparan sulfate or heparin out of multiple GAGs tested display high affinity for bFGF; 2) heparinase selectively disrupts the GAG component of binding (34,38,44). Two known heparan sulfate proteoglycans produced by neurons might play a role in binding bFGF. The first which consists of an 80 kD core protein and multiple heparan sulfate side chains has previously been studied in association with laminin (47,48). The second is the amyloid beta precursor protein, related to the amyloid protein of Alzheimer's disease, which has been reported to bear heparan sulfate (49). Possible participation of these glycoproteins in bFGF binding requires further investigation.

The bFGF receptors have been initially characterized by affinity labeling with disuccinimidyl suberate (DSS). Hippocampal neurons show a major receptor-[^{125}I]bFGF complex of about 150-160 kD and a minor one of about 100-110 kD. Allowing for the contribution of [^{125}I]bFGF, these bands would correspond to membrane proteins of 135-145 and 85-95 kD. The two bands were detected in cultures of neurons from many regions of the CNS (16). The larger neuronal band comigrates with a receptor species from fibroblasts (16), and probably is similar to receptors characterized on PC12 cells and a variety of mesenchymal cells (37,50-53). Preliminary studies suggest that astrocytes bear only a single receptor type which co-migrates with the larger neuronal receptor. The smaller neuronal receptor has not as yet been reported on other cell types. Recently, 150 and 100 kD receptors have been purified from adult brain tissue (54), which might suggest that the smaller receptor is not an artifact of tissue culture.

The 85-100 kD receptor is likely to be either a fragment of the larger receptor or a relatively specific neuronal form of bFGF receptor. Attempts to increase the proportion of small receptor by allowing increased intervals for lysis by endogenous proteases were not successful (16). The possibility that the small receptor was a hypoglycosylated form of the larger was also investigated, but both forms appeared to be glycoproteins recognized by wheat germ agglutinin (55,56). The true relationship between the two receptor proteins should soon be clarified since both have been isolated from brain (54). The possible existence of a distinct form of bFGF receptor relatively specific for neurons could have important implications for potential design of pharmacological agents and therapeutic strategies related to bFGF.

INTERNALIZATION AND METABOLISM OF bFGF

Evidence for internalization of bFGF comes from both histological and biochemical studies. Immediately after exposure to [^{125}I]bFGF, autoradiography shows grains present outlining both the neuronal soma and processes (9). After several hours at 37°C, most of the label appears to lie over perinuclear cytoplasm. Electron microscopic autoradiography demonstrates the presence of the majority of label in cytoplasmic vesicles (Fig 1). Occasional grains appeared to be associated with nuclear chromatin (Fig. 1A). The possibility that a portion of internalized bFGF maybe transported into the nucleus has also been raised in studies with endothelial cells (57).

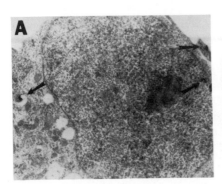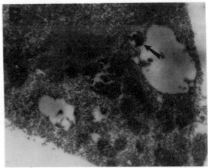

Fig. 1 Electron microscope autoradiography for localization of [^{125}I]bFGF after internalization by hippocampal neurons _in vitro_. Arrows mark grains. A) 7,000 x; B) 20,000 x.

Intracellular localization was further supported by biochemical studies showing progressive sequestration of [^{125}I]bFGF into a cellular compartment where it was protected from extracellular high salt and proteases. After internalization, bFGF is metabolized into three smaller peptides of 15, 9.5 and 4 kD. These peptides are quite stable and can be found in association with neurons for 2-3 days after initial exposure to [^{125}I]bFGF. Preliminary characterization suggests that the 9.5 kD peptide includes at least residues 30-80, and the 4 kD peptide contains at least residues 106-120 (17). The 106-120 region appears to contain a domain recognized by the bFGF receptor, and synthetic peptides containing this sequence have been shown be mixed agonists/antagonists in bioassay (58). Whether the endogenous metabolites of bFGF are biologically active is an interesting question for speculation.

SYNTHESIS AND DISTRIBUTION OF bFGF

The presence of bFGF in brain was clearly established by extraction and identification by both immunological criteria and N-amino terminal sequencing (22). Estimates of its concentration range between 15 and 60 ng/gm. Since biological responses _in vitro_ occur with as little as 0.05 ng/ml, bFGF appears to be extremely abundant. However, the concentration of bFGF in brain is only about 10% of that in pituitary and 1% of that in kidney (8,43,59). In these extra-neural tissues, nearly all of the bFGF is postulated to be sequestered in storage sites in the ECM (10,60), where it is not actively participating in regulation of growth or mitosis.

Immunohistochemical studies of brain show bFGF-like material in basement membranes around blood vessels and the meninges. staining is observed in a significant number of neurons, particularly the large pyramidal neurons of the cortex and hippocampus (18-21,60). We have obtained consistent results with three polyclonal antisera raised against synthetic peptides from different regions of the bFGF sequence, a polyclonal raised against intact bFGF, and a monoclonal raised against intact bFGF. On Western blots, these antibodies, like those from other laboratories, also bind to proteins of 22 and 25 kD in addition to the 16-18 kD bands for bFGF (61). The 22 and 25 kD proteins have been purified from brain tissue and reported to be large forms of bFGF (62,63). Whether these different molecular weight forms are sequestered in different cells, and how they contribute to the immunohistochemical pattern are as yet unknown.

Brain bFGF does appear to be locally produced, because its mRNA can be detected in extracts from several brain regions (23,24). To determine which CNS cells produce bFGF, mRNA was prepared from highly enriched cultures of astrocytes or telencephalic neurons. Glia contained high levels of bFGF mRNA but message was barely detectable in neurons (23). Astrocytes have further been demonstrated to synthesize bFGF protein in vitro (14,25). _In situ_ hybridization studies employing sections of adult rat brain surprisingly showed that the highest levels of bFGF mRNA were to be found in a few populations of neurons. These neurons occur in region CA2 and portions of CA1 in the hippocampus, the fasciola cinereum, the indusium griseum and portions of the cingulate cortex (23). Since the Northern blots indicated that total amounts of bFGF mRNA were roughly comparable in the hippocampus and other regions such as hypothalamus which lacked intensely labeled neurons, other sites of bFGF transcription must exist. Perhaps widely distributed astrocytes synthesizing bFGF at low but fairly constant levels provide most of brain bFGF (23).

The neurons which contain bFGF mRNA hybridization are among the most intensely stained on immunohistochemistry for bFGF, but many other cortical and hippocampal neurons also react for bFGF protein (18-21). If the immunohistochemistry reliably reflects localization of bFGF, then these neurons presumably obtain bFGF from other sources. The presence of bFGF immunoreactivity is consistent with the interpretation that these neurons likely internalize and concentrate bFGF which is derived from another cell, possibly astrocytes.

Although bFGF protein can be found in many tissues, bFGF mRNA is only readily detected in brain. This is consistent with the hypothesis that, in most tissues, bFGF predominantly exists in an inert storage form. Unlike neurons, mesenchymal cells do not require a constant supply of trophic factor for survival. In intact stable tissue, endothelial cells and other mesenchymal cells probably use little bFGF. The site of storage is believed to be predominantly extracellular, based on both biochemical and immunohistochemical studies demonstrating the presence of bFGF in basement membranes and ECM in many tissues. The ability of heparan sulfate to stabilize and protect bFGF from proteolytic enzymes is likely important during potentially prolonged periods of extracellular storage. Injury is believed to cause mobilization of bFGF stores through one of several mechanisms: 1) direct damage to the basal lamina; 2) stimulation of secretion of heparinases and proteases which degrade the ECM and liberate bFGF; 3) stimulation of secretion of small heparan sulfate bFGF carrier glycoproteins. Released bFGF then interacts with cell receptors to stimulate mitosis and the process of wound healing. The term "stormone" has been proposed to describe this unusual handling of bFGF (7,8,10,60,64-66).

The presence of bFGF mRNA solely in intact brain tissue suggests unusually high rates of bFGF synthesis in brain. However, the concentration of bFGF protein in brain is relatively low. Together these observations imply that bFGF turn over is more rapid in brain than in other tissues. Perhaps this only reflects the relative paucity of ECM in the brain, which prevents formation of typical stable extracellular stores. It is interesting to note that, unlike other cell types, neurons are thought to require a constant supply of trophic factor for survival (2,6,11). It is also interesting that the 100 kD receptor seen only on neurons _in vitro_ exists in adult brain (54). The unusually high rate of turn over would be consistent with bFGF acting as a NTF, though it would also be consistent with other roles as, for example, a neuromodulator.

Although little bFGF mRNA is present in intact somatic tissues, it can be easily extracted from cultures of mesenchymal cells. In fact, many cells which respond to bFGF, like endothelial cells or smooth muscle cells, appear to be capable of producing bFGF as an autocrine factor, at least _in vitro_ (43,67,68). In the telencephalic neuronal cultures employed for mRNA extraction a sizeable minority of neurons, on the order of 20-30%, would be expected to be responsive to bFGF (30). Yet bFGF mRNA was scarcely detectable (23). This might suggest that the majority of neurons are not capable of bFGF synthesis even under conditions where it would be induced in astrocytes (14,23,25) or mesenchymal cells. Therefore, with the exception of the limbic neurons seen in the _in situ_ hybridization studies, CNS neurons might be predicted to be dependent on external sources of bFGF. Dependence on external supplies of bFGF could be envisioned to make neurons more vulnerable to shortages, particularly during times of increased utilization after injury.

Reliance on bFGF derived from other cells appears particularly precarious in light of evidence that bFGF is not released very efficiently. The bFGF gene lacks a typical signal sequence (24), which implies that bFGF is not secreted by the normal cellular mechanism. Since bFGF is found in ECM both in vitro and in vivo it does appear to get out of cells (7,8,60,64,69,70), but how is unknown. Potentially, release may be an important point for regulation of bFGF availability to neurons in the CNS. It should also be noted that brain contains other members of the FGF family which do have signal sequences (8). Possibly some of the actions attributed to bFGF in this paper may actually be mediated by FGF-5 or other related peptides in situ.

EFFECTS OF EXOGENOUSLY APPLIED bFGF ON NEURONS

Several studies have suggested that administration of exogenous bFGF through osmotic pumps or slow release pellets can enhance neuronal survival in vivo. The fimbria-fornix transection model has been widely employed for demonstration that application of NGF can support survival of cholinergic septal neurons after axotomy and separation from their source of NTF in the hippocampus (4,71-73). Recent studies have shown that bFGF can also increase survival of cholinergic septal neurons in this paradigm, although a somewhat smaller proportion may respond to bFGF than to NGF (27). With recent evidence for production of bFGF by some hippocampal neurons (23), it might be argued that bFGF could function as a typical retrogradely transported NTF for a subpopulation of septal neurons, acting in this situation quite analogously to NGF.

Administration of bFGF has also been shown to increase survival of retinal ganglion cells after section of the optic nerve (26), and of some dorsal root ganglion sensory neurons after lesions of the posterior roots (74). Influence on neurite elongation in vivo is suggested by studies in which bFGF has been shown to enhance the rate of peripheral nerve regeneration (8,10,75).

These studies demonstrate that positive effects of bFGF on neuronal survival and growth are not limited to the unusual conditions seen in vitro but also occur in vivo. Whether these responses reflect direct and exclusive action of the applied bFGF on the responding neurons is far from clear. bFGF application is angiogenic in many tissues (7,10,22,76), and increased neovascularization has been reported in both brain and peripheral nerve after bFGF infusion (8,21,75,76). Besides altering cellular constituents, prolonged infusions of bFGF would be expected to produce compensatory changes in rates of synthesis of other endogenous trophic factors. Truly comprehending the mechanism through which an administered multifunctional factor produces a change in one particular cell population is likely to be a formidable task.

bFGF AS A NTF IN NORMAL AND PATHOLOGICAL BRAIN

Although there are many gaps to be filled in the experimenta data, an outline of possible functions of bFGF in the CNS are beginning to emerge. A distinction should probably be made between possible actions of bFGF in the few regions where it is made by neurons and in the rest of the brain. For the few neurons labeled by in situ hybridization, bFGF may potentially function as an autocrine NTF. It is interesting that the neurons of region CA2 appear to better resist global insults like

ischemia than other hippocampal neurons (23). Possibly some of
the bFGF made by hippocampal neurons functions as a traditional
retrogradely transported NTF for a subclass of septal
cholinergic neurons. In this one particular situation, bFGF may
act in a manner analogous to NGF. The possibility that bFGF
might be used as a neurotransmitter or neuromodulator in
synaptic circuits related to memory should also be considered.

It appears likely that many other regions of the brain
contain neurons responsive to bFGF. These neurons do not
appear to synthesize bFGF, and would be expected to be
dependent on supplies from an external source. Astrocytes
would appear to be the most likely source (14,23,25). Since
macrophages make bFGF (8,77), microglia should be considered
as a potential source. Although preliminary evidence suggests
that these neurons appear to internalize and concentrate bFGF
from their environment, these interactions may occur locally
rather than in the context of retrograde transport from
distant target regions. Substantiating these hypotheses will
of course require much more experimental investigation.

Whatever the function of bFGF in the intact brain, its role
in the damaged or pathological brain is likely different and
potentially more complex. After perturbation of the normal CNS,
changes might be expected to occur in both the sources and
targets of bFGF. After some types of injury, it is likely that
bFGF synthesis will be induced in mesenchymal cells like
endothelial cells (67) which are participating in the repair
process. Invading macrophages (8,77) or possibly activated
microglia might be other sources of bFGF. There is evidence to
suggest that bFGF synthesis may be up-regulated in reactive
astrocytes (18). The failure of most neurons to produce bFGF
mRNA _in vitro_ might suggest that they will also not induce its
synthesis after injury _in vivo_.

Neurons are not the only cells to alter their behavior after
injury. Many other cell types from brain tissue also participate
in reparative changes. Extrapolating from _in vitro_ studies, bFGF
could be hypothesized to participate in several processes,
including: 1) neovascularization; 2) scar formation by
fibroblasts and connective tissue cells; 3) gliosis; 4) neuronal
atrophy and death (deficiency); 5) sprouting by some neuronal
types. Participation in these processes is not mutually
exclusive, and possibly bFGF might help mediate several of these
degenerative and reparative responses. Attempting to generate
models of bFGF function in these complex alterations in tissue
brings up a central question: how is the activity of a
pleiotropic factor regulated and directed to certain cellular
targets? Several possible mechanisms will be presented in the
remainder of this chapter.

It should be noted, however, that several of the rather
distinctive features in the interaction of bFGF with neurons
versus mesenchymal cells may have implications for
neuropathology. The sparse ECM characteristic of neural
tissues will limit the amount of bFGF which can be stored in
the vicinity of CNS neurons compared to other cells like
endothelial cells. The relatively low affinity of the
neuronal bFGF receptor may further worsen the ability of
neurons to take advantage of available bFGF. As endothelial

cells or astrocytes increase their bFGF consumption in response to injury, they may compete more intensively with neurons for available bFGF. Unlike most mesenchymal cells and astrocytes, many neurons do not appear to be capable of synthesizing autocrine bFGF and so are dependent on external sources. Together these properties appear consistent with the greater vulnerability and less successful regenerative responses of neurons after CNS injury.

POTENTIAL CONTROL MECHANISMS FOR PLEIOTROPIC FACTORS

Strict control of spatial availability is one obvious method to limit the number of responsive cells which are exposed to a pleiotropic agent. To some extent, distribution can be controlled at the level of cellular release by restriction to specialized structures or junctions such as synapses. It may be more than coincidental that several novel NTFs besides bFGF appear to bind to heparin and related ECM constituents (5). This property will greatly limit their range of diffusion in tissues. The ECM is already recognized to play a significant role in ordering the cellular microenvironment. Regulating availability and distribution of trophic factors may be another dimension of this role.

A second level of control could occur at the level of activation of the factor by its potential target cell. In the specific case of bFGF, it has been suggested that target cells may need to release heparinases or proteases to release bFGF from the ECM (10,70). Small heparin-like polymers or more traditional binding proteins provide other alternatives for mobilizing stored bFGF and transporting it to the target cell (45,66). Although less relevant to bFGF, other mechanisms in this category would include separation of an active moiety from an inactive complex as seen with TGF beta 1, and the proteolytic activation of zymogen proteases.

A third level of control could occur at the level of release. For trophic factors secreted through the normal vesicular pathway, a variety of hormonal or chemical signals could be anticipated to influence release. bFGF is not unique in its lack of a typical signal sequence for secretion. This property is shared by IL-1 and some forms of TGF beta. Possibly particular types of cellular interactions may be involved in the as yet unknown mechanisms leading to release of these factors.

A fourth level of control could occur at the level of receptors on the target cell. Potentially responsive targets do not necessarily express receptors for a trophic factor at all times and under all circumstances. Receptor levels are likely influenced by a variety of stimuli including hormonal signals, past history of exposure to the trophic factor, and interactions with other trophic factors. The affinity of the receptor may differ among different cell types. Evidence for differences in the kinetics of neuronal and mesenchymal bFGF receptors was presented above. Other studies suggest that neuronal insulin and IGF receptors may also differ somewhat

from those of mesenchymal cells (78-84). Differences in the
domains of laminin and fibronectin preferred by neurons and
mesenchymal cells might also suggest some receptor
heterogeneity (5,85,86). Variations in receptor function might
reflect permanent structural differences from, for example,
differential splicing of mRNA or altered glycosylation.
Differences in kinetics could also reflect transient
modification by processes like phosphorylation. The amount of
second messenger generated by the receptor after interaction
with its ligand is obviously influenced by many other ongoing
cell processes. Among these should be considered actions of
traditional neurotransmitters which likely have important
functions as growth modulators (87).

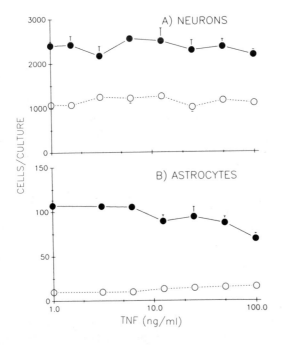

Fig. 2 Effects of TNF alpha on neurons (A) and astrocytes (B) in hippocampal cultures. Astrocytes were identified by immunohistochemistry for glial fibrillary acidic protein. Open circles: control conditions. Solid circles: + 1 mg/ml bFGF.

Finally the interactions among individual agents in
complexes of trophic factors are likely to be extremely
important (12). An illustrative example uses tumor necrosis
factor alpha (TNF alpha), a factor which among its many
actions inhibits endothelial cell proliferation in response to
bFGF (88,89). Over the same concentration range, TNF appears
to have no deleterious effects on either neuronal survival or
process outgrowth in response to bFGF (Figs. 2A and 3).

But like endothelial cells, astrocytes appear to be inhibited by TNF so that less proliferation occurs in response to bFGF (Fig 2B). Thus under these particular culture conditions, the combination of TNF and bFGF appears to be a more specific stimulus for neuronal growth than bFGF alone.

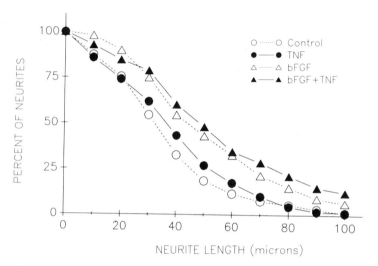

Fig. 3 Effects of TNF alpha on process outgrowth. Neurons were grown for 24 hours in the presence of TNF (100 ng/ml) or bFGF (1 ng/ml) as appropriate. Neurite length was measured on 150 cells grown under each condition. bFGF vs. control, $P<0.01$, chi square. No significant differences with TNF.

The recognition that pleiotropic factors might serve as NTFs greatly increases the number of NTFs available for investigation. Studies on the function of these factors are likely to lead to new insights into pathology, including both degenerative and reparative responses. The number of agents available for consideration as potential experimental therapies also increases greatly. However, application of multifunctional trophic factors in neurobiology and neurology may have to wait until methods can be developed for restricting and controlling the potential range of action of pleiotropic agents.

REFERENCES

1. Stewart, S.S. and Appel, S.H. (1988) Trophic factors in neurologic disease. Ann. Rev. Med. 39: 193-201.
2. Thoenen, H. and Edgar, D. (1985) Neurotrophic factors. Science 229: 238-242.
3. Levi-Montalcini, R. (1987) The nerve growth factor 35 years later. Science 237: 1154-1162.
4. Whittemore, S.R. and Seiger, A. (1987) The expression, localization and functional significance of B-nerve growth factor in the central nervous system. Brain Res. Rev. 12: 439-464.
5. Walicke, P.A. (1989) Novel neurotrophic factors, receptors and oncogenes. Ann. Rev. Neurosci. 12: 103-126.
6. Barde, Y.A. (1988) What, if anything, is a neurotrophic factor?. TINS 11: 343-346.
7. Gospodarowicz, D., Neufeld, G. and Schweigerer, L. (1986) Molecular and biological characterization of fibroblast growth factor, an angiogenic factor which also controls the proliferation and differentiation of mesoderm and neuroectoderm derived cells. Cell Differ 19: 1-17.
8. Baird, A. and Bohlen, P. (1989) Fibroblast growth factors. In: Handbook of Experimental Pharmacology, edited by Sporn,M. and Roberts, A. New York: Springer-Verlag,in press.
9. Walicke, P.A. and Baird, A. (1988) Trophic effects of fibroblast growth factor on neural tissue. Prog. Brain Res. in press.
10. Baird, A. and Walicke, P.A. (1989) Fibroblast growth factors. Brit. Med. Bull. 45: 438-452.
11. Davies, A.M. (1988) Role of neurotrophic factors in development. Trends in Genetics 4: 139-143.
12. Sporn, M.B. and Roberts, A.B. (1988) Peptide growth factors are multifunctional. Nature 332: 217-219.
13. Walicke, P.A. and Baird, A. (1988) Neurotrophic effects of basic and acidic fibroblast growth factors are not mediated through glial cells. Dev. Brain Res. 40: 71-79.
14. Hatten, M.E., Lynch, M., Rydel, R.E., Sanchez, J., Joseph-Silverstein, J., Moscatelli, D. and Rifkin, D.B. (1988) In vitro neurite extension by granule neurons is dependent upon astroglial-derived fibroblast growth factor.Dev. Biol. 125: 280-289.
15. Unsicker, K., Reichert-Preibsch, H., Schmidt, R., Pettmann, B., Labourdette, G. and Sensenbrenner, M. (1987) Astroglial and fibroblast growth factors have neurotrophic functions for cultured peripheral and central nervous system neurons. Proc. Natl. Acad. Sci. USA 84: 5459-5463.
16. Walicke, P.A., Feige, J.J. and Baird, A. (1989) Characterization of the neuronal receptor for basic fibroblast growth factor (bFGF): Comparison to mesenchymalcell receptors. J. Biol. Chem. 264: 4120-4126.
17. Walicke, P.A., Harrison, C. and Baird, A. (1989) Basic fibroblast growth factor is internalized and metabolized into specific peptides by CNS neurons and glia. Submitted.
18. Finklestein, S.P., Apostolides, P.J., Caday, C.G., Prosser, J., Philips, M.F. and Klagsbrun, M. (1988) Increased basic fibroblast growth factor (bFGF) immunoreactivity at the site of focal brain wounds. Brain Res. 460: 253-259.

19. Pettmann, B., Labourdette, G., Weibel, M. and Sensenbrenner, M. (1986) The brain fibroblast growth factor (FGF) is localized in neurons. Neurosci. Lett. 68: 175-180.

20. Janet, T., Miehe, M., Pettmann, B., Labourdette, G. and Sensenbrenner, M. (1987) Ultrastructural localization of fibroblast growth factor in neurons of rat brain. Neurosci. Lett. 80: 153-157.

21. Walicke, P.A. (1989) New neurotrophic agents: Fibroblast growth factor. Rev. Esp. Neurol. 4: 253-259.

22. Esch, F., Baird, A., Ling, N., Ueno, N., Hill, F., Denoroy, L., Klepper, R., Gospodarowicz, D., Bohlen, P. and Guillemin, R. (1985) Primary structure of bovine pituitary basic fibrolast growth factor (FGF) and comparison with the amino-terminal sequence of bovine brain acidic FGF. Proc. Natl. Acad. Sci. USA 82: 6507-6511.

23. Emoto, N., Walicke, P., Baird, A. and Simmons, D. (1989) Expression of Basic FGF RNA in Brain. Submitted.

24. Abraham, J.A., Mergia, A., Whang, J.L., Tumolo, A., Friedman, J., Hjerrild, K.A., Gospodarowicz, D. and Fiddes, J.C. (1986) Nucleotide sequence of a bovine clone encoding the angiogenic protein, basic fibroblast growth factor. Science 233: 545-548.

25. Ferrara, N., Ousley, F. and Gospodarowicz, D. (1988) Bovine brain astrocytes express basic fibroblast growth factor, a neurotropic and angiogenic mitogen. Brain Res. 462: 223-232.

26. Sievers, J., Hausmann, B., Unsicker, K. and Berry, M. (1987) Fibroblast growth factors promote the survival of adult rat retinal ganglion cells after transection of the optic nerve. Neurosci. Lett. 76: 157-162.

27. Anderson, K.J., Dam, D., Lee, S. and Cotman, C.W. (1988) Basic fibroblast growth factor prevents death of lesioned cholinergic neurons in vivo. Nature 332: 360-361.

28. Walicke, P.A., Cowan, W.M., Ueno, N., Baird, A. and Guillemin, R. (1986) Fibroblast growth factor promotes survival of dissociated hippocampal neurons and enhances neurite extension. Proc. Natl. Acad. Sci. USA 83: 3012-3016.

29. Morrison, R.S., Sharma, A., de Vellis, J. and Bradshaw, R.A. (1986) Basic fibroblast growth factor supports the survival of cerebral cortical neurons in primary culture. Proc. Natl. Acad. Sci. USA 83: 7537-7541.

30. Walicke, P.A. (1988) Basic and acidic fibroblast growth factors have trophic effects on neurons from multiple CNS regions. J. Neurosci. 8: 2618-2627.

31. Ferrari, G., Minozzi, M.-C., Toffano, G., Leon, A. and Skaper, S.D. (1989) Basic fibroblast growth factor promotes the survival and development of mesencephalic neurons in culture. Dev. Biol. 133: 140-147.

32. Hefti, F. (1989) Function of neurotrophic factors in the adult and aging brain and their possible use in the treatment of neurodegenerative diseases. Neurobiol. of Aging, in press.

33. Lipton, S.A., Wagner, J.A., Madison, R.D. and D'Amore, P.A. (1988) Acidic fibroblast growth factor enhances regeneration of processes by postnatal mammalian retinal ganglion cells in culture. Proc. Natl. Acad. Sci. USA 85: 2388-2392.

34. Schubert, D., Ling, N. and Baird, A. (1987) Multiple influences of a heparin-binding growth factor on neuronal development. <u>J. Cell Biol</u>. 108: 635-643.

35. Stemple, D.L., Mahanthappa, N.K. and Anderson, D.J. (1988) Basic FGF induces neuronal differentiation, cell division, and NGF dependence in chromaffin cells: A sequence of events in sympathetic development. <u>Neuron</u> 1: 517-525.

36. Rydel, R.E. and Greene, L.A. (1987) Acidic and basic fibroblast growth factors promote stable neurite outgrowth and neuronal differentiation in cultures of PC12 cells. <u>J. Neurosci</u>. 7: 3639-3653.

37. Neufeld, G., Gospodarowicz, D., Dodge, L. and Fujii, D.K. (1987) Heparin modulation of the neurotrophic effects of acidic and basic fibroblast growth factors and nerve growth factor on PC12 cells. <u>J. Cell. Physiol</u>. 131: 131-140.

38. Walicke, P.A. (1988) Interactions between basic fibroblast growth factor (FGF) and glycosoaminoglycans in promoting neurite outgrowth. <u>Exp. Neurol</u>. 102: 144-148.

39. Perraud, F., Labourdette, G., Miehe, M., Loret, C. and Sensenbrenner, M. (1988) Comparison of the morphological effects of acidic and basic fibroblast growth factors on rat astroblasts in culture. <u>J. Neurosci. Res</u>. 20: 1-11.

40. Morrison, R.S., de Vellis, J., Lee, Y.L., Bradshaw, R.A. and Eng, L.F. (1985) Hormones and growth factors induce the synthesis of glial fibrillary acidic protein in rat brain astrocytes. <u>J. Neurosci. Res</u>. 14:167-176.

41. Eccleston, P.A. and Silberberg, D.H. (1985) Fibroblast growth factor is a mitogen for oligodendrocytes <u>in vitro</u>. <u>Dev. Brain Res</u>. 21: 315-318.

42. Saneto, R.P. and de Vellis, J. (1985) Characterization of cultured rat oligodendrocyhes proliferating in a serum-free, chemically defined medium. <u>Proc. Natl. Acad. Sci</u>. USA 82: 3509-3513.

43. Gospodarowicz, D., Neufeld, G. and Schweigerer, L. (1986) Fibroblast growth factor. <u>Molec. Cell. Endocrinol</u>. 46:187-204.

44. Moscatelli, D. (1987) High and low affinity binding sites for basic fibroblast growth factor on cultured cells: absence of a role for low affinity binding in the stimulation of plasminogen activator production by bovine capillary endothelial cells. <u>J. Cell. Physiol</u>. 131: 123-130.

45. Moscatelli, D. (1988) Metabolism of receptor-bound and matrix-bound basic fibroblast growth factor by bovine capillary endothelial cells. <u>J. Cell Biol</u>. 107: 753-759.

46. Carpenter, G. (1987) Receptors for epidermal growth factor and other polypeptide mitogens. <u>Ann. Rev. Biochem</u>. 56:881-914.

47. Matthew, W.D., Greenspan, R.J., Lander, A.D. and Reichardt, L.F. (1985) Immunopurification and characterization of a neuronal heparan sulfate proteoglycan. <u>J. Neurosci</u>. 5:1842-1850.

48. Chiu, A.Y., Matthew, W.D. and Patterson, P.H. (1986) A monoclonal antibody that blocks the activity of a neurite regeneration-promoting factor: studies on the binding site and its localization <u>in vivo</u>. <u>J. Cell Biol</u>. 102: 1383-1398.

49. Schubert, D., Schroeder, R., LaCorbiere, M., Saitoh, T. and Cole, G. (1988) Amyloid B protein precursor is possibly a heparan sulfate proteoglycan core protein. <u>Science</u> 241:223-226.

50. Neufeld, G. and Gospodarowicz, D. (1985) The identification and partial characterization of the fibroblast growth factor receptor of baby hamster kidney cells. J. Biol. Chem. 260:13860-13868.
51. Neufeld, G. and Gospodarowicz, D. (1986) Basic and acidic fibroblast growth factors interact with the same cell surface receptors. J. Biol. Chem. 261: 5631-5637.
52. Moenner, M., Chevallier, B., Badet, J. and Barritault, D. (1986) Evidence and characterization of the receptor to eye-derived growth factor I, the retinal form of basic fibroblast growth factor, on bovine epithelial lens cells. Proc. Natl. Acad. Sci. USA 83: 5024-5028.
53. Olwin, B.B. and Hauschka, S.D. (1986) Identification of fibroblast growth factor receptor of Swiss 3T3 cells and mouse skeletal muscle myoblasts. Biochem. 25: 3487-3492.
54. Imamura, T., Tokita, Y. and Mitsui, Y. (1988) Purification of basic FGF receptors from rat brain. Biochem. Biophys. Res. Commun. 155: 583-590.
55. Feige, J.J. and Baird, A. (1988) Glycosylation of the basic fibroblast growth factor receptor: The contribution of carbohydrate to receptor function. J. Biol. Chem. 263:14023-14029.
56. Walicke, P.A., Purcell, I. and Harrison, C. (1989) Glycosylation pattern of the neuronal basic fibroblast growth factor receptor. Submitted.
57. Bouche, G., Gas, N., Prats, H., Baldin, V., Tauber, J.-P., Teissie, J. and Amalric, F. (1987) Basic fibroblast growth factor enters the nucleolus and stimulates the transcription of ribosomal genes in ABAE cells undergoing Go-Gl transition. Proc. Natl. Acad. Sci. USA 84: 6770-6774.
58. Baird, A., Schubert, D., Ling, N. and Guillemin, R. (1988) Receptor and heparin binding domains of basic fibroblast growth factor: Design and synthesis of peptides with partial antagonist activities of an angiogenic factor. Proc. Natl. Acad. Sci. USA 85: 2324-2328.
59. Mormede, P., Baird, A. and Pigeon, P. (1985) Immunoreactive fibroblast growth factor (FGF) in rat tissues: molecular weight forms and the effects of hypohysectomy. Biochem. BiophYs. Res. Commun. 128: 1108-1113.
60. Folkman, J., Klagsbrun, M., Sasse, J., Wadzinski, M., Ingber, D. and Vlodavsky, I. (1988) A heparin-binding angiogenic protein--basic fibroblast growth factor--is stored within basement membrane. Am. J. Pathol. 130:393-400.
61. Presta, M., Foiani, M., Rusnati, M., Joseph-Silverstein, J., Maier, J.A.M. and Ragnotti, G. (1988) High molecular weight immunoreactive basic fibroblast growth factor-like proteins in rat pituitary and brain. Neurosci. Lett. 90: 308-313.
62. Moscatelli, D., Joseph-Silverstein, J., Manejias, M. and Rifkin, D.B. (1987) Mr25,000 heparin-binding protein from guinea pig brain is a high molecular weight form of basic fibroblast growth factor. Proc. Natl. Acad. Sci. USA 84:5778-5782.
63. Presta, M., Rusnati, M., Maier, J.A.M. and Ragnotti, G. (1988) Purification of basic fibroblast growth factor from rat brain: identification of a Mr 22,000 immunoreactive form. Biochem. Biophys. Res. Commun. 155: 1161-1172.

64. Baird, A., Ueno, N., Esch, F. and Ling, N. (1987) Distribution of fibroblast growth factors (FGFs) in tissues and structure-function studies with synthetic fragments of basic FGF. J. Cell. Physiol. Suppl. 5: 101-106.

65. Gospodarowicz, D. and Cheng, J. (1986) Heparin protects basic and acidic FGF from inactivation. J. Cell. Physiol. 128: 475-484.

66. Saksela, O., Moscatelli, D., Sommer, A. and Rifkin, D.B. (1988) Endothelial cell-derived heparan sulfate binds basic fibroblast growth factor and protects it from proteolytic degradation. J. Cell Biol. 107: 743-751.

67. Schweigerer, L., Neufeld, G., Friedman, J., Abraham, J.A., Fiddes, J.C. and Gospodarowicz, D. (1987) Capillary endothelial cells express basic fibroblast growth factor, a mitogen that promotes their own growth. Nature 325: 257-259.

68. Gospodarowicz, D., Ferrara, N., Haaparanta, T. and Neufeld, G. (1988) Basic fibroblast growth factor: expression in cultured bovine vascular smooth muscle cells. Eur. J. Cell Biol. 46: 144-151.

69. Vlodavsky, I., Fridman, R., Sullivan, R., Sasse, J. and Klagsbrun, M. (1987) Aortic endothelial cells synthesize basic fibroblast growth factor which remains cell associated and platelet-derived growth factor-like protein which is secreted. J. Cell Physiol. 131: 402-408.

70. Baird, A. and Ling, N. (1987) Fibroblast growth factors are present in the extracellular matrix produced by endothelial cells in vitro: implications for a role of heparinase-like enzymes in the neovascular response. Biochem. Biophys. Res. Commun. 142: 428-435.

71. Williams, L.R., Varon, S., Peterson, G.M., Wictorin, K., Fischer, W., Bjorklund, A. and Gage, F.H. (1986) Continuous infusion of nerve growth factor prevents basal forebrain neuronal death after fimbria fornix transection. Proc. Natl. Acad. Sci. USA 83: 9231-9235.

72. Kromer, L.F. (1987) Nerve growth factor treatment after brain injury prevents neuronal death. Science 235: 214-235.

73. Hefti, F. (1986) Nerve growth factor promotes survival of septal cholinergic neurons after fimbrial transections. J. Neurosci. 6: 2155-2162.

74. Otto, D., Unsicker, K. and Grothe, C. (1987) Pharmacological effects of nerve growth factor and fibroblast growth factor applied to the transectioned sciatic nerve on neuron death in adult rat dorsal root ganglia. Neurosci. Lett. 83: 156-160.

75. Danielsen, N., Pettmann, B., Vahlsing, H.L., Manthorpe, M. and Varon, S. (1988) Fibroblast growth factor effects on peripheral nerve regeneration in a silicone chamber model. J. Neurosci. Res. 20: 320-330.

76. Hayek, A., Culler, F.L., Beattie, G.M., Lopez, A.D., Cuevas, P. and Baird, A. (1987) An in vivo model for study of the angiogenic effects of basic fibroblast growth factor. Biochem. Biophys. Res. Commun. 147: 876-880.

77. Joseph-Silverstein, J., Moscatelli, D. and Rifkin, D.B. (1988) The development of a quantitative RIA for basic fibroblast growth factor using polyclonal antibodies against the 157 amino acid form of human bFGF. J. Immunol. Methods 110: 183-192.

78. Burgess, S.K., Jacobs, S., Cuatrecasas, P. and Sahyoun, N. (1987) Characterization of a neuronal subtype of insulin-like growth factor receptor. J. Biol. Chem. 262: 1618-1622.

79. Lowe, W.L.Jr., Boyd, F.T., Clarke, D.W., Raizada, M.K., Hart, C. and LeRoith, D. (1986) Development of brain insulin receptors: structural and functional studies of insulin receptors from whole brain and primary cell cultures. Endocrinology 119: 25-35.

80. McElduff, A., Poronnik, P. and Baxter, R.C. (1987) The insulin-like growth factor-II (IGF II) receptor from rat brain is of lower apparent molecular weight than the IGF II receptor from rat liver. Endocrinology 121: 1306-1311.

81. Gammeltoft, S., Staun-Olsen, P., Ottesen, B. and Fahrenkrug, J. (1984) Insulin receptors in rat brain cortex. Kinetic evidence for a receptor subtype in the central nervous system. Peptides 5: 937-944.

82. Shemer, J., Raizada, M.K., Masters, B.A., Ota, A. and LeRoith, D. (1987) Insulin-like growth factor I receptors in neuronal and glial cells. J. Biol. Chem. 262: 7693-7699.

83. Roth, R.A., Morgan, D.O., Beaudoin, J. and Sara, V. (1986) Purification and characterization of the human brain insulin receptor. J. Biol. Chem. 261: 3753-3757.

84. Ciaraldi, T., Robbins, R., Leidy, J.W., Thamm, P. and Berhanu, P. (1985) Insulin receptors on cultured hypothalamic cells: functional and structural differences from receptors on peripheral target cells. Endocrinology 116: 2179-2185.

85. Edgar, D., Timpl, R. and Thoenen, H. (1984) The heparin-binding domain of laminin is responsible for its effects on neurite outgrowth and neuronal survival. EMBO J. 3: 1463-1468.

86. Rogers, S.L., McCarthy, J.B., Palm, S.L., Furcht, L.T. and Letourneau, P.C. (1985) Neuron-specific interactions with two neurite-promoting fragments of fibronectin. J. Neurosci. 5: 369-378.

87. Mattson, M.P. (1988) Neurotransmitters in the regulation of neuronal cytoarchitecture. Brain Res. Rev. 13: 179-212.

88. Schweigerer, L., Malerstein, B. and Gospodarowicz, D. (1987) Tumor necrosis factor inhibits the proliferation of cultured capillary endothelial cells. Biochem. Biophys. Res. Commun. 143: 997-1004.

89. Frater-Schroeder, M., Risau, W., Hallmann, R., Gautschi-Sova, P. and Bohlen, P. (1987) Tumor necrosis factor-alpha, a potent inhibitor of endothelial cell proliferation in vitro, is angiogenic in vivo. Proc. Natl. Acad. Sci. USA 84: 5277-5281.

GROWTH FACTOR AND LYMPHOKINE EFFECTS ON BRAIN CHOLINERGIC SYSTEMS

Dalia M. Araujo, Paul A. Lapchak[*], Jean-Guy Chabot, and Remi Quirion

Douglas Hospital Research Center and Dept. of Psychiatry, McGill University, and *Neuroanatomy Lab., Montreal Neurological Institute, Montreal Quebec, Canada

INTRODUCTION

The localization of various growth factors (GFs) and lymphokines in the mammalian brain (1) has expanded the list of possible roles for these substances. The identification of specific binding sites for GFs such as nerve GF (NGF), epidermal GF(EGF), and the insulin-like GFs (IGF-1 and IGF-2) (2), and for IL-1 (3-5), on cells of glial and neuronal origin have underlined further the importance of GFs and ILs in the mammalian CNS. However, the precise function of these substances in the brain has not been completely elucidated.

The GFs were originally thought to function only as trophic and maintenance factors in the CNS, but it is now evident that GFs display a multitude of functions in the CNS. Under certain circumstances, some GFs have been suggested to act as modulators of neuronal activity. For example, IGF-1 has been shown to alter the release of various neurohormones and neurotransmitters (6-9). IL-1, which was thought to be restricted to the immune system, has been shown to exist in the CNS(1, 10, 11), where it functions as a potent neuromodulator of CNS activity (12-16). In contrast, no such role has been postulated for IL-2. Thus, it is of the utmost importance to determine the significance of GFs and ILs in the brain, and whether they interact with their respective receptors to exert some regulation of neuronal activity.

IGFs AND IGF BINDING SITES IN THE MAMMALIAN BRAIN

Previous studies have demonstrated that IGF-like immunoreactive (IR) material and IGF mRNA can be detected in both fetal (17-20) and adult (21-24) brain tissue. In addition, using either membrane binding (17, 25-28) or receptor autoradiographic techniques (29-31), it has become evident that specific binding sites for IGF-1 and IGF-2 are also present in both fetal and adult brain, although brain structures which are enriched with these sites do not necessarily contain high levels of IGF-like IR material.

Distribution of IGF-1 binding sites in the rat brain

Using autoradiographic analysis of [125I]IGF-1 binding to 20 um thick sections of rat brain tissue, we have shown that specific IGF-1 sites are widely distributed throughout the adult (3-month old) rat brain (Table 1). In the neonatal rat brain (P1), the relative density of specific [125I]IGF-1 binding sites is higher than in the adult, although the distribution of sites appears to be less extensive, with only a few structures labeled (Table 1). The pattern of [125I]IGF-1 labeling in the superficial cortical layers and in the hippocampus is similar in the neonatal compared to the adult rat brain. In contrast, other brain structures such as the striatum and various thalamic nuclei differ in their pattern of distribution of IGF-1 sites in the neonate compared to the adult. In these brain areas in the neonatal rat, specific [125I]IGF-1 binding sites re extremely low or even undetectable (Table 1). Thus, it appears that there is a broader distribution of IGF-1 sites in the adult compared to the neonatal rat brain. Our studies to date indicate that this modification of brain IGF-1 sites that occurs during development may be the result of a change in the apparent affinity or may be due to an increase in the density of sites in certain brain structures. At present, we cannot distinguish between these two possibilities, although recent evidence (28) suggests that the latter is more likely to occur. Furthermore, the differential pattern of localization of IGF-1 sites that appears to occur during brain development and maturation may be indicative of a concomitant modification in the function of these sites. Therefore, in the adult brain, IGF-1 can be classified as more than a trophic and maintenance factor.

TABLE 1. [125I]IGF-1 binding sites in selected regions of the rat brain

Brain region	IGF-1 binding (fmol/mg tissue wet wt.)	
	Adult (3-month old)	Neonate (P1)
Cortical laminae	8.2 + 0.7	32.4 + 6.4
Caudate/putamen	4.6 + 0.9	ND
Nucleus accumbens	8.4 + 1.8	25.6 + 0.7
Hippocampus	12.7 + 1.0	25.8 + 0.7
Thalamus	10.0 + 1.2	0.7 + 0.3

Quantitaive analysis of autoradiographic data using computerized densitometry. Sections (20 um) were incubated with 50 pM [125I]IGF-1. Non-specific binding, assessed using 100 nM unlabeled IGF-1, was subtracted from all readings. Values are the mean + S. E. M. of 3-9 determinations. ND= not determined.

EGF BINDING SITES IN THE RAT BRAIN

In contrast to IGF-1, we found that specific binding of
[125I]EGF appears to be restricted to a few regions of the
early post-natal (P3) rat brain (not shown). [125I]EGF
binding sites seem to be localized mostly to cortical areas,
with few sites observed in the striatum and septum, and
fewer still in the hippocampus. Similarly, only low densities of EGF sites were seen in the adult rat brain (not
shown). However, using antibodies specific for the EGF
receptor, it has been shown that EGF receptors are present
in the adult rat brain, although in much lower densities
than in younger animals (32). The apparent discrepancy
between this finding and our results using the autoradiographic analysis of [125I]EGF binding is not clear but is
the subject of future studies.

IL-2 and IL-2 BINDING SITES IN THE RAT BRAIN

IL-1 has been suggested to be synthesized and released
from within brain structures (33-36). In addition, a widespread distribution of specific IL-1 sites within the mammalian brain has been clearly demonstrated (3-5). However,
the localization of other ILs, such as IL-2, and their
respective specific receptor sites within the rat brain have
not been extensively investigated.

Using a radioimmunoassay (RIA) with antibodies specific
for IL-2, we showed the presence of IL-2-like IR material in
various regions of the rat brain (37). Of the extracts of
brain tissue tested, IR material was most concentrated in
hippocampus and striatum and least in the cerebral cortex
(Table 2). Autoradiographic analysis of the distribution of
[125I]IL-2 binding sites revealed a pattern of binding that
was limited to a few regions of the rat brain. Quantitative
analysis of the binding data showed relatively dense
[125I]IL-2 labeling in the hippocampus, where there was a
discrete pattern of IL-2 sites (Table 3). Low densities of
IL-2 sites were observed in other brain structures such as
the cerebral cortex, striatum, cerebellum, septum, and
thalamus. In rats unilaterally lesioned with kainic acid,
so as to destroy intrinsic innervation, the density of IL-2
sites was significantly increased in the lesioned compared
to the contralateral (control) hippocampi (Table 3). Thus,
it is apparent that lesioning may up-regulate the density of
specific IL-2 sites in the hippocampus.

TABLE 2. IL-2-like IR material in the rat brain

Brain region	IR material (ng/mg tissue)
Hippocampus	0.72 + 0.06
Striatum	0.65 + 0.07
Cortex	0.12 + 0.01

IL-2-like IR material was measured in extracts of
brain tissue. Results are the mean + S.E.M. of 10
determinations.

TABLE 3. IL-2 binding sites in the rat brain

Brain region	IL-2 binding (fmol/mg tissue wet wt.)
Intact rats	
Hippocampus	1.7 ± 0.1
Kainate-lesioned rats	
Lesioned hippocampus	2.7 ± 0.2
Intact contralateral hippocampus	1.6 ± 0.2

Quantitative analysis of the autoradiographic distribution of [125I]IL-2 binding to sections (20 um) of rat brain. Sections were incubated with 50 pM [125I]IL-2 and non-specific binding was assessed in the presence of 10 nM unlabeled IL-2. Specific binding in other brain regions was excessively low or non-detectable. Values are the mean ± S.E.M. of 4-8 determinations.

In the hippocampus, there appears to be a positive correlation between the level of IL-2 sites and that of IL-2-like IR material. This suggests that IL-2, by acting on its specific receptor, may be involved in the modulation of hippocampal activity. Similarly, in the frontal cortex, where low levels of IL-2-like IR material were measured, low densities of specific IL-2 sites were also seen. However, there appears to be an apparent discrepancy between the measured IL-2-like IR material (high) and the density of IL-2 sites (not detectable) in the striatum. The reasons for this apparent discrepancy are not clear, but it is possible that the IL-2 contained within the rat striatum is not involved in the local regulation of neuronal activity (see below).

ACUTE EFFECTS OF GFs ON ACETYLCHOLINE (ACh) RELEASE FROM RAT BRAIN SLICES

Presently, the significance of and possible function of GFs in the adult brain are not clear, although there is increasing evidence for a possible neuromodulatory role for GFs in adult brain. IGF-1, for example, has been shown to enhance ACh release from slices of rat cerebral cortex (8), to inhibit the in vivo release of growth hormone from hypothalamus (6), and to alter somatostatin release from hypothalamic cell cultures (7).

Effects of IGF-1 on ACh release

In our study, we investigated the possible effects of IGF-1 on cholinergic nerve terminal activity in slices of rat brain. The rationale for this study was that the hippocampus, which is enriched with cholinergic nerve terminals (38, 39) and ACh receptors (40), is also densely labeled with [125I]GF-1 (see above). Our results demonstrate that IGF-1 significantly reduces the release of endogenous ACh evoked by a high concentration of potassium (25 mM) from slices of adult rat hippocampus (Table 4). Moreover, the IGF-1-induced decrease in ACh release is not seen in slices

TABLE 4. Effects of various GFs on ACh release from slices of adult rat brain

GF (uM)	Evoked ACh release (%control)	
	Hippocampus	Frontal cortex
IGF-1		
0.5	84 + 8	104 + 5
1	77 + 3	109 + 8
IGF-2		
0.1	103 + 7	ND
0.5	111 + 10	ND
Insulin		
1	98 + 8	ND
100	115 + 12	ND
EGF		
0.5	78 + 6	96 + 6
1	73 + 6	101 + 9
5	68 + 7	114 + 16
NGF		
0.1	104 + 10	ND
0.5	101 + 6	ND

Slices were depolarized with high-potassium (25 mM) Krebs medium and incubated in the presence or absence (control) of GF. Values are the mean + S.E.M. of 5-8 experiments.

of frontal cortex (Table 4), implying a regional specificity for the IGF-1 reduction of ACh release.

Analysis of the data obtained from the binding of [125I]IGF-1 to sections of rat brain clearly demonstrated that some modifications in the site distribution occur with development and maturation (see Table 1). However, it was not completely evident whether these changes would be reflected in altered receptor function. Thus, we determined whether the effect of IGF-1 on hippocampal ACh release was also apparent in immature rat brain. In hippocampal slices from 6- and 18-day old rats, IGF-1 did not affect evoked ACh release (range: 94-118 % of control). Therefore, it appears that at least some modifications in IGF-1 receptor site function occur with brain maturation. Specifically, it seems clear that the ability of the IGF-1 receptor to regulate the stimulated release of ACh from hippocampus occurs only in the adult rat brain.

Effects of EGF on ACh release

Although EGF receptor sites have been found in the cortex of adult rats (32), the existence of receptor sites specific for EGF in the adult hippocampus have not yet been conclusively demonstrated (29). However, we found exogenous EGF to decrease the potassium-evoked release of ACh from hippocampal, but not cortical, slices of adult rat; this effect was dependent of the concentration of EGF tested (Table 4). Whether this effect of EGF is mediated by a specific EGF receptor awaits the development of more sensitive probes with which to visualize the receptor. Clearly though, the EGF-induced reduction of ACh release from adult rat hippocampus cannot be considered a non-specific artefact since the GF did not affect ACh release from hippocampal slices of 6- and 18-day old rats (range: 96-108% of control). Therefore, the list of functions attributable to EGF, such as acting as a trophic and maintenance factor (42), can be enlarged to include a neuromodulatory function, at least in the adult rat brain.

Effects of other GFs on ACh release

IGF-2 and insulin, both of which are weak competitors for the type-1 IGF-1 receptor site (26, 41) did not affect ACh release from either adult or immature rat brain slices (Table 4). Thus, the reduction of evoked ACh release from hippocampus induced by IGF-1 appears to be mediated by a receptor specific for IGF-1, the type-1 IGF receptor (41). Similarly, NGF was ineffective in altering either the basal or the evoked release of ACh from hippocampal slices (Table 4).

EFFECTS OF ILs ON ACh RELEASE FROM RAT BRAIN

An increasing body of literature points to the ILs as mediators of brain-immune interactions (3, 33-35, 43). The co-localization of high levels of IL-2-like IR material and IL-2 sites in the hippocampus provided the first evidence that neuronal-immune interaction might occur in this structure of the rat brain (37). Moreover, IL-2 significantly depressed the potassium-evoked release of ACh from hippocampal slices (Table 5). This IL-2 effect was apparent with nanomolar concentrations of the lymphokine (Table 5). In slices of rat cerebral cortex or striatum, IL-2 did not significantly change ACh release (range: 91-119% of control). Other lymphokines tested, such as IL-1, IL-4 (Table 5) and γ-interferon (γ-IFN) did not affect ACh release from hippocampal slices. Thus, in rat hippocampus, IL-2 inhibits ACh release by interacting with its specific receptor.

TABLE 5. Effects of various lymphokines on ACh release from rat hippocampal slices

Lymphokine (nM)	Evoked ACh release (%control)
IL-2	
1	71 + 5
5	64 + 5
10	57 + 2
IL-1	
10	97 + 8
100	109 + 7
IL-4	
10	91 + 10
100	102 + 8

Slices were incubated with or without (control) an IL. Values are the mean ± S.E.M. of 5 experiments.

158

Our results support the hypothesis that in the hippocampus, IL-2 may function as a modulator of presynaptic
cholinergic function. However, it remains to be determined
under what physiological conditions such regulation of hippocampal ACh release might be of significance. There is
some evidence that in response to injury, there is an
increase in glial mitogenic activity and in IL-2 content of
brain and microglia (44, 45). The exact mechanism of this
effect and the importance of IL-2-induced reductions in
hippocampal ACh release in this remain to be elucidated.

FUTURE FOR GFs AND ILs IN THE POTENTIAL DIAGNOSIS AND THERAPY OF CNS DISEASES

At present, the potential benefit of GF therapy in the
treatment of degenerative diseases of the CNS is a subject
of controversy. So far, NGF seems to be most likely candidate for clinical trials in Alzheimer's disease (AD). NGF
has been shown to promote survival of forebrain cholinergic
neurons in vivo (46), prevent some effects of chemical
lesions on cortical cholinergic markers (47), and ameliorate
spatial memory impairment in aged rats (48). Fibroblast GF
(FGF) has also been shown to prevent the death of lesioned
cholinergic neurons in vivo in the rat basal forebrain (49).
Thus, the enthusiasm with which potential use of NGF or FGF
therapy in AD is being approached seems warranted. However,
a certain amount of caution needs to be exercised as well
because recent studies have suggested that the resultant
nerve sprouting generated by GFs such as NGF and FGF may be
detrimental rather than helpful in AD (50).

The possible benefits of other GFs in the treatment of
CNS diseases have not been characterized extensively.
Although both EGF (41) and IGF-1 (19, 51) act as mitogens in
CNS cultures, their effects on neuronal survival and/or
regeneration require further study. Our results on the
reduction of hippocampal ACh release by IGF-1 and EGF sug-
gest that the possibility of chronic treatment with either
GF may present certain difficulties.

Although IL-1 and -2 have been implicated in the body's
response to CNS trauma (44, 45), it is not apparent whether
the ILs may be beneficial in the treatment of CNS degenerative diseases. In a recent study, microglia reactive to
monoclonal antibodies against IL-2 receptors were shown to
be particularly concentrated around senile plaques and
around degenerating tissue in post-mortem AD brains (52).
Thus, identifying regions of the human brain that are highly
concentrated with IL-2 sites may provide a useful diagnostic
tool with which to study the severity and the progression of
AD.

Acknowledgments

This work was supported by the Medical Research Council
of Canada and the Fonds de Recherches en Sante du
Quebec.

References

1. Pimentel, E.: Hormones, Growth Factors and Oncogenes. CRC Press Inc., Boca Raton, Florida, 1987.
2. Herschmann, H. R.: Polypeptide growth factors and the CNS. Trends Neurosci. 9, 53-57, 1986.
3. Farrar W. L., Hill J. M., Harel-Bellan A., Vinocur M.: The immune logical brain. Immunol. Rev. 100 361-378, 1987.
4. Farrar W. L., Kilian P. L., Ruff M. R., Hill J. M., Pert C. B.: Visualization and characterization of interleukin 1 receptors in brain. J. Immunol. 139 459-468, 1987.
5. Hill J. M., Lesniak M. A., Pert C. B.: Co-localization of IGF-II receptors, IL-1 receptors and Thy 1.1 in rat brain. Peptides 9, suppl. 1 in press.
6. Berelowitz M., Szabo M., Frohman L. A., Firestone S., Chu L., Hintz R. L.: Somatomedin-C mediates growth hormone negative feedback by effects on both the hypothalamus and the pituitary. Science 212 1279-1281, 1981.
7. Tannenbaum G. S., Guyda H. J., Posner B. I.: Insulin-like growth factors: a role in growth hormone negative feedback and body weight regulation. Science 220 77-79, 1983.
8. Nilsson L., Sara V. R., Nordberg A.: Insulin-like growth factor 1 stimulates the release of acetylcholine from rat cortical slices. Neuroscience Lett. 88 221-226, 1988.
9. Araujo D. M., Lapchak P. A., Collier B., Chabot J.-G., Quirion R.: Insulin-like growth factor-1 (somatomedin C) rceptors in the rat brain: distribution and interaction with the hippocampal cholinergic system. Brain Res. 484: 130-138, 1989.
10. Claman, H. N.: The biology of the immune response. JAMA 258 2834-2840, 1987.
11. Dinarello C. A., Mier J. W.: Lymphokines. New Eng. J. Med. 317 940-945, 1987.
12. Dinarello C. A., Bernheim H.: Ability of human leukocytic pyrogen to stimulate brain prostaglandin synthesis in vitro. J. Neurochem. 37 702-708, 1981.
13. Dinarello, C. A.: Interleukin 1. Rev Infect. Dis. 6, 51-95, 1984.
14. Bernton E. W., Beach J. E., Holaday J. W., Smallridge R. C., Fein H. G.: Release of multiple hormones by a direct action of interleukin 1 on pituitary cells. Science 238 519-521, 1987.
15. Sapolsky R., Rivier C., Yamamoto G., Plotsky P., Vale W.: Interleukin 1 stimulates the secretion of hypothalamic corticotropin-releasing factor. Science 238 522-524, 1987.
16. Berkenbosch F., van Oers J., del Rey A., Tilders F., Besedovsky H.: Release of multiple hormones by a direct action of interleukin 1 on pituitary cells. Science 238 524-526, 1987.
17. Sara V. R., Hall K., Von Holtz H., Misaki M., Pryklund L., Christensen N., Wetterberg L.: Ontogenesis of somatomedin and insulin receptors in the human fetus. J. Clin. Invest. 71 1094-1097, 1983.
18. Sara V. R., Carlsson-Skwirut C., Andersson C., Hall E., Sjogren B., Holmgren A., Jornvall H.: Characterization of somatomedins from human fetal brain: identification of a variant form of insulin-like growth factor-I. Proc.

Natl. Acad. Sci. USA <u>83</u> 4904-4907, 1986.

19. Han V. K. M., Lauder J. M., D'Ercole A. J.: Characterization of somatomedin/insulin-like growth factor receptors and correlation with biologic action in cultured neonatal rat astroglial cells. J. Neurosci. <u>7</u> 501-511, 1987.

20. Rotwein P., Burgess S. K., Milbrandt J. D., Krause J. E.: Differential expression of insulin-like growth factor genes in rat central nervous system. Proc. Natl. Acad. Sci. USA <u>85</u> 265-269, 1988.

21. Lund P. K., Moats-Staats B. M., Hynes M. A., Simmons J. G., Jansen M., D'Ercole A. J., Van Wyk J. J.: Somatomedin-C/insulin-like growth factor-I and insulin-like growth factor-II mRNAs in rat fetal and adult tissues. J. biol. Chem. <u>261</u> 14539-14544, 1986.

22. Mathews L. S., Norstedt G., Palmiter R. D.: Regulation of insulin-like growth factor I gene expression by growth hormone. Proc. Natl. Acad. Sci. USA <u>83</u> 9343-9347, 1986.

23. Noguchi T., Kurata L. M., Sugisaki T.: Presence of a somatmedin-C-immunoreactive substance in the central nervous system. Neuroendocrinol. 46 277-282, 1987.

24. Hansson H. A., Nilsson A., Isgaard J., Billig H., Isaksson O., Skottner A., Andersson I. K., Rozell B.: Immunohistochemical localization of insulin-like growth factor I in the adult rat. Histochem. <u>89</u> 403-410, 1988.

25. Goodyer C. G., de Stephano L., Lai W. H., Guyda H. J., Posner B. I.: Characterization of insulin-like growth factor receptors in rat anterior pituitary, hypothalamus, and brain. Endocrinology <u>114</u> 1187-1195, 1984.

26. Gammeltoft S., Haselbacher G. K., Humbel R. E., Fehlman M., Van Obberghen E.: Two types of receptor for insulin-like growth factors in mammalian brain. EMBO J. <u>4</u> 3407-3412, 1985.

27. Rosenfeld R. G., Pham H., Keller B. T., Borchardt R. T., Pardridge W. M.: Demonstration and structural comparison of receptor for insulin-like growth factor-I and -II (IGF-I and -II) in brain and blood-brain barrier. Biochem. Biophys. Res. Comm. <u>149</u> 159-166, 1987.

28. Pomerance M., Gavaret J.-M., Jacquemin C., Matricon C., Toru-Delbauffe D., Pierre M.: Insulin and insulin-like growth factor 1 receptors during postnatal development of rat brain. Dev. Brain Res. <u>42</u> 77-83, 1988.

29. Quirion R., Araujo D., Nair N. V. P., Chabot J.-G.: Visualization of growth factor receptor sites in rat forebrain. Synapse <u>2</u>: 212-218, 1988.

30. Baskin D. G., Wilcox B. J., Figlewicz D. P., Dorsa D. M.: Insulin and insulin-like growth factors in the CNS. Trends Neurosci. <u>11</u>, 107-111, 1988.

31. Bohannon N. J., Corp E. S., Wilcox B. J., Figlewicz D. P., Dorsa D. M., Baskin D. G.: Localization of binding sites for insulin-like growth factor I (IGF-I) in the rat brain by quantitative autoradiography. Brain Res. <u>444</u> 205-213, 1988.

32. Gomez-Pinilla F., Knauer D. J., Nieto-Sampedro M.: Epidermal growth factor receptor immunoreactivity in rat brain. Development and cellular localization. Brain Res. <u>438</u> 385-390, 1988.

33. Fontana A., Kristensen F., Dubs R., Gemsa D., Weber E.: Production of prostaglandin E and an interleukin-1 like factor by cultured astrocytes and C6 glioma cells. J. Immunol. <u>129</u> 2413-2419, 1982.

34. Fontana A., Grob P., Lymphokine Res. 3 11-25, 1984.
35. Giulian D., Baker T. J., Shih L.-C. N., Lachman L. B.: Interleukin 1 of the central nervous system is produced by ameboid microglia. J. Exp. Med. 164 594-604, 1986.
36. Breder C. D., Dinarello C. A., Saper C. B.: Interleukin 1 immunoreactive innervation of the human hypothalamus. Science 240 321-324, 1988.
37. Araujo D., Lapchak P. A., Collier B., Quirion R.: Interleukin-2-like immunoreactivity and interleukin-2 receptors in the rat brain: interaction with the cholinergic system. Brain Res. in press.
38. Fibiger, H. C.: The organization and some projections of cholinergic neurons of the mammalian forebrain. Brain Res. Rev. 4 327-388, 1982.
39. Mesulam M. M., Mufson E. J., Wainer B. H., Levey A. I.: Central cholinergic pathways in the rat: an overview based on an alternative nomenclature (Ch1-Ch6). Neuroscience 10 1185-1201, 1985.
40. Quirion R., Araujo D., Regenold W., and Boksa P.: Characterization and quantitative autoradiographic distribution of [3H]acetylcholine muscarinic receptors in mammalian brain. Apparent labelling of an M2-like receptor sub-type. Neuroscience 29: 271-289, 1989.
41. Rechler M. M., Nissley S. P.: The nature and regulation of the receptors for insulin-like growth factors. Annu. Rev. Physiol. 47 425-442, 1985.
42. Morrison R. S., Kornblum H. I., Leslie F. M., Bradshaw R. A.: Trophic stimulation of cultured neurons from neonatal rat brain by epidermal growth factor. Science 238 72-75, 1987.
43. Ballieux R. E., Heijnen C. J.: Brain and immune system: a one-way conversation or a genuine dialogue. In: de Kloet E. R., Wiegant V. M., de Wied D. (eds) Progress in Brain Research vol. 72. Elsevier Science Publishers, Netherlands, 1987, pp 71-77.
44. Nieto-Sampedro M., Chandy K. G.: Interleukin-2-like activity in injured rat brain. Neurochem. Res. 12 723-727, 1987.
45. Nieto-Sampedro M., Saneto R. P., de Vellis J., and Cotman C. W.: The control of glial populations in brain: changes in astrocyte mitogenic and morphogenic factors in response to injury. Brain Res. 323: 320-328, 1985.
46. Hefti, F. J.: Nerve growth factor (NGF) promotes survival of septal cholinergic neurons after fimbrial transections. J. Neurosci. 6 2155-2162, 1986.
47. Haroutunian V., Kanof P. D., Davis K. L.: Partial reversal of lesion-induced deficits in cortical cholinergic markers by nerve growth factor. Brain Res. 386 397-399, 1986.
48. Fischer W., Wictorin K., Bjorklund A., Williams L. R., Varon S., Gage F. H.: Amelioration of cholinergic neuron atrophy and spatial memory impairment in aged rats by nerve growth factor. Nature 329 65-68, 1987.
49. Anderson K. J., Dam D., Lee S., Cotman C. W.: Basic fibroblast growth factor prevents death of lesioned cholinergic neurons in vivo. Nature 332 360-361, 1988.
50. Uchida Y. and Tomonaga M.: Neurotrophic action of Alzheimer's disease brain extract is due to the loss of inhibitory factors for the survival and neurite

formation of cerebral cortical neurons. Brain Res. 481: 190-193, 1989.

51. Shemer J., Raizada M. K., Masters B. A., Ota A., LeRoith D.: Insulin-like growth factor I receptors in neuronal and glial cells: characterization and biological effects in primary culture. J. biol. Chem. 262 7693-7699, 1987.

52. Itagaki S., McGeer P. L., Tago H., McGeer E. G.: Expression of HLA-DR and interleukin-2 receptor on reactive microglia in senile dementia of the Alzheimer type. Soc. Neurosci. Abst. 13 366.15, 1987.

METABOLIC SUPPORT OF NEURAL PLASTICITY:

IMPLICATIONS FOR THE TREATMENT OF ALZHEIMER'S DISEASE

James E. Black and William T. Greenough

Beckman Institute, College of Medicine, Departments of Psychology and
Cell & Structural Biology, and the Neural & Behavioral Biology Program
University of Illinois at Urbana-Champaign, Urbana, IL 61801

Imagine a "magic bullet" for Alzheimer's Disease, i.e., a therapy that would do more than just halt the degeneration--this novel treatment would restore the atrophied neocortex and perhaps even replace some of the lost information. Such a glamorous cure for Alzheimer's disease carries with it a hidden requirement, one that has been relatively neglected in this area of research. The addition of cortical tissue late in life will impose new metabolic demands for synthesis of synaptic connections and the associated dendritic and axonal material. In addition, the volume expansion will tend to dilute metabolic support as the existing capillaries are spread apart. For these reasons any significant restoration of functional cortex will have to include some improvement in its metabolic support.

Over the last few years we have examined the metabolic support of neural plasticity by using the paradigm of differential environmental complexity. This paradigm essentially compares the brains of animals given complex experience with those merely provided the standard laboratory environment. The animals given extensive opportunities to learn typically produce new synaptic connections, as well as new dendritic and axonal processes, all of which are attributed to the storage of learned information. In association with this manifestation of neural plasticity are some changes in glial and microvascular support, particularly the growth of new capillaries. However, the robust angiogenesis of weaning-age animals appears to be substantially impaired by the time they reach middle age, and we suspect that the impaired ability to support neural plasticity may restrict any therapeutic efforts to heal the damage done by Alzheimer's disease.

ANGIOGENESIS IN YOUNG RATS

Our first efforts to study the vascular support of neural plasticity examined weaning-age animals, an age at which the synaptogenesis and cortical volume differences among experimental groups are quite substantial (1). In this study eleven sets of male triplet littermate rats were assigned at weaning age (23-25 days) to one of three experimental conditions for 30 days. Eleven rats were housed together in a complex environment (EC) that consisted of a large cage filled with toys that were changed daily in order to provide an optimal environment for learning. In addition, these rats were placed for an hour each day in a large playpen filled with different toys while the home cage was cleaned. Another 11 rats were paired off in standard cages (SC) without any toys, and the remaining 11 rats were kept individually (IC) in similarly barren cages. Tissue blocks from the occipital cortex were prepared for conventional light and electron microscopy. A prior study of these animals (1) showed that the number of synapses per neuron in the EC rats exceeded that in the IC rat by about 20%. The SC rats had intermediate values significantly different from the EC rats. The increased number of synapses-per-neuron and the lower neuronal density in the EC rats reflect the addition of neuropil and the expansion of cortical volume.

For the microvasculature portion of this large study (2), we used coronal 0.5-μm-thick sections that were stained with toluidine blue and that allowed reliable identification of the empty lumens of blood vessels against the stained tissue background. The upper half of each section and all of the vessel profiles were drawn at a total magnification of x1250. The diameter of each vessel was then measured perpendicular to the longer dimension of the contour, excluding those vessels with irregular or cutoff profiles. Vessels with diameters larger than 10 μm were excluded from the sample, so that nearly all of the remaining vessels were capillaries. Grid overlays were then used to count the number of points over the vessel lumens and the number within the sample areas. The ratio of these two numbers corresponds to the volume fraction of blood in the tissue (3). Because the tissue was fixed while perfused under pressure and essentially all capillaries were open, this value is an estimate of the *maximum* amount of blood that can be in the tissue. Many cerebral capillaries are not perfused in the quietly resting animal, thereby providing the animal with a substantial vascular reserve to call upon when metabolic demands are increased (4). Volume fraction is determined by the distribution of vessel diameters and the spacing of the vessels, two other important vascular parameters. Assuming that the smaller vessels are randomly oriented (5), the mean distance from a random point in tissue to the nearest capillary can calculated from the density of profiles in the sample area (6). This measure is comparable to physiologically meaningful parameters, such as the tissue diffusion distance for metabolites.

The effect of complex experience on the cortical vasculature is summarized in Figure 1. The EC animals had greater blood volume fraction than the SC or IC animals. The mean distance to the nearest capillary was smaller for EC rats than for SC or IC rats. Both large

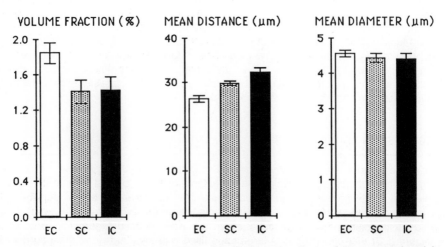

Fig. 1   Group means and standard error bars. Significant main effects of group were found for volume fraction (EC>SC,IC), mean distance from a random point to the nearest capillary (EC<SC<IC), and mean vessel diameter (EC>SC,IC).

and small capillaries contributed to the decreased distance between vessels, as reflected by the density of capillary profiles as a function of vessel diameter (Fig. 2). All of the experimental groups showed very similar distributions of vessel diameter, but mean vessel diameter was slightly greater for EC rats than for SC or IC rats.

The literature suggests that neural plasticity, with its increased metabolic demand, would be supported by hemodynamic changes in these animals rather than by the growth of new vessels. Vascular sprouting in rat cerebral cortex falls off to nearly zero by 21 days of age (7), well before the onset of complex experience and the related synaptogenesis. Furthermore, the blood volume fraction in visual cortex of rats raised in standard laboratory conditions does not increase much from 20 to 55 days, and the density of vessels in upper cortex increases only 5% (5), possibly reflecting the normal shrinkage of neuropil during that period. The finding that EC rats had more dense packing of capillaries in the face of expanding tissue volume was thus unexpected. Previous studies have used rats raised in standard laboratory conditions that may not have imposed additional metabolic demand in visual cortex after weaning, leaving some residual capacity for vascular proliferation unobserved. In contrast, complex experience appears to have stimulated an increase in cortical thickness and synapse production, as well as extension of dendrites, axons, and glia (1, 8,9). The addition of neuropil, with its own very high metabolic requirements (10), also spreads the pre-existing vessels further apart and effectively reduces the quality of vascular support. In these young animals this metabolic challenge was met by substantial production of new capillaries, as suggested by the smaller distance between vessels and the increased density of branch points in the EC rats.

In an extension of this work (11), we examined the branching pattern of the visual cortex capillaries of another set of EC, SC, and IC rats placed in the environments at weaning. By perfusing them with an india ink solution, the elaborate and graceful arcades of vessels can be visualized in 120-μm-thick brain sections. As any new capillary segment starts out as two sprouts that join together, the formation of new capillary branches can be inferred from changes in the volume density of capillary branch points. As predicted from the earlier study, the EC rats had a greater density of branch points, and

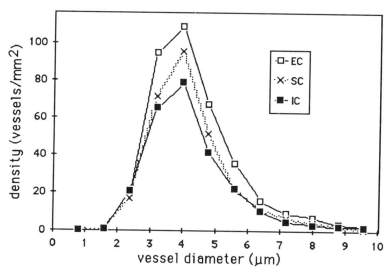

Fig. 2.   Group distributions of vessel density by diameter. EC rats generally have a tighter packing of both large and small vessels.

these branches were spaced closer together along capillary segments, than those of the SC and IC rats. Thus, these young EC rats generated many new capillary segments to infiltrate the expanding cortical volume.

We have also examined the vascular support of neural plasticity in young adult rats (12). These 3-month-old rats were placed in either EC or IC conditions for 10-, 30-, or 60-day periods. The vascular parameters were similar to those described above (2), with the addition of a simple measure of visual cortex thickness. The cortical thickness of the EC rats was significantly thicker after 10 days, corresponding to the earlier findings of synaptogenesis in these animals (13), both of which suggest an expanding tissue volume. The mean distance from a random point in tissue to the nearest capillary, however, was not affected by complex experience. Because vessel spacing was maintained in the face of expanding tissue volume, we suspect that these young adult rats were able to infiltrate the additional neuropil by adding new capillaries. This interpretation is further supported by the finding of many small vessels after 10 days of experience, along with the gradual expansion in vessel size after 30 and 60 days. Apparently new, smaller-diameter vessels were introduced within 10 days, but they had not matured in size until after 30 days. These young adult rats apparently were able to generate new capillaries in response to metabolic demands, but in a less vigorous fashion than was observed in the weanling animals.

IMPAIRED VASCULAR SUPPORT IN MIDDLE AGE

Although synaptogenesis in response to complex experience can occur in old animals, its magnitude appears to be substantially impaired (14,15,16). In order to examine the possible role of angiogensis in this phenomenon, we examined the microvasculature of eight middle-aged (12 months old) and nine old (22 months old) rats kept in EC or SC for 50 days (17). The visual cortex of the middle-aged EC rats was significantly thicker than that of the SC cohorts, and the density of vessels was unaffected (Fig. 3). This pair of findings suggests that new capillaries had infiltrated the expanding tissue while pre-existing vessels were pushed apart. This inference is supported by a dramatic change in vessel size, in which the middle-aged EC rats had many more small-diameter capillaries than the SC cohorts (Fig. 4), much as if immature capillaries had infiltrated the tissue. And the decreased density of large-diameter vessels in the middle-aged EC rats reflects the tissue expansion that spread pre-existing vessels apart. Although the general trends in these parameters were preserved in the older animals, essentially no change had occurred in tissue volume or microvasculature. It appears that the middle-aged animals were perhaps installing new vessels after 50 days, while the younger animals had finished the task in just 30 days. Of course, synaptogenesis and cortical expansion in the old animals may have failed because its metabolic support was inadequate, or it may be that angiogenesis was not called upon because the aging neural plasticity mechanisms had failed for some other reason. This unresolved issue of causality will become important in therapies attempting to reverse the pathology of Alzheimer's disease.

CAN VASCULAR SUPPORT IMPROVE WITHOUT VOLUME CHANGE?

It is not clear at this point whether increased metabolic demand in the absence of volume expansion will similarly elicit angiogenesis. A study in progress is examining the capillaries in the paramedian lobule (PML) of the cerebellum of middle-aged rats (18,19). The cerebellar cortex in this region substantially expands in rats given extensive acrobatic training, but it retains its original volume in rats given considerable repetitive physical exercise. In fact, the most athletic rats in the exercise group had run about 40 kilometers during the one-month experiment, but their PML closely resembled

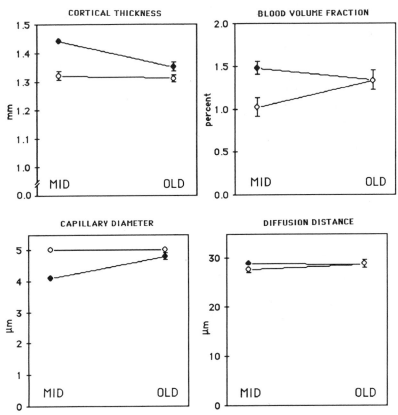

Fig. 3. Group means and standard error bars for cortical thickness, maximum blood volume fraction, capillary diameter, and distance from a random point in tissue to the nearest capillary. Standard error bars were not plotted if they were smaller than the group symbol. EC filled circles; SC open circles.

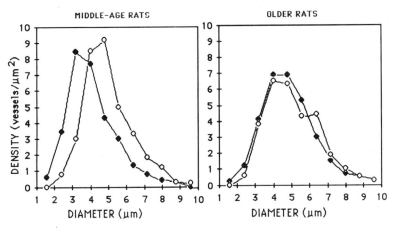

Fig. 4 Distributions of vessel diameter for middle-aged and older rats. EC filled circles; SC open circles.

those of the control rats, which were allowed no exercise at all. Our earlier work with middle-aged rats (17) suggests that angiogenesis in the PML of the acrobatic rats will be impaired, such that the capillary density may be decreased in the expanded cortex or there may be evidence of immature vessels. An intriguing possibility is suggested by the rats that were given considerable physical exercise and did not add many new synapses to this region. They most likely used the existing PML synapses more often than the rats given acrobatic training, and as increased synaptic activity leads to increased sodium transport, for example, the PML of thse animals may have had greater metabolic demands imposed on it without any increase in tissue volume. The increased demand may have been met by hemodynamic changes (e.g., perfusing a greater number of capillaries) or by altering some physical parameter of the microvasculature. It is the latter possibility that we are presently investigating.

SOME IMPLICATIONS FOR THERAPY

In summary, hypertrophy associated with synaptogenesis apparently can elicit angiogenesis in adult rat visual cortex, presumably because such expansion imposes new metabolic demands on the microvasculature. However, the capacity to create new capillaries is impaired substantially by middle age. From our reading of the literature the microvasculature does not appear to be responsible for any aspect of Alzheimer's disease itself. However, we believe that an age-associated impairment of vascular plasticity may severely limit any therapeutic attempts to reverse the pathological changes. Additional studies of vascular adaptation in senescence thus may be an important adjunct to this area of research.

ACKNOWLEDGEMENTS

This research was supported by the Retirement Research Foundation, NIMH 35321 & 43830, and a student scholarship from the Stroke Council of the American Heart Association. We thank the undergraduate students who helped with these studies: Christine Gorman, Devin Shafron, Anthony Zelazny, Michael Polinsky, and Lisa Vinci.

REFERENCES

1. Turner, A. M. and Greenough, W. T. (1985) Differential rearing effects on rat visual cortex synapses. I. Synaptic and neuronal density and synapses per neuron. Brain Research **329**, 195-205.
2. Black, J. E., Sirevaag, A. M. and Greenough, W. T. (1987) Complex experience promotes capillary formation in young rat visual cortex. Neuroscience Letters **83**, 351-355.
3. Weibel, E. R. (1979) Stereological Methods, Vol. 1. Academic Press, New York.
4. Weiss, H. R., Buchweitz, E., Murtha, T. J. and Auletta, M., (1985) Quantitative regional determination of morphometric indices of the total and perfused capillary network in the rat brain. Circulation Research **51**, 494-503.
5. Bar, T. (1980) The Vascular System of the Cerebral Cortex. Springer-Verlag, Berlin.
6. Homer, L. D. (1984) Moments of distributions of distances to the nearest capillary in tissue. Microvascular Research **27**, 114-116.
7. Rowan, R. A. and Maxwell, D. S. (1981) Patterns of vascular sprouting in the postnatal development of the cerebral cortex of the rat. American Journal of Anatomy **160**, 247-255.

8. Sirevaag, A. M. and Greenough, W. T. (1985) Differential rearing effects on rat visual cortex synapses. II. Synaptic morphometry. <u>Developmental Brain Research</u> **19**, 215-226.

9. Sirevaag, A. M. and Greenough, W. T. (1987) Differential rearing effects on rat visual cortex synapses. III. Neuronal and glial nuclei, boutons, dendrites, and capillaries. <u>Developmental Brain Research</u> **424**, 320-332.

10. Mata, M., Fink, D. J., Gainer, H., Smith, C. B., Davidsen, L., Savaki, H., Schwartz, W. J. and Sokoloff, L. (1980) Activity-dependent energy metabolism in rat posterior pituitary primarily reflects sodium pump activity. <u>Journal of Neurochemistry</u> **34**, 213-215.

11. Sirevaag, A. M., Black, J. E., Shafron, D. and Greenough, W. T. (1988) Direct evidence that complex experience increases capillary branching and surface area in visual cortex of young rats. <u>Developmental Brain Research</u> **43**, 299-304.

12. Black, J. E., Zelazny, A. M. and Greenough, W. T. (1988) Complex experience induces capillary formation in visual cortex of adult rats. <u>Society for Neuroscience Abstracts</u> **14**, 1135.

13. Hwang, H.-M. and Greenough, W. T. (1986) Synaptic plasticity in adult occipital cortex following short-term, long-term and reversal of differential housing complexity. <u>Society for Neuroscience Abstracts</u> **12**, 1284.

14. Black, J. E., Parnisari, R., Eichbaum, E. and Greenough, W. T. (1986) Morphological effects of housing environment and exercise on cerebral cortex and cerebellum of old rats. <u>Society for Neuroscience Abstracts</u> **12**, 1579.

15. Conner, J. R., Melone, J. H., Yeun, A. and Diamond, M. C. (1981) Dendritic length in aged rat's occipital cortex: An environmentally induced response. <u>Experimental Neurology</u> **73**, 827-830.

16. Diamond, M. C., Johnson, R. E., Protti, A. M., Ott, C. and Kajisa, L. (1985). PLasticity in the 904-day-old male cerebral cortex. <u>Experimental Neurology</u> **87**, 309-317.

17. Black, J. E., Polinsky, M. and Greenough, W. T. (1989) Progressive failure of cerebral angiogenesis supporting neural plasticity in aging rats. <u>Neurobiology of Aging</u>, in press.

18. Black, J. E., Jones, A. L., Anderson, B. J., Isaacs, K. R., Alcantara, A. A. and Greenough, W. T. (1987) Cerebellar Plasticity: Preliminary evidence that learning, rather than repetitive motor exercise, alters cerebellar cortex thickness in middle-aged rats. <u>Society for Neuroscience Abstracts</u> **13**, 1596.

19. Anderson, B. J., Isaacs, K. R., Black, J. E., Vinci, L., Alcantara, A. A. and Greenough, W. T. (1988) Synaptogenesis in cerebellar cortex after less than 15 hours of visuomotor training over 30 days. <u>Society for Neuroscience Abstracts</u> **14**, 1135.

BRAIN-ENHANCED DELIVERY OF ANTI-DEMENTIA DRUGS

Marcus E. Brewster, Cynthia Robledo-Luiggi[a]
Akio Miyake[b], Emil Pop and Nicholas Bodor[c]

Center for Drug Design and Delivery,
College of Pharmacy, University of Florida
Gainesville, FL 32610

INTRODUCTION

Senile dementia of the Alzheimer's type (SDAT) is a slowly progressive neurological disorder which is characterized by severe and debilitating memory loss. This insidious and pernicious malady is expected to strike 20% of all individuals over the age of eighty (Bartus et al., 1982), an important and growing demographic block. At present the etiological basis of SDAT is unknown and work has been aimed at palliative treatments to increase the quality of life of those individuals stricken with the disease. In SDAT, numerous biochemical/physiological observations have suggested that a cholinergic deficit is in some way related to the disease (Becker and Giacobini, 1988 and references cited therein). Such evidence includes selective degeneration of cholinergic neurons in the basal forebrain, decreased activity and concentration of acetyl choline (ACh), choline acetyltransferase, the enzyme responsible for synthesizing ACh and acetyl cholinesterase (AChE), the enzyme responsible for ACh degradation (Sims et al., 1983). Given this biochemical basis for dementia, therapeutic approach have concentrated on bolstering the impaired cholinergic system either by agonist administration (Corkin, 1981) or by developments of AChE inhibitors. Compounds resulting from the latter scheme have offered the most potential in SDAT and include physostigmine, aminopyridines and 9-amino-1,2,3,4-tetrahydroacridine (THA).

In the case of physostigmine, human clinical experiences have been varied at best (Becker and Giacobini, 1988). While significant improvement in various symptoms has been observed, these ameliorations are not sufficient to return patients to an unsupervised arrangement. In addition, this drug has potent and unpleasant side effects associated with peripheral cholinesterase inhibition and the drug is characterized by a short duration of action. Other AChE inhibitors such as THA offer some advantages over physostigmine but these compounds are also associated with peripheral dose-limiting toxicities and a limited duration of action. Clearly, many of the toxicological aspects of these agents could be

----

*Contribution No. 44 in the series "Improved Delivery Through Biological Membranes.
[a]Present address: University of Puerto Rico, Mayaguez, P.R.
[b]Present address: Takeda Pharmaceuticals, Inc., Osaka, Japan.
[c]To whom all correspondence should be addressed.

avoided or mitigated if the compounds of interest could be selectively delivered to their site of action, i.e., the brain. Such selectivity would decrease untoward peripheral reactions by lowering extratarget tissue drug levels and could increase the efficacy of the administered agent by shunting a larger portion of the administered dose to the central nervous system (CNS). Work by Mattio et al. (1986) in the dog has shown in fact that when physostigmine is introduced directly into the CNS via intrathecal (i.t) administration, peripheral AChE activity is minimally effected compared with intravenous (i.v.) dosing. This administration also produced significantly fewer peripheral side effects. In addition, recent work by Mesulam et al (1987) suggests that AChE inhibitors may behave in qualitatively different ways in the CNS of demented patient compared with normal individuals. This postulate arises from the potent effects of these agents on cholinesterase associated with neuritic plaques and neurofibrillary tangles, the histological hallmarks of SDAT. Given this, the selective delivery of AChE inhibitor becomes even more important. Methods for achieving this type of selectivity without the pain and inconvenience of i.t. dosing would, therefore, be beneficial.

Physostigmine (eserine)   THA

One general method which has proven useful in selectively enhancing drug delivery to the CNS is the chemical delivery system (CDS) (Bodor et al., 1981; Bodor and Brewster, 1983a; Bodor, 1988). The CDS is a carrier-mediated delivery approach in which the drug of interest is transiently attached to a organ-targeting moiety. In the case of CDS designed for the CNS, derivatives of dihydronicotinic acid have been shown to be quite useful as carriers. In practice, an amine or hydroxy containing drug is condensed with a nicotinic acid derivative giving rise to the corresponding nicotinate or nicotinamide. These intermediates are then alkylated with methyl iodide to give the quaternary salt and reduced giving the 1-methyldihydronicotinates or nicotinamides which are termed CDS's. The attachment of this reduced carrier to the drug imparts to the resulting conjugate relatively high lipophilicity and membrane permeability. Upon systemic administration, the lipophile can rapidly and extensively distribute in the body entering many compartments, such as the CNS, some of which may be inaccessible to the unmanipulated drug. With time, the drug-carrier conjugate undergoes an enzymatically-mediated oxidation to generate the quaternary salt form of the drug-carrier conjugate (Figure 1). This derivative is now highly polar and is as much as 100,000-fold more hydrophilic than its dihydro precursor. When this conversion takes place, the peripheral clearance of the carrier complex is accelerated as the charged conjugate becomes an excellent substrate for elimination by the kidney and liver. Paradoxically, this conversion acts to trap the conjugate in the CNS. This occurs because the oxidized carrier drug combination poorly penetrates lipid barriers such as the blood-brain barrier and as a result the species is depoted or "locked-in" the brain. This conversion of the lipophilic membrane permeable transport molecule to a hydrophilic, membrane impermeable form is crucial for CDS operation and is the step which imparts CNS selectivity. In the brain, the trapped conjugate can degrade through hydrolytic means to release the active principle in a slow and sustained fashion. In this scheme, manipulation of the parent compound generally results in a diminution or abolition of pharmacological potency. Thus the transport forms of the drug lack the toxicological potential of the parent compound. This aspect of the CDS provides for the improved therapeutic index afforded by the approach. The overall effect of this method is then to reduce peripheral dose
-related toxicities by providing for rapid elimination of the compounds of interest and at the

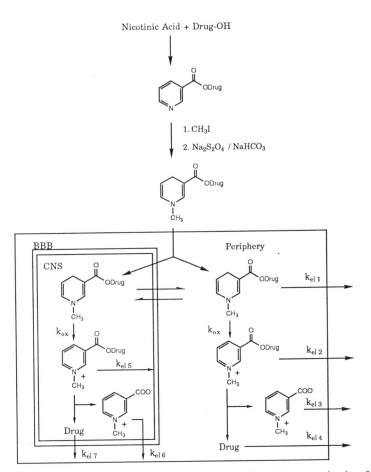

Figure 1. In the CDS, a drug is condensed with nicotinic acid, quaternized to form trigonellinate salt and reduced to give the CDS. Systemic administration of this CDS results in extensive tissue distribution. In all locations, the labile CDS is converted to the trigonellinate salt (k_{ox}). This more polar species is rapidly eliminated from the periphery but retained in the CNS ($k_{el1} \gg k_{el5}$) because of its charge and size and its inability to readily back-diffuse through the BBB. In the CNS, the "locked-in" salt is slowly hydrolyzed liberating the manipulated drug and the carrier salt. The drug can then interact with bioreceptors while the nontoxic trigonellinate salt is actively eliminated from the CNS (k_{el6}).

same time tying up the active principle as much as possible as an inactive conjugate. In the CNS, toxicity may also be abated since the majority of the delivery drug is present in the form of the inactive depot conjugate which must hydrolyze prior to receptor interaction. This carrier-based system has been extensively applied to various drug classes including neurotransmitters such as dopamine, aminobutyric acid and tryptamine (Bodor and Farag 1983; Anderson et al., 1987; Bodor et al., 1986), sex steroids including estradiol, ethinyl estradiol, testosterone and norethindrone (Bodor et al.,.1987; Brewster et al., 1986; Bodor and Farag, 1984), glucocorticoids including dexamethasone (Anderson et al., 1989), antiepileptic agents, anticancer agents (Raghavan et al., 1987; Bodor et al., 1989) and others. Safety evaluations of these systems have indicated that they are not associated with neurotoxicological manifestations when administered on either an acute or subchronic basis (Brewster et al., 1988). Other predictions including the rapid elimination of the spent carrier molecules, trigonelline, have also been experimentally confirmed (Bodor et al., 1986). Based on these and other studies, one of the CDS has entered human clinical trials and is presently being evaluated in a Phase I protocol (Howes et al., 1988).

A second corollary to the CDS postulate involves compounds which contain in their structure a potential delivery moiety such as a reducible pyridinium substructure (Brewster and Bodor, 1983a). In these cases, the transport carrier does not disassociate from the drug after CNS deposition as it is an integral portion of it. Successful applications of this technology include 2-pralidoxime chloride (2-PAM), a potent reactivator of inhibited AChE (Bodor et al., 1975; Bodor et al, 1976) and berberine, an anticancer alkaloid (Brewster and Bodor 1983b).

RESULTS AND DISCUSSION

The ability of the CDS to target drugs to the CNS and to attenuate toxicity provided a logical extension of these systems to anti-dementia drugs including inhibitors of AChE as well as certain phenethylamine derivatives. Certainly, the most highly studied AChE inhibitor has been physostigmine (eserine). Unfortunately, the chemical structure of this compound is not amenable to simple synthetic manipulation thus prompting a search for AChE inhibitors which could serve as lead compounds. Of the available derivatives, two structurally related compounds were selected as targets: pyridostigmine (Taylor, 1980) and benzstigmine (Wuest and Sakal, 1951). Both of these agents are pyridinium salts and as such would not be expected to penetrate the BBB restricting them to peripheral uses. Application of the CDS to these compounds would therefore be expected to alter their spectrum of activity. Reduction of these salts to their corresponding dihydropyridines should allow for brain uptake and at the same time should mitigate the biological potency of these compounds since the charged nitrogen is an essential requirement for AChE interaction. Attempts to reduce pyridostigmine were unsuccessful using a variety of reducing agents and experimental conditions. This may be related to the observation that electron-withdrawing groups which are capable of conjugation are required in the 3 and/or 5 position of pyridine derivatives to yield stable products upon reduction (Eisner and

Pyridostigmine   Benzstigmine   1,4-Dihydrobenzstigmine

Kuthan, 1972). Electron-withdrawing functionalities in the 1-position also stabilize dihydropyridines. Thus while pyridostigmine could not be readily reduced to a isolable product, the 1-benzyl moiety of benzstigmine did provide for a stable adduct upon sodium dithionite reduction. The CDS, 1,4-dihydrobenzstigmine, was found to readily oxidize in various biological matrices to regenerate the parent compound. The ability of benzstigmine and its CDS to inhibit AChE was investigated using the well known Ellman method (Ellman et al., 1961). In this assay, the dihydrobenzstigmine was shown to inhibit AChE activity 35.4% at a concentration of 13 μg/mL while the parent compound inhibited the enzyme 48.4% at 0.3 μg/mL. The inhibition ratio of the CDS to the parent compound was less than 0.015 corroborating the expected decrease in activity associated with CDS formation. Further distributional and pharmacological evaluations of this and other structurally related analogs is ongoing.

A second structural type of AChE inhibition are derivatives of aminopyridine including 4 aminopyridine (AP), 3,4-diaminopyridine (DAP) and 9-amino-1,2,3,4-tetrahydroacridine (THA). THA and AP have been used in human clinical trials as a treatment for SDAT (Summers et al., 1986; Wesseling et al., 1986; Kaye et al., 1982) and DAP has been examined in various animal models (Gibson et al., 1983; Peterson and Gibson, 1982). All of these compounds appear to possess activity although the report by Summers et al., (1986) that THA produced substantial improvements in patients suffering from SDAT has generated by far the most interest. A CDS for aminopyridine derivatives has been described by Allen et al., (1986). In this approach, 4-aminopyridine was condensed with trigonellonyl chloride to give the AP-Q + (Scheme I). This nicotinamide salt was then reduced giving the AP-CDS. Similar manipulations are possible for derivatization of DAP. These derivatives have been examined for their ability to restore cholinergically deficient memory in a dark avoidance assay. In the model, mice are placed in a chamber which contains a dark compartment and one which can be lighted. A strong light then forces the test animal into the dark portion of the box where it receives an electrical shock. If an anticholinergic agent such as scopolamine is given, the ability of the mouse to remember the unpleasant experience is compromised. Administration of the AP-CDS lead to an antagonism of this effect.

Scheme I

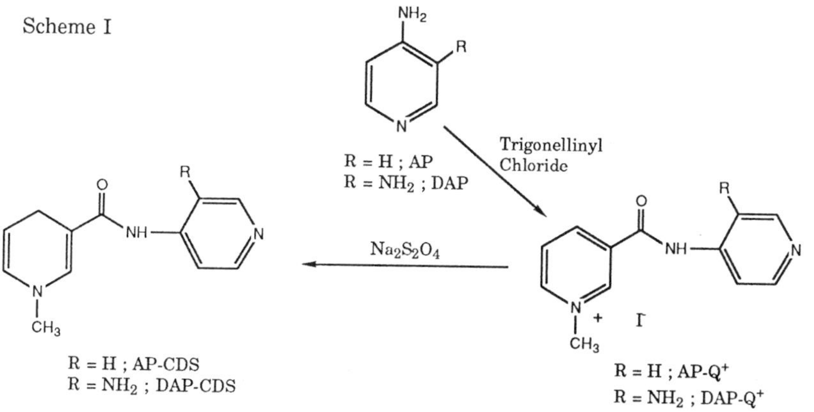

R = H ; AP
R = NH$_2$; DAP

R = H ; AP-CDS
R = NH$_2$; DAP-CDS

R = H ; AP-Q$^+$
R = NH$_2$; DAP-Q$^+$

In applying the CDS to THA, a nicotinamide type derivative was designed. The chemical manipulation of the amino group of THA and indeed of the aminopyridines in general is difficult because of resonance interaction which decreases nucleophilicity of the amino functionality. In the case of THA, rather harsh conditions (refluxing pyridine) were required to acylate the 9-amino position with nicotinic anhydride. Once the nicotinamide was obtained, it was quaternized with methyl iodide to give THA-Q$^+$ and reduced with aqueous basic sodium dithionite to give the THA-CDS (Scheme II).

In vitro studies on the THA-CDS indicated that the dihydronicotinamide readily converted to the "lock-in" quaternary salt in various matrices including rat brain and liver homogenates and rat whole blood. As with the benzstigmine, the biological potency of the CDS was examined and compared to that of its parent. Table I, which indicates percent AChE inhibition as a function of drug concentration, shows that derivatization of THA increases its IC$_{50}$ from 0.072 μm to 65 μm, a decrease in potency of almost 1000-fold. Again this inactivation of the transport form is consistent with the CDS approach.

Prior to initiating tissue distribution analysis, the tolerance of rats to the CDS and THA was assayed. In the protocol, the drugs were dissolved in dimethyl sulfoxide (DMSO) and given i.v. in the tail vein. The maximum tolerated dose of the THA-CDS was approximately 30 mg/kg while animals could routinely survive i.v. dose of only 2.8 mg/kg

177

Scheme II

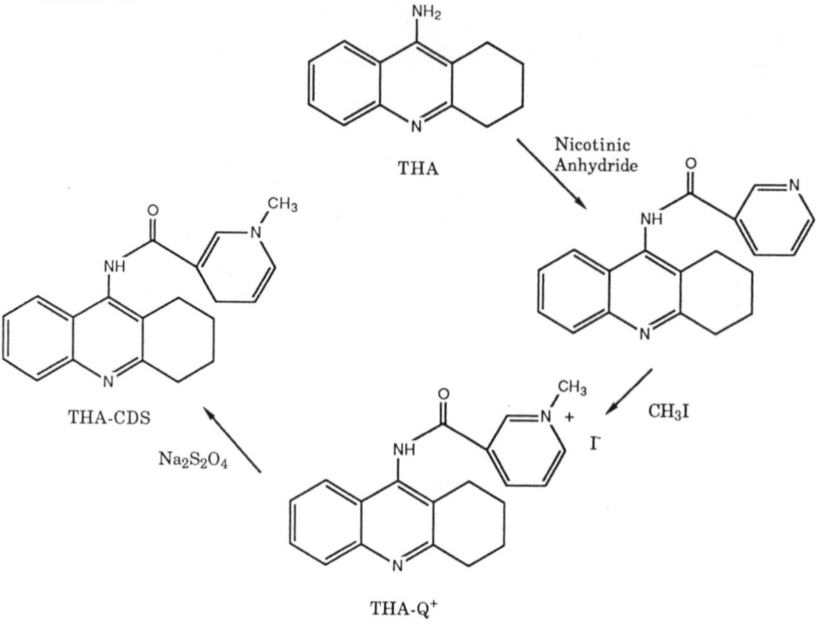

Table I. Effect of THA and THA-Q⁺ on the cholinesterase activity of purified acetyl cholinesterase (EC 3.1.1.7, Type III obtained from the Electric Eel)

Compound	Drug Concentration	Percent Inhibition
THA	2.93 μM	97.8%
	0.293 μM	81.3%
	0.0585 μM	44.0%
	0.0293 μM	29.3%
	0.0146 μM	5.5%
THA-Q⁺	888 μM	93.8%
	178 μM	73.9%
	35.5 μM	31.6%
	17.8 μM	23.1%
	8.88 μM	6.2%

of the THA. This mitigated toxicity is clearly related to a decrease cholinergic effect as THA-treated animals demonstrated classic signs of cholinergic excess including lacrimation, salivation and convulsion. These effects were not observed after THA-CDS administration. In the distribution studies, these doses of THA and the THA-CDS were administered (i.v., tail vein) to conscious, restrained Sprague-Dawley rats (BW=250 g). At various times post-drug administration (0.25, 0.5, 1, 2, 6 and 24 hr in the case of THA-CDS, 0.5, 2 and 6 h in the case of THA) animals were sacrificed and organs and trunk blood collected and rapidly frozen on dry ice until processed for analysis. Organs were homogenized in isotonic phosphate buffered saline to generate 20% w/v organ suspensions and blood was diluted 1:1 with buffer. The homogenates were then deproteinized and extracted with cold acetonitrile. In the protocol, one volume of the organ or blood homogenates was mixed with two volumes of cold acetonitrile, vortexed and centrifuged at 13,000x (Beckman Microfuge12). The organic layer which separated under these conditions was collected and stored in vials prior to analysis. The method use found to be 90% efficient in extracting the compounds of interest. Assay of the samples was by high performance liquid chromatography (HPLC) using a Spectra-Physics SP 8810 pump, an SP 8780 autosampler, an SP 4290 integrator, a LDC/Milton Roy Spectromonitor D variable wavelength detector and a Kontron SFM 23/B spectrofluorometric detector. The compounds were assayed on an Alltech 8744 Spherisorb C8 5 25 cm x 4.6 mm i.d. analytical column which was jacketed and maintained at 30°C. The mobile phase consisted of acetonitrile:KH_2PO_4 0.05 M, pH 5.4 35:65 and 0.1 mM tetrabutyl ammonium perchlorate. The flow rate was 1.2 mL/min. The THA and THA-Q$^+$ were detected at 242 nm while the THA was also assayed by fluorescence using an excitation band at 310 nm and an emission frequency of 360 nm. The UV and fluorescence detectors were connected in series. The use of fluorescence detection increased the sensitivity of the assay for THA by over an order of magnitude. THA could be reliably detected in amounts as low as 1.25 ng injected by UV and 130 pg injected by fluorescence. In the assays, UV detection was used in the quantitation of the THA-Q$^+$ while fluorescence was used in the quantitation of THA.

When THA is given i.v. to animals it is rapidly lost from both brain and blood (Figure 2). The first order half-life of THA in brain was found to be 0.77 h while in the blood this value was 0.48 h. At 6 h only 5.3 ng of THA/g could be detected in brain, while in blood no THA was present. Administration of the THA-CDS gave a different distribution. After a 30 mg/kg dose of the delivery system, high levels of the corresponding quaternary salt could be detected in the brain. This compound was present in the CNS for relatively prolonged periods compared to THA after THA dosing. The half-life of this quaternary salt in the brain was 10.7 h. This "lock-in" salt was associated in a small but sustained release of THA which reached levels of 15 ng/g by 24 h. No THA was found in the CNS 24 h after THA administration. We are presently examining the pharmacological significance of this delivery.

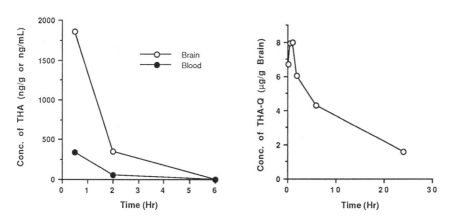

Figure 2. Concentration of THA in brain and blood after an i.v. dose of 2.8 mg/kg THA in the rat (left panel) and the disappearance of THA-Q$^+$ from rat brain after a 30 mg/kg dose of THA-CDS (right panel). At 24 hours, no THA was detected in the brain of animals dosed with THA while levels of 10-15 ng/g were detected in animals receiving the THA-CDS. In both panels the data point represents the mean of five animals.

In addition to the compounds thus far described, a series of benzoic acid derivatives containing a phenethylamino substructure has been found to be useful agents for facilitatory learning and memory. One compound from this series, m-[2-(benzylmethylamino)ethyl] benzoic acid methyl ester (BAB), has been studied for its ability to restore memory and various intellectual skills in both man and experimental animals (Hansl, 1975; Hansl, 1974; Hansl and Mead, 1978). In rats, BAB facilitates acquisition and increase memory retention. In man, improvements in learning and retention of verbal information are evident. These studies seem to indicate that BAB was particularly useful in improving performance for subjects over the age of 30 compared to younger individuals. Thus a CDS was considered for this derivative. Since BAB itself can not be directly manipulated, an analog was considered in which the benzyl group was replaced with the nicotinamide targeting moiety. The synthesis of this analog is given in Scheme III. BAB was prepared according to reported procedures (Hansl, 1975) with minor modification. Its analog, BAB-CDS, was generated by debenzylation of BAB followed by acylation with nicotinic acid and quaternization of the nicotinamide with methyl iodide (BAB-Q$^+$). Attempts to reduce this secondary amide using sodium dithonite or sodium cyanoborohydride were unsuccessful. The 1,6-dihydro isomer was obtained by reducing BAB-Q$^+$ with sodium borohydride in methanol and this reaction occurred without further reduction to the tetrahydropyridine species. The structural assignments for the BAB-CDS were based on its UV ((MeOH) 270, 356 nm) and the 1-H NMR spectra. The CDS could be quantitatively converted to the quaternary salt by oxidation in alcoholic silver nitrate. The in vitro stability of the CDS is summarized in Table II and indicates facile conversion of BAB-CDS to its depot form.

Scheme III

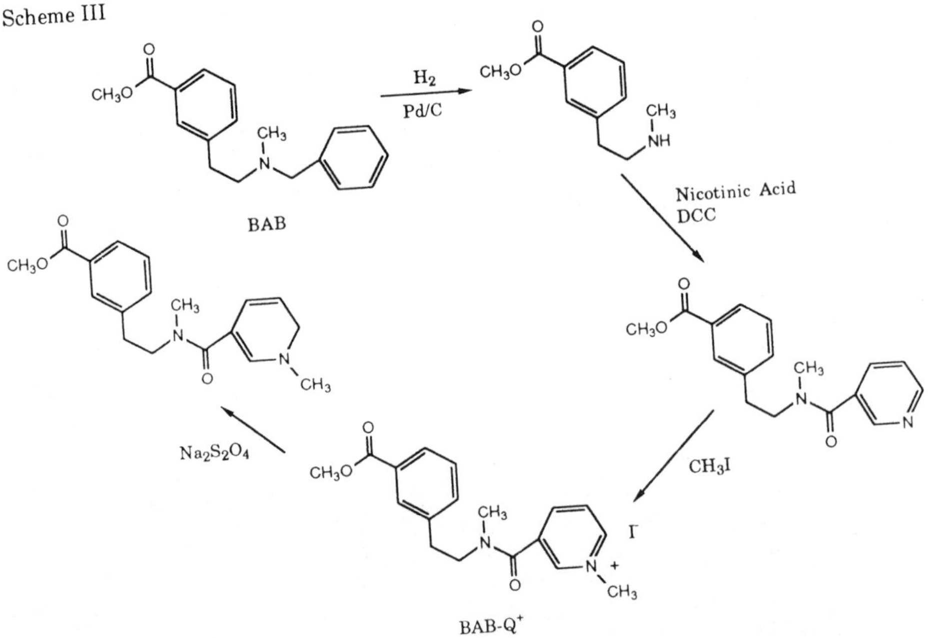

Table II. Stability of the BAB-CDS in various tissue homogenates and blood. All matrices were maintained at 37°C and were prepared in phosphate buffered saline.

Medium	$t_{1/2}$ min	r
Plasma	34.7	0.995
Whole Blood	17.0	0.950
Brain Homogentate	16.3	0.997
Liver Homogentate	3.1	0.988

In vivo tissue distribution studies used Sprague-Dawley rats which has been anesthetized with Inovar (i.m.). These animals were then underwent a minor surgical procedure to expose the external jugular vein. BAB-CDS in DMSO was then infused at a rate of 55 μL/min using a calibrated syringe pump (Sage). The dose administered was 75 mg/kg. At various times after the end of drug infusion, 1 mL of blood was withdrawn from the heart by cardiac puncture and animals were perfused with 20 mL of normal saline, decapitated and organs were collected and weighed. Blood and organs were then homogenized in 1 mL of water followed by addition of 3 mL of cold acetonitrile. The suspension was then centrifuged, filtered and analyzed by HPLC. The chromatographic system configuration included a Waters U6K injector, Model 6000 pump and Model 440 fixed wavelength UV detector. The BAB-Q$^+$ was separated and analyzed in a 30 cm x 3.9 i.d. mm 10 particle size reversed phase μBondapak C$_{18}$ column operating at ambient temperature. The mobile phase contained 70:30 acetonitrile:0.001 M NH$_3$H$_2$PO$_4$. The flow rate was 2 mL/min and, under these conditions, BAB-Q$^+$ had a retention time of 6.4 min. The in vivo study is summarized in Figure 3. As shown, there is a rapid distribution phase of the BAB-CDS resulting in relatively high initial levels of BAB-Q$^+$ in brain, lung and kidney. This is followed by a rapid decrease in the concentration of the quaternary salt in both lung and kidney but brain levels are maintained throughout the time frame of the experiment. At 5 hours, blood and liver levels were low and brain concentration exceeded the level in all other tissues by at lease 3-fold. Thus, the lock-in aspect of the CDS is clearly demonstrated and the rapid peripheral elimination confirmed.

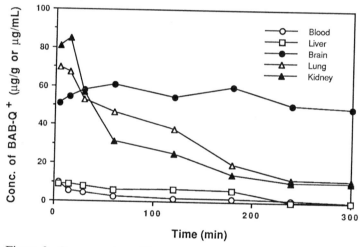

Figure 3. Concentration of BAB-Q$^+$ in various tissues and blood after a 75 mg/kg dose of BAB-CDS. The vehicle used in this study was DMSO. Each data point represents the mean of five animals.

In conclusion, the application of the CDS to delivery of anti dementia drugs was examined. While the data is clearly preliminary, enhanced drug uptake and retention in the CNS has been demonstrated. This approach is potentially useful for improving the pharmacokinetic/pharmacodynamic profiles of known drugs and should be included in the design process for new entities.

ACKNOWLEDGMENTS

The authors are indebted to J. Scott, K. Prokai and J. Simpkins for their helpful discussions and technical assistance. The expert editorial skills of J. Martignago are also acknowledged. This work was supported by the NIH (GM 27167) and by a grant from Pfizer, Inc.

REFERENCES

1. Allen, R., Effland, R. and Klein, J., U.S. Patent 4,578,394 (1986).

2. Anderson, W., Simpkins, J., Woodard, P., Winwood, D., Stern, W. and Bodor, N., Anxiolytic activity of a brain delivery system for GABA. Psycopharmacol. 92 (1987) 157-163.

3. Anderson, W., Simpkins, J., Brewster, M. and Bodor, N., Evidence for prolonged suppression of stress-induced release of ACTH and corticosterone with a brain¬enhanced dexamethasone redox delivery system. Neuroendocrinol. 00 (1989) 0000.

4. Bartus, R. T., Dean, R., Beer, B. and Lippa, A., The cholinergic hypothesis of geriatric memory dysfunction. Science, 217 (1982) 408-417.

5. Becker, R. and Giacobini, E., Mechanisms of cholinesterase inhibition in senile dementia of the Alzheimer type: Clinical, pharmacological and therapeutic aspects. Drug Develop. Res., 12 (1988) 163-195.

6. Bodor, N., Redox drug delivery systems for targeting drugs to the brain. Ann. N. Y. Acad. Sci., 507 (1988) 289-306.

7. Bodor, N., Shek, E. and Higuchi, T., Delivery of a quaternary pyridinium salt across the blood-brain barrier as its dihydropyridine derivative. Science, 190 (1975) 155-156.

8. Bodor, N., Shek, E. and Higuchi, T., Improved delivery through biological membranes 1. Synthesis and properties of 1-methyl-1,6-dihydropyridine-2¬carbaldoxime, a prodrug of N-methyl pyridinium-2-carbaldoxime chloride. J. Med. Chem., 19 (1976) 102-108.

9. Bodor, N., Farag, H. and Brewster M., Site-specific, sustained release of drugs to the brain. Science, 214 (1981) 1370-1372.

10. Bodor, N. and Brewster, M., Problems of delivery of drugs to the brain. Pharmacol. Ther., 19 (1983a) 337-386.

11. Bodor, N. and Brewster, M., Improved delivery through biological membranes 15. Sustained brain delivery of berberine. Eur. J. Med. Chem., 18 (1983b) 235-240.

12. Bodor, N. and Farag, H., Improved delivery through biological membranes 13. Brain specific delivery of dopamine with a dihydropyridine-pyridinium salt type redox delivery system. J. Med. Chem., 26 (1983) 528-534.

13. Bodor, N. and Farag H., Improved delivery through biological membranes 14. Brain specific, sustained delivery of testosterone using a redox chemical delivery system. J. Pharm. Sci., 73 (1984) 385-389.

14. Bodor, N., El Kommos, M. and Nath, C., In vivo elimination of dihydropyridine drug delivery carriers from brain and blood of rats. Bull. Pharm. Sci., Assiut Univ., 9 (1986) 14-29.

15. Bodor, N., Nakamura, T. and Brewster, M., Improved delivery through biological membranes 23. Synthesis, distribution and neurochemical effects of a tryptamine chemical delivery system. Drug Design Del., 1 (1986) 51-64.

16. Bodor, N., McCornack, J. and Brewster, M., Improved delivery through biological membranes 22. Synthesis and distribution of brain-selective estrogen delivery systems. Int. J. Pharm., 35 (1987) 47-59.

17. Bodor, N., Venkatraghavan, V., Winwood, D., Estes, K. and Brewster, M., Improved delivery through biological membranes 41. Brain-enhanced delivery of chlorambucil. Int. J. Pharm., 00 (1989) 0000.

18. Brewster, M., Estes, K. and Bodor, N., Improved delivery through biological membranes 24. Synthesis, in vitro studies and in vivo characterization of brain¬specific and sustained progestin delivery system. Pharm. Res., 3 (1986) 278-285.

19. Brewster, M., Estes, K. S., Perchalski, R. and Bodor, N., A dihydropyridine conjugate which generates high and sustained levels of the corresponding pyridinium salt in the brain does not exhibit neurotoxicity in cynomolgus monkeys. Neurosci. Lett., 87 (1988) 277-282.

20. Corkin, S., Acetylcholine, aging and Alzheimer's disease. Trends Neuro Sci., 12 (1981) 287-290.

21. Eisner, U. and Kuthan, J., The chemistry of dihydropyridines. Chem. Rev., 72 (1972) 1-42.

22. Ellman, G., Courtney, K., Andres, V. and Featherstone, R., A new and rapid colorimetric determination of acetylcholinesterase activity. Biochem. Pharmacol., 7 (1961) 88-95.

23. Gibson, G., Pelmas, C. and Peterson, E., Cholinergic drugs and 4-aminopyridine after hypoxic induced behavior deficits. Pharm. Biochem. Behav., 18 (1983) 909-916.

24. Hansl, N., A novel spasmolytic and CNS active agent: 3-(2-benzyl-methylamino ethyl) benzoic acid methyl ester hydrochloride. Experientia, 30 (1974) 271-272.

25. Hansl, N., U. S. Patent 3,870,715 (1975).

26. Hansl, N. and Mead, B., PRL-8-53: Enhanced learning and subsequent retention in humans as a result of low oral doses of new psychotropic agent. Pschopharmacol. 56 (1978) 249-253.

27. Howes, J., Bodor, N., Brewster, M., Estes, K. and Eve, M., A pilot study with PR-63 in post-menopausal volunteers. J. Clin. Pharmacol., 28 (1988) 951.

28. Kaye, W., Sitaram, N., Weingartner, H., Ebert, M., Smallberg, S. and Gillin, J., Modest facilitation of memory in dementia with combined lecithin and anticholinesterase treatment. Biol. Psyciat., 17 (1982) 275-280.

29. Mattio, T., McIlhany, M., Giacobini, E. and Hallak, M., The effect of physostigmine on acetylcholinesterase activity of CSF, plasma and brain. A comparison of intravenous and intraventricular administration to beagle dogs. Neuropharmacol., 25 (1986) 1167-1177.

30. Mesulam, M., Geula, C. and Moran A., Anatomy of cholinesterase inhibition in Alzheimer's disease: Effect of physostigmine and tetrahydroaminoacridine on plaques and tangles. Ann. Neurol., 22 (1987) 683-691.

31. Peterson, C. and Gibson, G., 3,4-Diaminopyridine alters acetylcholine metabolism and behavior during hypoxia. J. Pharm. Exp. Ther., 222 (1982) 576-582.

32. Raghavan, K., Shek, E. and Bodor, N., Improved delivery through biological membranes 30. Synthesis and biological aspects of 1,4-dihydropyridine based chemical delivery system for brain-sustained delivery of hydroxy-CCNU. Anti¬Cancer Drug Design, 2 (1987) 25-36.

33. Sims, N., Bower, D., Allen, S., Smith, C., Neary, D., Thomas D. and Davison, A., Presynaptic cholinergic dysfunction in patients with dementia. J. Neurochem., 40 (1983) 503-509.

34. Summers, W., Majouski, L., Marsh, G., Tachiki, K. and Kling, A., Oral tetrahydroaminoacridine in long term treatment of senile dementia, Alzheimer's type. New Engl. J. Med., 315 (1986) 1241-1245.

35. Taylor, P., Anticholinesterase agents. In Gilman, A., Goodman, L. and Gilman, A. (Eds). The Pharmacological Basis of Therapeutics. Macmillan Publishing Co., Inc., New York, N.Y., 1980, pp. 100-119.

36. Wesseling H., Agostan, S., VanDam, G., Pasma, J., DeWit, D. and Hauinga, H., Effects of 4-aminopyridine in elderly patients with Alzheimer's disease. New Engl. J. Med., 310 (1986) 988-989.

37. Wuest, H. and Sakal, E., Some derivatives of 3-pyridol with parasympathomimetic properties. J. Am. Chem. Soc., 73 (1951) 1210-1216.

DEVELOPMENT OF A PYRROLIDINONE DERIVATIVE (CYCLIC GABA) FOR MODULATING BRAIN GLUTAMATE TRANSMISSION

Kenji Matsuyama, Choichiro Miyazaki and Masataka Ichikawa

Department of Hospital Pharmacy, Nagasaki University Hospital
7-1 Sakamoto-machi, Nagasaki 852, Japan

INTRODUCTION

Senile Dementia of Alzheimer Type (SDAT) is a debilitating neurological disease that affects about one in six persons past the age of sixty (1,2). In spite of numerous hypotheses concerning the etiology of SDAT, e.g., abnormal blood aluminum levels (3), viral agents (4), genetic factors (5) and selective vulnerability of specific neuronal systems (6,7), its precise cause or causes remain unknown.

In 1976, Davies and Maloney (8) reported the selective loss of choline acetyltransferase (CAT), the synthesizing enzyme for acetylcholine, in the cortex of patients with SDAT. Since then, neurochemical studies have increased tremendously in scope and number. Alterations in the cholinergic (9,10), serotonergic (11), noradrenergic (12) and glutamatergic systems (13,14) have been reported. Recently, the potential roles of gamma-aminobutyric acid (GABA), glutamate (Glu) and aspartate (Asp) in neural functions have become an additional center of attraction in this disease process.

The amino acids Glu and Asp are major excitatory transmitters in the central neurons system. When present in high concentration, they are neurotoxic and could play a role in ischemic damage in the brain, suggesting their potential participation in vascular dementia. Furthermore, Greenamyre et al. (14) proposed that high levels of Glu are closely involved in the development of SDAT from the observation that neurofibrillary tangles, senile plaques and granulovacuolar degeneration selectively occurred in the hippocampal CA1 region to which Glu neurons project.

As illustrated in Fig. 1, the release of glutamate can be modulated at several distinct sites. Receptors for GABA (15) and adenosine (16) have been localized in the presynaptic glutamate terminal, and have been shown to modulate Glu release (17,18). Furthermore, GABA has been reported to enhance acetylcholine release from hippocampal nerve endings (19). From that point of view, we developed GABAergic derivatives in the form of prodrugs for the transmitter. The use of prodrug therapy is discussed in detail in other chapters of this book.

Shashoua et al. (20) has demonstrated increased permeability of GABA derivatives into the brain in the form of various aliphatic and steroidal esters. Each ester was taken into the brain faster than GABA itself after peripheral administration; however, only the cholesteryl ester of GABA exerted a pharmacological response. This observation demonstrates that the rate of hydrolysis in the brain can be another important factor for prodrug-potency.

With these observations in mind, three kinds of aromatic acids, isonicotinic acid, nicotinic acid and anisic acid, were used for the pro-moieties of GABA because these groups attributed different electron states on amido bonds formed between these acids and the amino group of GABA. In the present study, we determined the GABA levels in the mouse whole brain after the intraperitoneal administration of the same dose of isonicotinoyl-GABA (IG), nicotinoyl-GABA (NG), anisoyl-GABA (AG), isonicotinoyl-2-pyrrolidinone (IP), nicotinoyl-2-pyrrolidinone (NP), and anisoyl-2-pyrrolidinone (AG) to determine if the brain GABA-elevating effect of GABAergic derivatives reflected the difference in the electron state of the amido bond of IG, NG, AG, IP, NP and AP. The structures of these compounds are shown in Fig. 2.

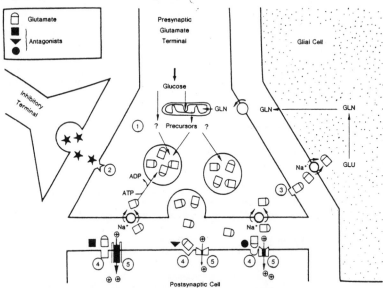

Fig 1 Schematic diagram for pre- and postsynaptic glutamate neuron.
(1) Synthesis of neurotransmitter pool of glutamate. (2)
Presynaptic GABA and adenosine receptors. (3) Glutamate
autoreceptors. (4) Antagonists of postsynaptic receptors
(represented by solid synbols). (S) Receptor ion channel blockers.
GLU indicates glutamate; GLN glutamine; ADP, adenosine diphosphate;
ATP, adenosine triphosphate; and Na, sodium.
From Greenamyre (14).

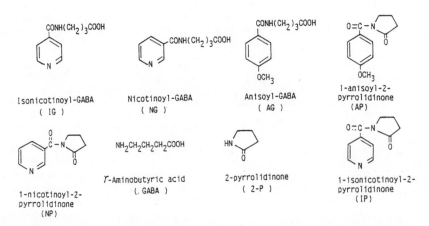

Fig. 2 The structures of IG, NG, AG, IP, NP, AP, 2-P and GABA

EXPERIMENT

Apparatus Fluorescence HPLC of o-phthalaldehyde (OPA) derivatives was performed with a model 510 pump (Waters, Milford, USA) equipped with a model 420-AC fluorescence detector (Waters). Gradient separations utilized a Model 680 automated gradient controller (Waters), a Waters 740 data module and a WISP 710B Waters Resolve 5 um C-18 column (150 x 3.9 mm) was used at 40°C.

Reagents Sodium valproate (VPA) was a gift from Kyowa Hakko Kogyo, Co. Ltd., Tokyo, Japan. OPA, 5-amino-n-valeric acid (AVA), 2-mercaptoethanol and amino acids were obtained from Tokyo Kasei Kogyo Co. Ltd., Tokyo, Japan. Reagent-grade isoniazid, 2-pyrrolidinone (2-P) and anisoylchloride were purchased from Wako Pure Chemical Ind. Co., Ltd., Osaka, Japan. Reagent-grade nicotinic acid hydrazide was obtained from Aldrich Chemical Company, Inc., Milwaukee, WI.

Borate Buffer: A total of 9.5 g of sodium tetraborate decahydrate was dissolved with heating in 250 ml of distilled water. The pH was adjusted to 10.0 with 1 M sodium hydroxide.

OPA Buffer Reagent: A total of 50 mg of OPA solution, 300 ul of 2-mercaptoethanol were added and the solution was mixed and diluted to 10 ml with pH 10.0 borate buffer.

Syntheses of IG, NG, AG, IP, NP and AP were performed according to our previous methods (21-23).

Animal Experiments Male mice (20 to 30 g) were fed a commercial diet (Clea Japan, Ind. Co. Ltd.,Tokyo, Japan) but fasted for 12 h prior to the experiment. Water was given <u>ad libitum</u>. Solutions of VPA, IG, NG, AG, GABA, and 2-P were prepared using 0.9% (W/V) NaCl, and the pH was adjusted to pH 7.0. Solutions of IP, NP and AP were pre- pared in DMSO. Each solution was administered intraperitoneally in a volume of 0.1 ml/10 g body weight. After administration, the mouse brain was weighed and homogenized in 4 ml of 0.2 M trichloroacetic acid con- taining 500 ug of AVA as an interal standard for HPLC determination. The process described above was done within 3 min. The homogenate was filtered to remove brain tissues and protein using a membrane filter (Centriflo CF-25, Amicon). Ten ul of the filtrate were diluted with 300 ul of pH 10 borate buffer.

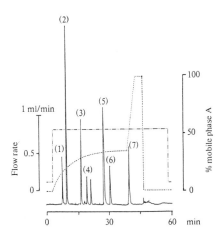

Fig. 3. Elution of OPA-2-mercaptoethanol Amino Acid Derivatives by a Step Gradient. The organic component of mobile phase A was 65% methanol and a mixture of 3% THF, 2% methanol and 95% $Na_2HPO_3-NaOAc$ buffer, pH 6.7, was the mobile phase B. The dotted line and the chain line represent the gradient pattern and the new rate, respectively. Numbered peaks were identified as follows: (I) Asp; (2) Glu; (3) Gln; (4) Gly; (S) Tau; (6) GABA; (7) AVA.

HPLC Assay   According to our previous paper (24), gradient elution was performed by using phase A and phase B. Five μl of OPA-2-mercaptoethanol reagent and 5 μl of sample were added to a WISP 710B Waters Intelligent Sample Processor at a flow rate of 0.1 ml/min for 2 min. Just after the 2 min reaction, the multistep gradient elution of the mobile phase was carried out as shown in Fig. 3 (dotted line). The column effluent was monitored with the fluorescence detector at 334 nm for excitation and 425 nm for emission. At the end of the separation, the column was washed with mixture A for 14 min.

Pentobarbital-Induced Hypnosis Male ddY mice weighing 20 to 25 g were used in this experiment. One hour after each compound tested was administered (4.81 mmol/kg), 45 mg/kg of pentobarbital was intraperitoneally administered to mice. The hypnotic effect was then evaluated by measuring the sleeping time, i.e., the time elapsed from loss to recovery of the righting reflex.

Reversal Activity of Scopolamine-Induced Amnesia of a Passive Avoidance Procedure in Rats   A step-through passive avoidance apparatus was used. The apparatus consisted of two compartments divided by a guillotine door into a darkened chamber (25x12x30cm) and an illuminated one (25x12x12 cm). The darkened chamber was made up of electrifiable grid floor and the shock was delivered to the animal's feet with a shock generator scrambler (SGS-004, BRS/LVE). One hour before acquisition of the passive avoidance response, rats (Wistar, male, 195-235 g) were trained to explore the step-through passive avoidance apparatus. Each rat was placed in the illuminated chamber and 10 sec later the door opened; as the rat stepped into the darkened chamber the door closed. The rat remained in the darkened chamber for 10 sec. The acquisition test was performed similarly to the training, with inescapable foot shock (4.5 mA, 1 sec) being administered to the rat's paws when it stepped through to the darkened chamber. Twenty-four hours after the acquisition test, the retention test was performed and the step-through latency was measured. This response latency was timed to an arbitary maximum of 300 sec. Thirty min before the acquisition test, each rat was injected with scopolamine (0.5 mg/kg, s.c.). Drugs were given immediately after the acquisition test.

Protective Effect Against Cerebral Anoxia in Mice   Groups of 10 mice (male, 28-34 g) were used for each drug-dose. At 1 hr after oral drug administration, all mice were placed into a transparent plastic container (13x13x16 cm) which have an inhalation and exhaust ports. They were exposed to a gas mixture of 4 % oxygen and 96 % nitrogen with a flow of 5 liters/min. The survival time, measured as the time from the induction of anoxia to the respiratory failure of the animals, was recorded.

RESULTS AND DISCUSSION

In fully developed animals the passage of polar substances from circulating blood to the brain parenchyma is very difficult because, unlike systemic capillaries, the endothelial cells of CNS capillaries have very

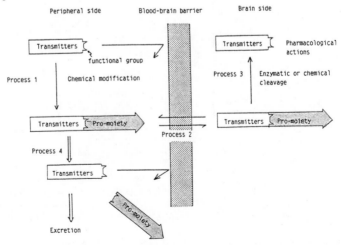

Fig. 4. Schematic representation of the use of prodrugs in topical therapy

tight junctions and are devoid of intracellular space (25,26). A promising approach to improve drug delivery to the brain is chemical modification of the polar active substances into prodrugs which convert to the active substances in the brain by enzymatic or chemical cleavage. In the case of GABA, high doses of GABA seem to penetrate the blood-brain barrier (BBB). The report from Frey and Loscher (27) demonstrated that the intraperitoneal administration of GABA to mice at a dose of 2 g/kg (19.4 mmol/kg) resulted in a significant increase in the brain GABA levels from 1.8 umol/g wet wt to 2.34 umol/g wet wt 1 h after administration. In the present study, administration of 4.81 mmol/kg of GABA increased brain GABA levels from 2.32 + 0.05 µmol/g wet wt in the control to 2.54 + 0.07 µmol/g wet wt (See Fig. 5A). However, 2-P only slightly elevated brain GABA concentrations in spite of being a potential prodrug for GABA (28,29) due to higher lipophilicity than GABA itself.

A weak enzymatic hydrolysis of 2-P in the brain seems to be rate limiting step in this process (process 3 in Fig.5). Any prodrug targeted for brain should have adequate lipophilicity and susceptibility to conversion to active form in the brain. In this respect, the development of an amido-type prodrug is always accompanied by the problem of slow hydrolysis in the brain because the amido bond is more resistant to carboxyl esterases than the ester bond is.

In the present study, we also compared electron-withdrawing and pushing pro-moieties. Isonicotinoyl groups withdraw electrons, resulting in a low density of electrons on the amido bond of IG, whereas anisoyl groups give rise to a high density of electrons in the amido bond of AG due to its electron pushing character. The nicotinoyl group is thought to provide an intermediate level of electron-donor capacity between them.

As shown in Fig. 5B, brain GABA levels were increased in the order, IG, NG, and AG, with IG or NG being more hydrophilic than AG. The elevated GABA levels in the brain were also confirmed by pharmacological response on pentobarbital-induced hypnosis. The prolonged effect of IG, NG, AG, GABA and 2-P on pentobarbital -induced hypnosis was primarily parallel to the brain GABA levels seen 1 hr following each.

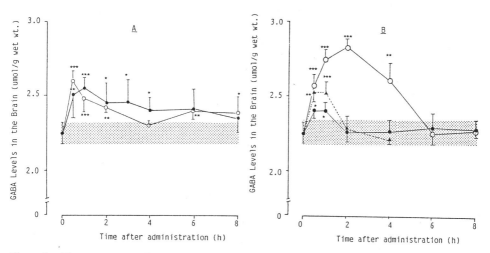

Fig. 5. Time course of GABA levels in the mouse brain. In the left figure (A), the closed and open circles represent the GABA levels after the intraperitoneal administration of GABA and 2-P (4.81 mmol/kg), respectively. In the right figure (B), the open circles, closed triangles, closed circles represent the GABA levels following the intraperitoneal administration of IG, NG and AG (4.81 mmol/kg) , respectively. The shadowed area represents the mean ± S.D. for the control level of GABA (n = 8). Vertical bars indicated S.D. ofthe mean of 6 animals. Statistical significance in the two-tailed Student's t-test: *** p <0.001, ** p <0.01, *p <0.05.

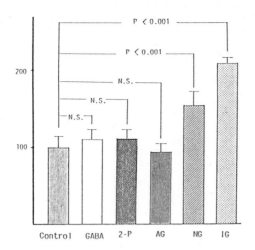

Fig. 6. Effects of GABA, 2-P, IG, NG and AG on pentobarbital-induced hypnosis in mice. Each compound (4.81 mmol/kg) was intraperitoneally administered 60 min before the injection of penotobarbital (45 mg/kg, i.p.).. Values are means of 10 mice and vertical bars indicate S.D.

compound as shown in Fig. 6. Olsen et al. (30) proposed that the GABA receptor was associated with a receptor for barbiturates and benzodiazepines as well as a chloride ionophore. According to this hypothesis, increased GABA transmission is expected to affect pentobarbital-induced hypnosis. As illustrated in Fig. 5, the brain GABA elevating action of IG was superior to that of GABA itself. However, the effect is not a fully satisfactory one. IG still contains the hydrophilic carboxyl group, in its structure. In order to mask the group, condensed-ring compounds were synthesized from IG, NG and AG by dehydration as shown in Fig. 7. Resulting compounds, IP, NP and AP were then used for the animal experiments. Following the intraperitoneal administration of IP, NP and AP at a dose of 4.81 mmol/kg, mouse brain GABA levels were increased in the order, AP, NP and IP (Fig. 8). In the case of the cyclic GABA derivative, the electron pushing anisoyl pro-moiety group contributes to the elevation of brain GABA levels in contrast to thecase of amido typed GABA-prodrugs. The GABA elevation effect of AP is better than that of IG. Whether the increased GABA is derived from AP or not is unknown in this point. The increased GABA may result from the inhibition of GABA-transaminase (GABA-T) by AP. However,

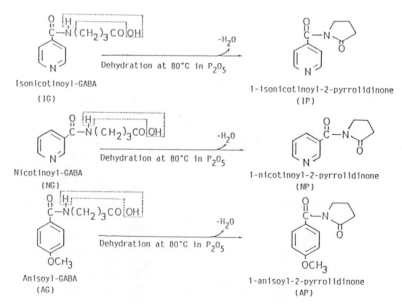

Fig, 7. Synthesis Procedure for IP, NP and AP. Each pyrrolidinone (cyclic GABA) derivative is prepared by dehydration of the corresponding GABA-prodrug.

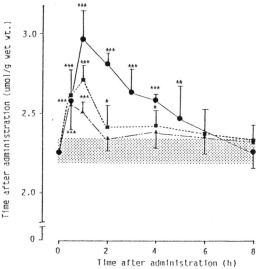

Fig. 8. Time course for GABA levels in mouse whole brain after
intra-peritoneal administration of 4.81 mmol/kg of AP (closed
circles), NP (closed squares) and IP (closed triangles),
respectively. Vertical bars indicate S.D. of the mean of 6 animals.
Statistical significance in two-tailed Student's t-test: *** p
<0.001, ** p <0.01; * p <0.05.

it is interesting that AP gives rise to more significant increments in
brain GABA levels than does GABA or IG judging from the report that GABA
inhibits the release of Glu presynaptically and stimulates acetylcholine
release as mentioned in the preface.

Giurgea (31) proposed a new class of drugs called nootropics that
act directly on the integrative activity of brain. Piracetam was the
model nootropic agent in that report; since then, the development of
pyrrolidinone derivatives as nootropics has accelerated. For example, AP
was been selected from a series of related compounds by the researchers
in Hoffmann-La Roche because of its interesting profile of activities in
preliminary cognition-related experiments. In this report, a
pyrrolidinone derivative with an electron pushing pro-moiety was found to
be suitable for the elevation of brain GABA.

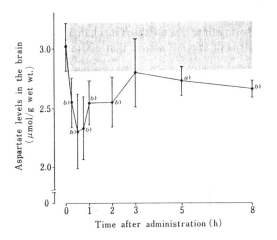

Fig. 9 Time Course of
Aspartate Levels in Mouse
Whole Brain after
Intraperitoneal
Administration of 200
mg/kg of VPA. The
shadowed area represents
the mean±S.D. for the
levels of control
aspartate (3.03 ± 0.20
μmol/g wet wt; n=6).
Vertical bars indicate
standard derivation of
the means of 6 animals.
Statistical significance
in two-tailed Student's
t-test: a) p<0.05. b)
p<0.01.

191

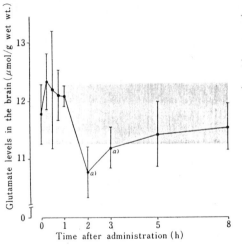

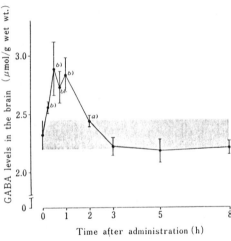

Fig. 10 Time Course for Glutamate
Levels in Mouse Brain after
Intraperitoneal Administration of
200 mg/kg of VPA. The shadowed
area represents the mean±S.D. for
the levels of control glutamate
(11.78±0.52 μmol/g wet wt; n=6).
Vertical bars indicate standard
deviation of the means of 6
animals. Statistical significance
in two-tailed Student's t-test:
a) p<0.05.

Fig 11 Time Course of GABA Levels
in Mouse Whole Brain after
Intraperitoneal Administration of
200 mg/kg of VPA. The shadowed
area represents the mean±S.D. for
the levels of control GABA
(2.32±0.12 μmol/g wet wt, n=6).
Vertical bars indicate standard
deviation of the means of 6
animals. Statistical significance
in two-tailed Student's t-test:
a) p<0.05. b) p<0.01.

Figure 12 shows the comparative effects of VPA and VP on the brain GABA
concentrations. VPA enhanced brain GABA levels more than VP did for the
first 1 hr. However, the VPA-induced elevations in GABA levels decreased
rapidly and returned to control levels by 4 hr. By contrast, VP caused a
more sustained elevation of brain GABA levels. This sustained elevation
may be due to the GABA formed from the hydrolyses of VP rather than to
inhibition of GABA-transaminase (GABA-T) by VPA formed by from VP.

$$CH_3CH_2CH_2 \diagdown \atop CH_3CH_2CH_2 \diagup CH\text{-}COOH \xrightarrow[\substack{\text{Reflux in} \\ \text{benzene}}]{SOCl_2} \quad CH_3CH_2CH_2 \diagdown \atop CH_3CH_2CH_2 \diagup CH\text{-}COCl$$

Valproic acid   Valproylchloride

$$\xrightarrow[\substack{\text{Stirring at} \\ \text{ambient temp}}]{\text{2-Pyrrolidinone}}$$

Valproyl-2-pyrrolidinone

Chart 1. Synthetic Procedure of Valproyl-2-pyrrolidinone (VP) from VPA.
Valproylchloride was obtained by reflux with VPA and thionyl chloride in
dried benzene. The valproylchloride reacts with 2-pyrrolidinone under
while being stirred at ambient temperature, resulting in VP formation.

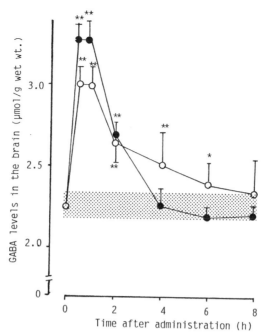

Fig. 12. Time Course of GABA levels in Mouse Whole Brain after
Intraperitoneal Administration of 2.40 mmol/kg of VPA (closed
circles) and VP (opened circles). The shadowed area shows the mean
± S.D. for the controls. Vertical bars indicate S.D. of the mean of
6 animals. Statistical significance in two-tailed Student's t-test:
** p<0.001, * p<0.05.

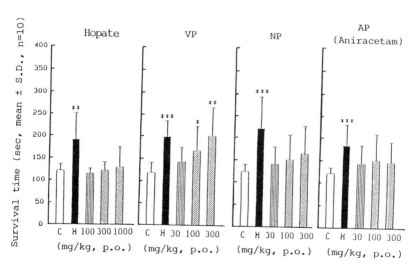

Fig. 13. Protective Effects of Hopate, VP, NP, AP Against Cerebral Anoxia
in Mice. Groups of 10 male ddY mice (30 g) were exposed to a gas mixture
of 4% oxygen and 96% nitrogen with a flow of 5 liters/min. The survival
time, measured as the time from the induction of anoxia to the
respiratory failure of the animals, was recorded. C; control (0.5% CMC
soln.), H; Hopate 300 mg/kg, i.p. Statistical analyses were performed
according to Student's t-test. *: p<0.05, **: p <0.01, ***: p <0.001.

In earlier studies, we observed that valproic acid (VPA) reduced brain concentrations of Asp (Fig. 9) and Glu (Fig. 10), whereas it enhanced GABA levels in the brain (Fig. 11) (32). Interestingly, the valproyl group also has an electron pushing character. On the basis of the findings described above, VPA was selected as a pro-moiety for 2-pyrrolidinone.

It is well accepted that brain metabolism is highly dependent on oxygen supply to the brain and that oxygen deficiency is one of the common and most damaging conditions affecting the brain function (33). When oxygen supply to the brain becomes deficient, cerebral function is compromised and neurological deficits can result from necrosis. Excitatory amino acids are thought to be involved in this process.

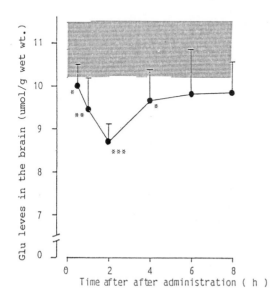

Fig 14. Time Course of Glu Levels in Mouse Whole Brain after Intraperitoneal Administration of 2.4 mmol/kg of VP. The shadowed area represents the mean ± S.D. for the control of Glu. Vertical bars indicate standard deviation of 5 animals. *: $p < 0.05$, **: $p < 0.01$, ***: $p < 0.005$

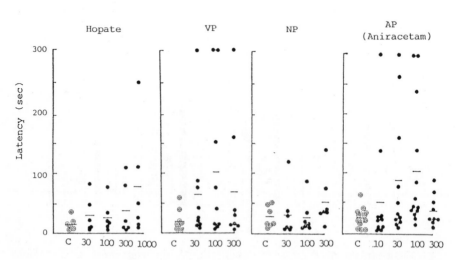

Fig. 15. Reversal of Scopolamine-Induced Transient Disruption of the of a Passive Avoidance Response in Rats. The amnesic agent scopolamine (0.5 mg/kg, s.c.) was injected 30 min before passive avoidance training. Specified drugs and doses (mg/kg) were administered orally immediately after exposure to electroconvulsive shock (ECS, 4.5 mA, 1.0 sec). The time elapsed between passive avoidance training and retention test was 24 hr.

Table I Acidic amino acid receptor subtypes

Class	Agonist	Alosteric agonist	Competitive antagonist	Non-competitive antagonist
NMDA in order of selectivity	NMDA Ibotanate L-Aspartate L-Glutamate Quisqualate	Glycine	D-AP5 D-AP7 CPP cis-2,3-PDA DGG	MK-801 PCP SKF10047 Mg^{2+}
Quisqualate (Q)	AMPA Quisqualate L-Glutamate L-Aspartate		No highly selective antagonists available for these receptor at present, but cis-2,3-PDA, DGG, GAMS show low potency and selectivity for K and Q	
Kainate (K)	Kainate Domoate L-Glutamate quisqualate			
L-AP4 (presynaptic receptors)	L-AP4		L-SOP	

Abbreviations: AMPA, α-amino-3-hydroxy-5-methylisoxazole-4-propionate; D-AP5, 2-amino-5-phosphonopentanoate; D-AP7, 2-amino-7-phosphonoheptanoate; CPP, 3-(2-carboxypiperazin-4-yl)-propyl-1-phosphonate; PDA, piperidine dicarboxylate; DGG, γ-D-glutamylglycine; GAMS, γ-D-glutamylaminomethylsulphonate; NMDA, N-metyl D-aspartate; PCP, phencyclidine; SKF10047, n-allylnormetazocine; L-AP4, L-2-amino-4-phosphonobutyrate; L-SOP, L-serine-O-phosphate.

The protective effect of VPA against cerebral anoxia was confirmed by our previous work (34). Figure 13 shows the protective effect of VP against cerebral anoxia compared to Hopate (Hopatenic acid), NP and AP. The intraperitoneal administration of Hopate (300 mg/kg) resulted in a significant prolongation of the mean survival time (closed bar). In the case of oral administration, it did not prolong the time even at 1000 mg/kg. Only VP prolonged the survival time against cerebral anoxia following the oral administration at a dose of 100 mg/kg . The effect was augmented at 300 mg/kg of AP (p.o.).

The protective effect of VP against the cerebral anoxia might be due to the significant decrease in Glu after VP as shown in Fig. 14. Figure 15 shows the comparative effect of Hopate, VP, NP and AP on the prolongation of latency time in a passive avoidance test. Both VP and AP showed a significant effect in the test . However, VP may be superior to AP judging from the result of the anoxia test.

The N-methyl-D-aspartate (NMDA)-type glutamate receptors appear to have special properties for synaptic transmission in the mammalian CNS, allowing them to play an important role in plasticity during development and learning. On the other hand, these receptors also appear to underlie the neurotoxic actions of Glu. Competitive and non-competitive antagonists of excitatory amino acid receptors are presented in Table I. These compounds seem to be effective against subsequent excess levels of excitatory toxins, e.g., Glu or Asp, after ischemia. We are currently planning to study the clinical efficacies of these compounds.

ACKNOWLEDGMENT
The authors thank Dr. J. Yamamoto and K. Toide of Taiho Pharmaceutical Co., for providing pharmacological data and Mr. T. Miyakawa, M. Okada, A. Mihara and F. Watanabe for their technical assistance.

REFERENCES

1) C. Mckhann, D. Drachman, M. Folstein, R. Katzman, D. Price and E. M. Stadlan, Neurology 34, 939-944 (1984).
2) Z. S. Khachaturian, Arch. Neurol. 42, 1097-1105 (1985).
3) D R. Crapper, S. S. Krishnan and S. Quittkat, Brain 99, 67-80 (1976).
4) S. B. Prusiner, N. Engl. J. Med., 310, 661-663 (1984).
5) J. Constantinidis, in Alzheimer's Disease: Senile Dementia and Related Disorders (R. Katzman, R. D. Terry and K. L. Bick, eds), pp.15-25 (Raven Press (1978).
6) P. J. Whitehouse, D. L. Price, A. W. Clark, J. T. Coyle and M. R. DeLong, Ann. Neurol. 10, 122-126 (1981).
7) P. L. McGeer, E. G. McGeer, J. Suzuki, C. E. Dolman and T. Nagai, Neurology 34, 741-745 (1984).
8) P. Davies and A. J. F. Maloney, Lancet, ii,1403 (1976).
9) T. D. Reisine, H. I. Yamamura, E. D. Bird, E. Spokes and S. J. Enna, Brain Res., 159, 477-481 (1977).
10) J. T. Coyle, D. L. Price and M. A. DeLong, Science, 219, 1184-1190 (1983).
11) D. M. Bowen, S. J. Allen, J. S. Benton, M. J. Goodhardt, E. A. Haan, A. M. Palmer, N. R. Sims, C. C. T. Smith, J. A. Spillance, M. M. Esiri, J. S. Snowdon, G. K. Wilcock and A. N. Davision, J. Neurochem. 41, 266-272 (1983).
12) B. E. Tomlinson, D. Irving and G. Blessed, J. Neurol. Sci. 49, 419-428 (1981).
13) J. T. Greenamyre, J. B. Penney, A. B. Young, C. J. D'Amato, S. P. Hicks, and I. Shoulson, Science 227, 1496-1499 (1985).
14) J. T. Greenamyre, Arch Neurol. 43, 1058-1063 (1986).
15) G. P. Wilkin, A. L. Hudson and D. R. Hill, Nature 294, 584-587 (1981).
16) R. R. Goodman, M. J. Kuhar and L. Hester, Science 220, 967-969 (1983).
17) S. J. Potashner and D. Gerard, J. Neurochem. 40, 1548-1557 (1983).
18) A. C. Dolphin and E. R. Archer, Neurosci Lett. 43, 49-54 (1983).
19) G. Bonanno and M. Raiteri, Neurosci. Lett., 70, 360-363 (1986).
20) V. E. Shashoua, J. N. Jacob, R. Ridge, A. Campbell and R. Baldessarini, J. Med. Chem. 27, 659-664 (1984).
21) K. Matsuyama, C. Yamashita, A. Noda, S. Goto, H. Noda, Y. Ichimaru and Y. Gomita, Chem. Pharm. Bull. 32, 4089-4095 (1984).
22) K. Matsuyama, C. Miyazaki, M. Ichikawa and S. Goto, Pharm. Res. submitted.
23) K. Matsuyama, C. Miyazaki, M. Ichikawa, S. Goto and J. Yamamoto, J Pharam. Dyn. submitted.
24) C. Miyazaki, M. Ogasawara, M. Ichikawa, K. Matsuyama and S. Goto, J. Pharm. Dyn. 11, 202-205, (1988).
25) M. W. Brightman and T. S. Reese, J. Cell. Biol. 40, 648-677 (1969).
26) J. D. Fenstermacher, R. G. Blasberg and C. S. Patlack, Pharmac. Ther. 14, 217-248 (1981).
27) H. H. Frey and W. Loscher, Neuropharmacology 19, 217-220 (1980).
28) P. S. Callery, L. A. Geelhaar, M. S. Balachandran, M. Stogniew and K. Gurudath Rao, J. Neurochem. 38, 1063-1067 (1982).
29) H. Bundgard, Design of Prodrugs, pp 64, Elsevier, Amsterdam (1985).
30) R. W. Olsen, J. Neurochem. 37, 1-13 (1981).
31) C. Giurgia, Actual Pharmacol. 25, 115-156 (1972).
32) C. Miyazaki, K. Matsuyama, M. Ichikawa and S. Goto, Chem. Pharm. Bull. 36, 3589-3594 (1988).
33) M. M. Cohen, Monogr. Neural Sci. 1, 1-49 (1973).
34) C.Miyazaki, K. Matsuyama and M. Ichikawa, The Kyushu Neuro-psychiatry, in press.

A BRAIN-ENHANCED CHEMICAL DELIVERY SYSTEM FOR GONADAL STEROIDS: IMPLICATIONS FOR NEURODEGENERATIVE DISEASES

James W. Simpkins[1,3], Mohamad H. Rahimy[1,3], and Nicholas Bodor[2,3]

Departments of Pharmacodynamics[1] and Medicinal Chemistry[2], College of Pharmacy and the Center for Drug Design and Delivery[3] University of Florida, Gainesville, FL 32610

INTRODUCTION

The brain is a primary target for the physiological and pharmacological actions of gonadal steroid hormones. These hormones exert two modes of action on the brain: (i) during the critical period of fetal/neonatal life these hormones affect permanently some features of the brain structure and function which result in neuronal differentiation and (ii) during the adult life exert their effects in a modulatory, reversible mode that influence adult brain function.

Evidence indicates that certain clinical problems arise when endogenous production of the gonadal hormones is decreased[1-3]. This results in brain deprivation of related hormones which leads to a number of central nervous system-mediated hormone withdrawal symptoms[1,2,4]. Though replacement therapy with currently available products (natural or synthetic) can alleviate the symptoms, their low efficacy and high peripheral toxicity limit their therapeutic application[5,6]. Therefore, an alternative and novel strategy to deliver the gonadal hormones preferentially to the brain is needed. The subjects of this review are: 1) to present some of the problems associated with the brain delivery of drugs; 2) to describe a novel design and methodology of achieving a brain-enhanced delivery of drugs; 3) to evaluate the application of the chemical delivery system (CDS) to an ovarian estrogen, 17-β estradiol (E_2); 4) to investigate the tissue distribution of the E_2-CDS after administration into rats and 5) to study the pharmacodynamic consequences and the potential clinical application of this delivery system.

THE BLOOD-BRAIN BARRIER AS AN OBSTACLE TO THE BRAIN DELIVERY OF DRUGS

Many drugs are excluded from entering the brain because of the existence of the blood-brain barrier (BBB). The BBB was first postulated by Ehrlich and based upon his observations that following systemic administration of various dyes, the brain remained uncolored while other organs were readily stained[7-9]. It was later discovered that many small molecules were similarly excluded from transport into the brain. This, then, led to the suggestion that the BBB was absolute; a concept which was soon thereafter dispelled when the nutrient requirements of the brain were elucidated[10]. It is now recognized that the BBB is a complex of morphological and enzymatic components which retard the passage of both large and small molecules which are not essential for cerebral function; however, it allows the movement of essential molecules via specific transport systems[11]. The morphological components of the BBB were defined using horseradish peroxidase (HRP). This relatively small enzyme has a high affinity for radiopaque substances and does not cross cerebral capillaries. When introduced into the brain, it readily diffuses throughout the extracellular space but does not pass between the endothelial cells of cerebral capillaries[12,13]. Unlike systemic capillaries, the endothelial cells of cerebral capillaries are joined by tight junctions[14]. These tight junctions form a zona occludes and provide, for molecules like HRP, an absolute barrier. Structurally, these junctions consist of aligned intra-membranous ridges and grooves which are in close opposition[9,15,16].

Two additional aspects of cerebral capillaries contribute to the BBB. First, cerebral endothelial cells have a paucity of vesicles and of vesicular transport capacity[17]. Second, astrocytic endfeet may be involved in the regulation of amino acid flux and in the absorption of proteins[18].

Finally, the enzymatic component of the BBB may be vital in protecting the brain from a variety of blood-borne chemicals, e.g., neurotransmitters[8,19-21]. Thus, catechol-o-methyltransferase, monoamine oxidase, aromatic amino acid decarboxylase and gamma-aminobutyric acid transaminase are located in the vicinity of cerebral vasculature. The presence of these enzymes in circumventricular areas, which lack a morphological barrier, may serve to exclude circulating neurotransmitters from these otherwise unprotected brain areas. The presence of butyryl-cholinesterase in cerebral, but not systemic capillaries, argues for the need to protect the brain from circulating neuroactive substances which are lipid soluble, such as butyrylcholine.

METHODS OF ACHIEVING THE ENHANCED DELIVERY OF DRUGS TO THE BRAIN

Drugs can gain access to the brain through one of several routes. First, if a drug has affinity for one of the carrier systems, it can diffuse across the BBB in association with that carrier. Second, drugs with intrinsic lipophilicity can diffuse passively through the phospholipid cellular matrix of capillary endothelial cells. The lipophilicity of drugs, as defined by their octanol-water partition coefficient correlates with their ability to penetrate the BBB for several classes of drugs, including narcotics[22], β-receptor antagonists[23], and barbiturates[24]. Third, drugs which cannot penetrate the BBB can gain access to limited areas around the circumventricular organs.

The BBB excludes a number of pharmacological agents from the brain because of their large size or low lipophilicity. Also the concentrations of other compounds are limited to brain concentrations which are subtherapeutic for the same reasons.

To increase the effectiveness of drugs against central maladies, the concentrations and/or transit time of the drug in the brain should be increased. Further, if selective drug delivery to the brain is achieved, the therapeutic index of the drug should increase for two reasons: (i) the increase in concentration and/or residence time of the agent at its receptor and (ii) of equal importance, the peripheral concentration of the drug would be reduced, thus decreasing its peripheral toxicity.

A general approach to enhance delivery of drugs to the brain is the prodrug approach[25-29]. Prodrugs are pharmacological agents which have been transiently modified to improve their water solubility and/or lipophilicity and to hinder their rapid metabolic inactivation. Ideally, the prodrug is biologically inactive but reverts to the active, parent compound <u>in vivo</u> at or around the site of action. This transformation can be mediated by an enzyme or may occur chemically as a result of designed instability in the agent. The purpose of these chemical modifications is to increase the concentration of the active compound at its site of action, thereby increasing its efficacy. By temporarily masking the polar groups of a drug, the lipophilicity of that drug can be increased and its ability to pass membranes is enhanced. This technique has been applied to a number of drugs including antibiotics[30,31], antineoplastic agents[32-34], miotics and mydriatics used in the treatment of glaucoma (Bodor and Visor, unpublished observation), anxiolytics and hypnotics, antiepileptic agents, and vitamins[11].

By increasing the lipid solubility of drugs non-specifically via the prodrug approach, all tissues are exposed to a greater drug burden. This is a major limiting factor in the use of these prodrugs, particularly those with cytotoxic activity.

One approach to eliminate this problem of general toxicity associated with enhanced lipophilicity of prodrugs has been the application of a dihydropyridine$\rightleftharpoons$pyridinium salt redox system to the delivery of drug specifically to the brain[26,35]. In this brain-specific delivery system, the lipoidal dihydropyridine moiety is attached to the drug, thus increasing its lipid solubility and thereby enhancing its permeability through the BBB. The reduced dihydropyridine can be oxidized to the pyridinium ion in the brain parenchyma as well as in the systemic circulation (See Chapter by Brewster <u>et al.</u>, this volume). The charged pyridinium-drug complex is thus locked into the brain while the peripheral ionized pyridinium-drug complex can be rapidly cleared by renal or biliary processes due to its increased hydrophilicity. Sustained release of the active drug from the charged pyridinium-drug complex occurs in the brain as a result of the enzymatic hydrolysis of the ester (or amide, etc.) linkage between the drug and the pyridinium moiety.

The redox chemical delivery system has been applied successfully to brain specific delivery of phenylethylamine[36,37], dopamine[38-40], antitumor drugs[41], antiepileptic agents, gamma-aminobutyric acid[42], antiviral agents, and antibiotics[11]. In the case of a highly polar compound, such as dopamine, which does not penetrate the BBB, we have been able to demonstrate specific brain delivery of the quaternary pyridinium complex of dopamine and an extended residence time of this molecule in the brain. In the peripheral circulation and in a variety of peripheral tissues, this charged moiety was quickly eliminated[38]. More recently, we have demonstrated dopamine release in the brain after systemic administration of the chemical delivery system[39]. In brief, we have documented previously the brain specific delivery and sustained release of a highly polar molecule, dopamine, following the peripheral administration of a dopamine-chemical delivery system.

APPLICATION OF THE CHEMICAL DELIVERY SYSTEM TO ESTRADIOL

An additional novel application of this redox chemical delivery system is to molecules with high intrinsic lipophilicity, which can themselves readily pass into and out of the brain. Their attachment to the dihydropyridine carrier encourages this brain-specific delivery by (i) locking them into the brain following the oxidation in the brain of the dihydropyridine carrier to the charged pyridinium moiety; and (ii) enhancement of the rate of elimination of the lipoidal drug, a still inactive form, from the periphery following its oxidation to the charged, more hydrophilic compound.

We applied this chemical delivery system to the naturally occurring female estrogen, estradiol-17-β, to achieve sustained local brain release of the steroid. Our purpose in this endeavor was to provide a sustained exposure of the brain to estradiol while reducing peripheral exposure to the steroid and hence peripheral estradiol toxicity. Presented in Figure 1 is a schematic representation of the proposed distribution in the body of the estradiol-chemical delivery system (E_2-CDS). Like the other drug-CDS's which we have evaluated, the brain enhanced delivery of estradiol requires a series of chemical processes, including oxidation of the dihydropyridine carrier of E_2-CDS to the corresponding quaternary pyridinium salt (E_2-Q^+), which provides the basis of locking the molecule in the brain, hydrolysis of the E_2-Q^+ by non-specific esterases at the C-17 position and the release of estradiol.

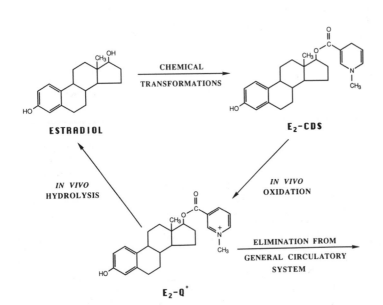

Fig. 1. Schematic representation of the synthesis and distribution of the estradiol-chemical delivery system (E_2-CDS). E_2-Q^+, the quaternary form of the E_2-CDS, is formed via enzymatic oxidation; it is locked into the brain but quickly eliminated from the peripheral tissues. Subsequent hydrolysis of the E_2-Q^+ provides sustained release of E_2 in the brain.

DISTRIBUTION OF THE E_2-CDS

We have undertaken a series of studies to describe the distribution of the oxidized and hydrolytic products of E_2-CDS, E_2-Q^+ and E_2, respectively, in brain and peripheral tissues to determine if the compound behaves as predicted on the basis of the physical and chemical properties designed into its structure. Male rats were treated by a single i.v. injection with 1 mg E_2-CDS/Kg B.W. or with the vehicle, hydroxypropylcyclodextrin and were killed by decapitation 1, 7 or 14 days later. Brain, serum, anterior pituitary, lung, liver, heart, kidney, and fat tissue were isolated and stored frozen for later assay of E_2-Q^+ and E_2 by the method previously described by us[43].

Brain concentrations of E_2-Q^+ increased to 318 ± 14 ng/g tissue (mean ± SEM) on day 1, followed by linear decline to 39 ± 2 ng/g by 14 days post-injection (Fig. 2). Brain E_2 concentrations increased to 8 ± 0.5 ng/g on day 1 and declined to 2 ± 0.1 ng/g on day 14 post-treatment. For both E_2-Q^+ and E_2, the half-life in the brain was approximately 8 days. This value is in agreement with a previous report by us of a $t_{1/2}$ of brain E_2-Q^+ of 9 days[44]. This long $t_{1/2}$ of brain E_2-Q^+ and E_2 is in contrast to their rapid clearance from serum and peripheral tissues[45]. The extent of the capture by the brain of the E_2-Q^+ is evident by our observation that over the time-course of this study brain E_2-Q^+ concentrations exceeded serum levels by 33- to 294-fold. The observed progressive increase in the brain to serum ratio of E_2-Q^+

reflects the relative rates of decline of brain and serum E_2-Q^+ levels. A similar observation was made with E_2. That is, brain E_2 concentrations exceeded serum concentrations by 39- to 82-fold over the 14 day time-course of this study. Collectively, these data support the concept of the brain-enhanced delivery of E_2 using the redox-based chemical delivery system.

For brain tissue, E_2-Q^+ concentrations exceeded E_2 concentrations by 18- to 22-fold and in plasma by 6- to 22-fold over the time-course of the evaluation. The dramatically lower concentrations of E_2 than E_2-Q^+ indicate that the hydrolytic cleavage of E_2 from E_2-Q^+ is a slow process, the rate of which in the brain is independent of the concentration of E_2-Q^+. To verify this relationship between brain E_2-Q^+ and E_2 concentrations, we administered 0, 10, 100 or 1000 μg E_2-CDS/KG B.W. to rats and are now assaying brain tissue for concentrations of E_2-Q^+ and E_2. We expect that brain concentrations of E_2-Q^+ and E_2 will be increased in a dose-dependent manner, but the ratio of E_2-Q^+ to E_2 will remain constant regardless of the dose administered.

These pharmacokinetic evaluations are consistent with our proposal that estradiol can be delivered to the brain using a redox-based chemical delivery

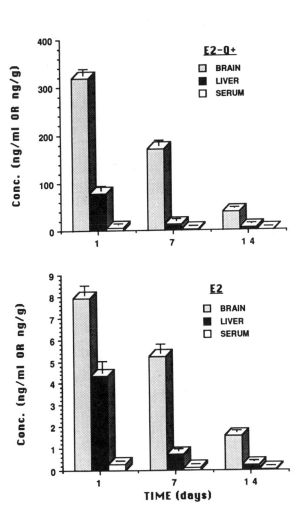

Fig. 2. Effects of a single dose of the E_2-CDS (1 mg/kg) on brain (▥), liver (■) and serum (□) concentrations of E_2-Q^+ (upper panel) and E_2 (lower panel) in adult male rats.

system in a manner which allows for the "lock-in" of the inactive, charged form of the delivery system, E_2-Q^+, and the slow and chronic release of the active steroid, E_2. On the basis of this pharmacokinetic behavior, following a single administration of the E_2-CDS, the compound should exhibit pharmacodynamic responses with long half-lives.

PHARMACODYNAMIC RESPONSES TO THE E_2-CDS

Pharmacodynamic responses to E_2-CDS were evaluated to determine if the long half-life of E_2-CDS in brain tissue correlated with the duration of action of the delivery system on brain mediated E_2 effects. We have conducted extensive evaluations of the E_2-CDS effects on secretion of luteinizing hormone (LH), on body weight and appetite regulation, and on the activity of specific neuronal systems which may be affected in neurodegenerative diseases. This strategy was used to evaluate the efficacy of the delivery system on responses which are known to be affected by estrogens (i.e. LH secretion and body weight) and to assess its efficacy on neuronal systems which are known to be affected in Alzheimer's disease (i.e. cholinergic and neuropeptide-containing neurons).

1. Effects of E_2-CDS on LH secretion

LH secretion is regulated by the release from the median eminence of the hypothalamus of a decapeptide, luteinizing hormone-releasing hormone (LHRH), and the feedback action of gonadal steroids on the anterior pituitary gland and the hypothalamus[46]. In the absence of gonadal steroids, e.g., following ovariectomy or the menopause, LH secretion increases due to the action of LHRH on the anterior pituitary gland[46]. A second condition in which gonadal steroids markedly affect LH secretion is during the preovulatory LH surge. Progressive increases in the titers of estradiol result in a surge of LH secretion which subsequently causes ovulation of the ovum from the graafian follicle. This preovulatory LH surge results from the transient increase in serum estradiol levels to levels of about 150 pg/ml or greater for 24 to 36 h during the late follicular phase[46]. Maintenance of elevated E_2 levels, however, prevents preovulatory surges of E_2 and represents the primary mechanism by which the estradiol component of contraceptives prevent ovulation.

Several studies were conducted to assess the efficacy of E_2-CDS in diminishing LH secretion in castrated rats. In an initial study, male rats were castrated and two weeks later were administered E_2-CDS (3 mg/Kg) or an equimolar dose of estradiol or the vehicle, dimethylsulfoxide (DMSO), by a single i.v. injection. Both estradiol and E_2-CDS reduced serum LH from 4 to 48 h (Fig. 3). From 4 to 12 days after drug treatment, LH levels increased progressively in the estradiol-treated rats to levels equivalent to those in DMSO-treated controls (Fig. 3). In contrast, LH concentrations in animals treated with the E_2-CDS remained low and were suppressed by 82, 88 and 90% compared to DMSO-treated rats at 4, 8 and 12 days after treatment, respectively (Fig. 3). Serum estradiol levels remained elevated through two days in both groups of rats treated with estradiol and E_2-CDS (Table I). By 4 days after drug administration, estradiol returned to levels observed in orchidectomized rats in both groups (Table I). At this 4-day time point, serum LH began to increase in the estradiol-treated group, but remained suppressed in the E_2-CDS treated animals. Thus, despite the peripheral clearance of E_2 in E_2-CDS treated rats, LH remained suppressed. This observation supports the local brain release of E_2 from the "locked-in" E_2-Q^+ as the mechanism for the sustained suppression of LH following administration of E_2-CDS.

Table I. Serum Estradiol Concentrations (pg/ml) in Serum Pools Following E_2-CDS, Equimolar Estradiol or Vehicle in Orchidectomized Rats.

Treatment Group	Time Post-Treatment							
	0 hr	4 hr	8 hr	24 hr	2 days	4 days	8 days	12 days
Vehicle	ND+	50	73	32	ND	19	47	ND
E_2-CDS	ND	>1000	>1000	637	285	59	22	20
Estradiol	ND	>1000	>1000	517	617	ND	15	ND

ND less than 10 pg/ml
Vehicle for all groups was DMSO.

An alternative approach to document the brain enhanced delivery of E_2 following E_2-CDS is to administer repeatedly, low doses of the drug and evaluate for a cumulative LH suppressing effect in castrated rats. In this study, we treated ovariectomized rats every 2 days for 7 injections (2 weeks) with E_2-CDS at doses of 10 to 333 μg/Kg, i.v. At 2 days after the last injection, rats were sacrificed for determination of serum LH and estradiol levels. Repeated treatment with E_2-CDS reduced serum LH by 32, 57, 72 and 76% of doses of 10, 33, 100 and 333 μg/Kg, respectively (Fig. 4). This LH suppression occurred without a significant increase in serum estradiol at the doses of 10 and 33 μg/Kg (Fig. 4). At higher doses of E_2-CDS, serum estradiol levels were elevated to levels equivalent to those observed after a single injection of the same dose. These data demonstrate that repeated dosing with low levels of E_2-CDS cause E_2 accumulation in the brain but not in the serum.

Collectively, the aforementioned data show that the chemical delivery system for estradiol cause a chronic suppression of LH secretion, the duration of which is consistent with the long half-life in the brain of the products of the E_2-CDS. In the face of rapid peripheral clearance of the drug and its two metabolic products, the chronic suppression of LH supports the concept of a brain-enhanced delivery of E_2, consistent with the scheme depicted in Fig. 1.

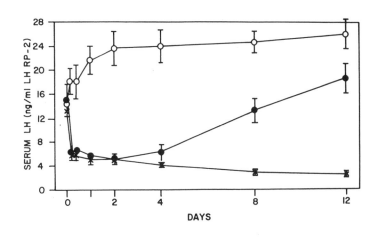

Fig. 3. Effects of a single dose of the E_2-CDS (3 mg/kg) or E_2 on serum LH concentrations in orchidectomized rats. (x) indicates E_2-CDS, (●) indicates equimolar dose of E_2 and (o) depicts vehicle-treated values.

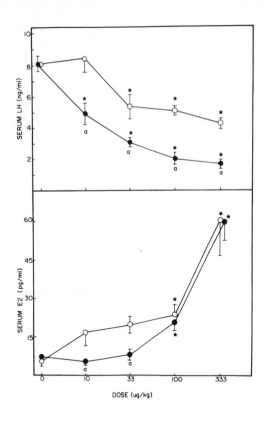

Fig. 4. Effects of single (o) or multiple doses (●) of E_2-CDS on serum LH (upper panel) and serum E_2 (lower panel) in ovariectomized rats.

2. Effects of E_2-CDS on Body Weight Regulation

Food intake and body weight vary during the estrous cycle of animals[47-49] and the menstrual cycle of primates[50,51] including women[52,53]. A consistent observation is that food intake and body weight decrease during the follicular phase of the estrous cycle when serum estradiol levels increase. In contrast, food intake and body weight increase during the luteal phase of the estrous cycle when estradiol levels decrease and progesterone levels increase. Similarly, food intake and body weight increase after ovariectomy, a state of gonadal steroid deprivation, and during pregnancy and pseudopregnancy, when progesterone levels are increased[54-56]. Collectively, these data indicate that the role of estradiol in body weigh regulation is common to many mammalian species and represents a fundamental role of estrogens in animals.

Although relatively few studies have evaluated steroid modulation of body weight regulation in human subjects, the available studies support a suppressory role of estradiol in appetite and body weight. Morton et al.[57] reported on a study of premenstrual syndrome (PMS) in prison inmates. Among the women studied, 37% reported craving sweets during the luteal phase of their menstrual cycles. Increased appetite was a frequently reported PMS symptom in 45 women studied by Fortin et al. (as reported by Smith et al.[58]). In a more quantitative analysis of the role of gonadal steroids in body weight regulation in human subjects, Dalvit[52] reported that the caloric intake of 8 women was significantly higher during the luteal phase than during the follicular phase of two consecutive menstrual cycles. Pliner et al.[53] studied 34 women and observed that the decreased food intake during the follicular phase was associated with significant weight loss and that the increased food intake during the luteal was concurrent with weight gain.

Thus in women, endogenously released estradiol has a consistent, albeit subtle, suppressory effect on food intake and body weight.

We evaluated the effects of E_2-CDS on food intake and body weight in male rats which were sexually mature and in 9 month old male rats whose obesity was age-related[59]. In each study, rats were treated with one of three doses of E_2-CDS or with the DMSO vehicle by a single i.v. injection. Body weights and 24 h food intake were determined prior to and daily for the next 12 to 14 days and at 3 to 7 day intervals thereafter. For adult male rats, E_2-CDS caused a dose-dependent reduction in the rate of body weight increase (Fig. 5). The dose-dependent reduction in body weight was maintained at each sampling time and by the last observation day (day 39) body weight of the 1 and 5 mg/kg doses were still significantly lower than the DMSO control animals (Fig. 5). These data indicate that E_2-CDS can suppress body weight chronically following a single administration, despite the clearance from the periphery of estradiol. The local release of estradiol from the E_2-CDS in the brain would appear to be responsible for the chronic reduction in body weight.

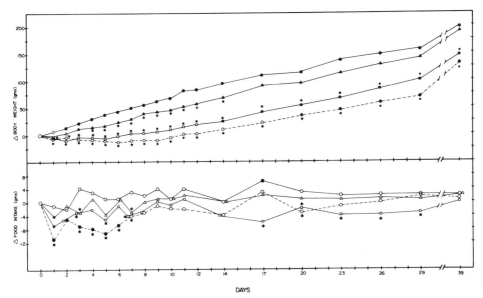

Fig. 5. Effects of E_2-CDS on body weight (upper panel) and daily food intake (lower panel) in lean male rats. Depicted are responses to E_2-CDS doses of o (vehicle, o——o), 0.2 mg/kg (△——△), 1.0 mg/kg (□——□) and 5.0 mg/kg (o----o). Darkened symbols indicate $p < 0.05$ versus day 0 and * indicates $p < 0.05$ versus vehicle controls.

Interestingly, a separation between the effects of E_2-CDS on body weight and food intake was observed. That is, despite body weight decreases at the 0.2 and 1 mg/kg doses of E_2-CDS, no consistent reduction in food intake was observed (Fig. 5) indicating that mechanisms other than reduced appetite are responsible for the weight loss observed.

Nine-month old male rats, whose body weights ranged from 632 ± 33 to 663 ± 43 gm at the onset of the experiment were treated by a single injection of various doses of E$_2$-CDS and the resulting changes in body weight and daily food intake were evaluated. In control, DMSO-treated rats, body weights (Fig. 6) and daily food intakes (data not shown) were stable throughout the course of the evaluation. E$_2$-CDS caused a dose-dependent increase in both the magnitude and duration of body weight loss (Fig. 6). Noteworthy is the duration of weight loss following a single exposure to the E$_2$-CDS. Body weight decline continued through 22, 36 and 57 days at the 0.2, 1 and 5 mg/kg doses. Thereafter, body weights gradually increased toward control levels through 64 days (the last observation point).

In obese males, the initial phase of weight loss was associated with a marked suppression in daily food intake (Fig. 6). The extent of the reduction in food intake may, during this initial weight loss phase, account for all or most of the weight loss observed.

It is interesting and may be clinically useful that the obese animals are more sensitive to both the body weight and food intake suppressory effects of E$_2$-CDS. Obese patients are a likely candidate for drug therapy in conjunction with voluntary reduction in food intake and enhanced energy expenditure to achieve weight loss.

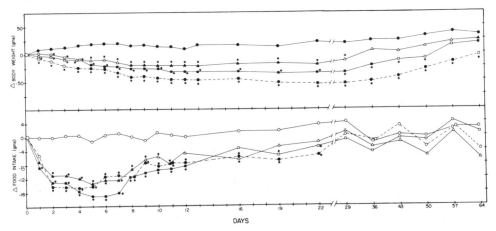

Fig. 6. Effects of E$_2$-CDS on body weight (upper panel) and daily food intake (lower panel) in obese male rats. Depicted are responses to E$_2$-CDS doses of 0 (vehicle, o—o), 0.2 mg/kg (△——△), 1.0 mg/Kg (□——□) and 5.0 mg/Kg (o- - -o). Darkened symbols indicate p<0.05 versus day 0 and * indicates p<0.05 versus vehicle controls.

3. Effects of E$_2$-CDS on Cholinergic Function

The biological basis for the involvement of estrogens in cognition comes from observations in laboratory animals. Estrogen receptors have been observed in the regions of the nuclei of the basal forebrain which are the major loci of cell bodies of cholinergic neurons which their fibers innervate the cerebral cortex, limbic system and hippocampus[60]. These brain regions are believed to be involved in the pathology of Alzheimer's Disease[61]. In rats, cholinergic neurons respond to peripheral administration of estrogen by increasing the activity of choline acetyltransferase,[62] acetylcholine synthesis[63] and high affinity choline uptake[63]. Estrogens may, therefore, serve a modulatory role in the function of cholinergic neurons and may serve as therapeutic agent in the stimulation of brain cholinergic neurons in patients with Alzheimer's Disease and other dementia which may be due to a cholinergic deficit.

While preliminary in nature, several studies have indicated that estrogens may be useful in the treatment of dementia, particularly when it is associated with the menopause. Elderly post-menopausal patients were evaluated for psychological function and behavior using the Hospital adjustment scale[64,65]. Premarin therapy did not significantly increase cognition but it prevented its further decline as compared to a placebo control group[64,65]. These studies suggest that chronic estrogen therapy may prevent the progression of loss in cognitive function in post-menopausal patients. In a second study[66], patients diagnosed as "probable Alzheimer's Disease" were subjected to a battery of tests to assess cognitive function and depression and were then treated with micronized estradiol for 6 weeks[66]. Modest improvements of scores on several tests of cognitive function were observed in one group of patients. In this group, the improvements were related primarily to improvements in attention, orientation, mood and social interaction. In only one patient improvement in memory noted.

Other studies have noted improvements in cognitive function, which were believed to be secondary to the antidepression actions of estrogen[67]. It is well known that emotional status affects memory and learning in both animals and man and that emotional disorders are frequently observed in Alzheimer's patients[68]. Thus, a primary effect of estrogens on mood could result in a secondary improvement in cognition.

E_2-CDS may be potentially useful in the treatment of dementia since currently there are no effective therapies for dementia and treatment regimens would have to be life-long. As such, peripheral estrogen toxicity would be a persistent problem for chronic administeration of estrogens peripherally. The brain-enhanced delivery of estradiol with the E_2-CDS may obviate this potential problem.

Given the aforementioned evidence for an effect of estrogen on cholinergic neuronal function, we evaluated the effects of E_2-CDS on neuronal systems which are known to be dysfunctional in Alzheimer's disease. In an initial study, female rats were ovariectomized (or received sham surgery) and 2 weeks later the ovariectomized rats were treated with the drug vehicle or E_2-CDS (1 mg/Kg, i.v.) and 5 days later all animals were sacrificed for a determination of high affinity choline uptake in the cerebral cortex, hippocampus and striatum. Ovariectomy reduced high affinity choline uptake in all three regions evaluated (Table II). Treatment with E_2-CDS increased high affinity choline uptake in the cortex and hippocampus to levels which were not different than intact control values (Table II). This single dose study, while preliminary, indicates that E_2-CDS can enhance the activity of cholinergic neurons in an ovariectomized animal model.

4. Effects of E_2-CDS on Brain Neuropeptides

Neuropeptide Y and somatostatin neurons show reduced peptide levels in the brain and/or CSF of patients with Alzheimer's Disease[69,70]. To determine the effects of estradiol on levels of these two peptides, we administered E_2-CDS and sacrificed animals at 0 (vehicle), 1, 7 or 14 days later. Tissue samples were obtained from the cortex, hypothalamus, hippocampus, striatum and brain stem and samples were assayed for NPY and somatostatin by specific RIA.

Table II. Effects of Ovariectomy and E_2-CDS on High Affinity Choline Uptake in Brain Regions

	Brain Region		
Group	Cortex	Hippocampus (cpm x 10^3/mg Protein)	Striatum
Intact females and vehicle[*]	176 ± 44	235 ± 33	657 ± 138
OVX and vehicle	100 ± 7	162 ± 2	392 ± 37
OVX and E_2-CDS	181 ± 14	198 ± 21	481 ± 33

[*] Vehicle for all groups was 2-β-hydroxypropylcyclodextrin

In response to E_2-CDS, NPY levels showed a progressive increase in the hypothalamus and cortex and a transient elevation in the hippocampus (Table III). Striatal and brain stem NPY levels were not affected by the E_2-CDS. In contrast to the effects of E_2-CDS on NPY levels, somatostatin concentrations did not change in response to administration of a single dose of the delivery system (data not shown).

Table III. Effects of E_2-CDS on Concentrations of NPY in Several Brain Regions

Brain Region	Days After E_2-CDS Treatment			
	0	1	7	14
	(pg/mg Protein)			
Hypothalamus	695 ± 101	730 ± 71	915 ± 137	1935 ± 371[*]
Cortex	97 ± 16	102 ± 25	107 ± 18	159 ± 25[*]
Hippocampus	104 ± 23	173 ± 24	118 ± 26	167 ± 29
Striatum	125 ± 11	105 ± 9	97 ± 13	125 ± 22
Brain Stem	28 ± 2	36 ± 5	33 ± 5	35 ± 4

[*] $p < 0.05$ vs. day 0 (vehicle injected) controls - ANOVA SNK tests

These data indicate that the chronic elevation of brain E_2 levels with the E_2-CDS can increase the activity of cholinergic neurons in ovariectomized rats and increased the concentrations of at least 1 neuropeptide which is deficient in patients with Alzheimer's Disease. These encouraging, albeit preliminary, results support the further evaluation of brain-enhanced delivery system for estrogen as a potential therapy for cognitive loss associated with estrogen decline at the menopause. The capacity of the chemical delivery system to deliver E_2 preferentially to the brain suggest that this delivery system should also be evaluated in conditions of cognitive impairment which may not be associated with overt declines in peripheral estrogen levels. Thus, if estrogen serve to maintain or enhance activity in cholinergic neurons or serve as a trophic substance which directly or indirectly act on cholinergic neurons, the result of enhanced brain exposure to E_2 may be an improvement in cognition. Further, since any therapy which is aimed at treating Alzheimer's disease must be chronic in its application to the patient, the sustained release of E_2 from the E_2-CDS is an additional useful benefit. As such, a careful evaluation of the E_2-CDS for the mechanism by which it improves cholinergic function and for its potential application to Alzheimer's Disease patients is clearly warranted.

CONCLUSIONS

The results described here support the view that the E_2-CDS may be potentially useful not only for the regulation of gonadotropin secretion but also in the treatment of certain other CNS-mediated estrogen withdrawal symptoms, e.g., hot flushes and cognitive impairment. In comparison to the currently used estrogen-esters, the E_2-CDS should achieve sustained stimulation of brain E_2 receptors at lower doses, or with less frequent dosing. Finally, the redox-based chemical delivery system can be useful in delivering and in "locking" a variety of drugs to the brain in a form which allows their slow and sustained release.

ACKNOWLEDGMENTS

The authors are indebted to Victoria Redd Patterson for her editorial review and typing of this manuscript. Supported in part by grants HD 22540, GM 27167 and a grant from Pharmatec, Inc.

REFERENCES

1. C. Lauritzen, The management of the pre-menopausal and the post-menopausal patient, in: "Aging and Estrogens," P.A. Van Keep and C. Lauritzen, eds., Karger, Basel (1973).
2. S. Campbell and M. Whitehead, Oestrogen therapy and the menopausal syndrome, Clin. Obstet. Gynaecol. 4:31 (1977).
3. H.L. Judd, Pathophysiology of menopausal hot flushes, in: "Neuroendocrinology of Aging," J. Meites, ed., Plenum press, New York (1983).
4. B.B. Sherwin, Estrogen and/or androgen replacement therapy and cognitive functioning in surgically menopausal women, Psychoneuroendocrinology 13:345 (1988).
5. I. Persson, The risk of endometrial and breast cancer after estrogen treatment, Acta. Obstet. Gynecol. Scand. 130 Suppl.:59 (1985).
6. D.B. Thomas, Steroid hormones and medications that alter cancer risks, Cancer 62:1755 (1988).
7. W.M. Pardridge, J.D. Connor and I.L. Crawford, Permeability changes in the blood-brain barrier: causes and consequences, CRC Crit. Rev. Toxic. 3:159 (1975).
8. E. Levin, Are the terms blood-brain barrier and brain capillary permeability synonymous, Exp. Eye Res. 25 Suppl.:191 (1977).
9. B. Van Duers, Structural aspects of brain barriers with special reference to the permeability of the cerebral endothelium and choroidal epithelium, Int. Rev. Cytol. 65:117 (1980).
10. H. Davson, The blood-brain barrier, J. Physiol. Lond. 255:1 (1976).

11. N. Bodor and M.E. Brewster, Problems of delivery of drugs to the brain, Pharmacol. Therapeut. 19:337 (1983).
12. M.J. Karnovsky, The ultrastructural basis of capillary permeability studies with peroxidase as a tracer, J. Cell Biol. 35:213 (1967).
13. T.S. Reese and M.J. Karnovsky, Fine structural localization of a blood-brain barrier to exogenous peroxidase, J. Cell Biol. 34:207 (1967).
14. M.W. Brightman and T.S. Reese, Junctions between intimately opposed cell membranes in the vertebrate brain, J. Cell Biol. 40:648 (1969).
15. W.H. Oldendorf, The blood-brain barrier, Exp. Eye Res. 25 Suppl.:177 (1977).
16. R.R. Shivers, The blood-brain barrier of a reptile, Anoli's Carolinensis. A freeze-fracture study, Brain Res. 169:221 (1979).
17. M.W. Brightman, Morphology of blood-brain interfaces, Exp. Eye Res. 25 Suppl.:1 (1977).
18. R.D. Broadwell and M. Saloman, Expanding the definition of the blood-brain barrier to protein, Proc. Soc. Acad. Sci. U.S.A. 78:7820 (1981).
19. J.E. Hardebo, B. Falck, C. Owman and E. Rosengren, Studies on the enzymatic blood-brain barrier: quantitative measurement of DOPA decarboxylase in the wall of microvessels as related to the parenchyma in various CNS regions, Acta Physiol. Scand. 105:453 (1979).
20. J.E. Hardebo and C. Owman, Barrier mechanisms for neurotransmitter monoamines and their precursors at the blood-brain interface, Ann. Neurol. 8:1 (1980).
21. G.P. Kaplan, B.K. Hartman and C.R. Creveling, Immunohistochemical localization of catechol-o-methyltransferase in circumventricular organ of the rat: potential variations in the blood-brain barrier to native catechols, Brain Res. 229:323 (1981).
22. W.H. Oldendorf, L. Braun, S. Hyman and S.Z. Oldendorf, Blood-brain barrier: penetration of morphine, codeine, heroin and methadone after carotid injection, Science 178:984 (1972).
23. J.M. Cruickshank, G. Neil-Dwyer, M.M. Cameron and J. McAinsh, β-adrenoreceptor-blocking agents and the blood-brain barrier, Clin. Sci. 59:453s (1979).
24. V.A. Levin, Relationship of octanol water partition coefficients and molecular weight to rat brain capillary permeability, J. Med. Chem. 23:682 (1980).
25. A.A. Sinkula and S.H. Yalkowsky, Rational for design of biologically reversible drug derivatives: Prodrugs, J. Pharm. Sci. 64:181 (1975).
26. N. Bodor, The soft drug approach, Chemtech Jan.:28 (1984).
27. N. Bodor, Novel approaches in prodrug design, Drugs of the future 6:165 (1981).
28. N. Bodor, Soft drugs: Principles and methods for the design of safe drugs, Med. Res. Reviews 4:449 (1984).
29. V. Stella, Pro-drugs: an overview and definition, in: "Prodrugs as Novel Drug Delivery Systems," T. Higuchi and V. Stella, eds., ACS Symposium Series Vol. 14, American Chemical Society, Washington, D.C. (1975).
30. R.D. Smyth, M. Pfeffer, D.R. Van Hanker, A. Cohen and G.H. Hottendorf, Human pharmacokinetics and disposition of sarmoxicillin, a lipophilic amoxicillin prodrug, Antimicrob. Ag. Chemother. 1004 (1981).
31. H. Ferres, Pro-drugs of β-lactam antibiotics, Chem. Ind. 11:436 (1980).
32. T.A. Connors, Possible pro-drugs in cancer chemotherapy, Chem. Ind. 11:447 (1980).
33. M. Masquelier, R. Baurain and A. Trouet, Amino acid and dipeptide derivatives of daunorubicin. 1. Synthesis, Physicochemical properties, and lysosomal digestion, J. Med. Chem. 23:1166 (1980).
34. P. Workman and J.A. Double, Drug Latentiation in Cancer Chemotherapy, Biomed. 28:255 (1978).

35. N. Bodor, E. Shek and T. Higuhi, Delivery of a quaternary pyridinium salt across the blood-brain barrier by its dihydropyridine derivative, Science 190:155 (1975).
36. N. Bodor, H. Farag and M.E. Brewster, site-specific sustained release of drugs to the brain, Science 214:1370 (1981).
37. N. Bodor and H. Farag, Improved delivery through biological membranes XI. A redox chemical drug delivery system and its use for brain specific delivery of phenethylamine, J. Med. Chem. 26:313 (1983).
38. N. Bodor and J.W. Simpkins, Redox delivery system for brain-specific, sustained release of dopamine, Science 221:65 (1983).
39. J.W. Simpkins, N. Bodor and A. Enz, Direct evidence for brain specific release of dopamine from a redox delivery system, J. Pharm. Sci. 94:1033 (1985).
40. N. Bodor and H. Farag, Improved delivery through biological membranes XIII. Brain specific delivery of dopamine with a dihydropyridine pyridinium salt type redox delivery system, J. Med. Chem. 26:528 (1983).
41. N. Bodor and M.E. Brewster, Improved delivery through biological membranes, XV. Sustained brain delivery of berberine, Eur. J. Med. Chem. 18:235 (1983).
42. W.R. Anderson, J.W. Simpkins, P.A. Woodard, D. Winwood, W.C. Stern and N. Bodor, Anxiolytic activity of a brain delivery system for GABA, Psychopharmacology 92:157 (1987).
43. M.H. Rahimy, N. Bodor and J.W. Simpkins, A rapid, sensitive method for the simultaneous quantitation of estradiol and estradiol conjugates in a variety of tissues: assay development and evaluation of the distribution of a brain-enhanced estradiol-chemical delivery system, J. Steroid Biochem. 33:000 (1989).
44. G. Mullersman, H. Derendorf, M.E. Brewster, K.S. Estes and N. Bodor, High-performance liquid chromatographic assay of a central nervous system (CNS)-directed estradiol chemical delivery system and its application after intravenous administration to rats, Pharm. Res. 5:172 (1988).
45. M.H. Rahimy, J.W. Simpkins and N. Bodor, Tissue distribution of a brain-enhanced chemical delivery system for estradiol, submitted for publication, Drug Design and Delivery (1989).
46. G.T. Ross, Disorders of the ovary and female reproductive tract, in: "Textbook of Endocrinology," J.D. Wilson and D.W. Foster, eds., W.B. Saunders Company, Philadelphia (1981).
47. J.A. Czaja, Body weight and growth rates throughout the guinea pig pregnancy: evidence for modulation by endogenous estrogens, Physiol. Behav. 30:197 (1975).
48. M.F. Tarttelin, Cyclical variations in food and water intake in ewes, J. Physiol. 195:29 (1968).
49. M.F. Tarttelin and R.A. Gorski, Variations in food and water intake in normal and acyclic female rats, Physiol. Behav. 7:847 (1971).
50. J.A. Czaja, Ovarian influence on primate food intake: assessment of progesterone actions, Physiol. Behav. 21:923 (1978).
51. J.A. Czaja, Food rejection by female rhesus monkeys during the menstrual cycle and early pregnancy, Physiol. Behav. 14:579 (1975).
52. S.P. Dalvit, The effects of the menstrual cycle on patterns of food intake, Am. J. Clin. Nutr. 34:1811 (1981).
53. P. Pliner and A.S. Fleming, Food intake, body weight and sweetness preferences over the menstrual cycle in humans, Physiol. Behav. 30:663 (1983).
54. T. Landau and I. Zucker, Estrogenic regulation of body weight in the female rats, Horm. Behav. 7:29 (1976).
55. J.F. McElroy and G.N. Wade, Short- and long-term effects of ovariectomy on food intake, body weight, carcass composition and brown adipose tissue in rats, Physiol. Behav. 39:361 (1987).

56. M.F. Tarttelin and R.A. Gorski, The effects of the ovarian steroids on food and water intake and body weight in the female rats, <u>Acta Endronol.</u> 72:551 (1973).

57. J.H. Morton, H. Additon, R.G. Addison, L. Hunt, J.J. Sullivan, A clinical study of premenstrual tension, <u>Am. J. Obstet. Gynecol.</u> 65:1182 (1953).

58. S.L. Smith and C. Sauder, Food cravings, depression and premenstrual problems, <u>Psychosom. Med.</u> 31:281 (1969).

59. J.W. Simpkins, W.R. Anderson, R. Dawson, Jr., A. Seth, M. Brewster, K.S. Estes and N. Bodor, Chronic weight loss in lean and obese rats with a brain-enhanced chemical delivery system for estradiol, <u>Physiol. Behav.</u> 44:573 (1988).

60. V.N. Luine, R.I. Khylchevskaya and B.S. McEwen, Effect of gonadal steroids on activity of monoamine oxidase and choline acetylase in rat brain, <u>Brain Res.</u> 86:293 (1975).

61. J.T. Coyle, D.L. Price and M.R. Delong, Alzheimer's disease: a disorder of cortical cholinergic innervation, <u>Science</u> 219:1184 (1983).

62. V.N. Luine, Estradiol increases choline acetyltransferase activity in specific basal forebrain nuclei and projection areas in female rats, <u>Exp. Neurol.</u> 89:484 (1985).

63. C.A. O'Malley, R.D. Hautamaki, M. Kelley, E.M. Meyer, Effects of ovariectomy and estradiol benzoate on high affinity choline uptake, Ach synthesis, and release from rat cerebral cortical synaptosomes, <u>Brain Res.</u> 403:389 (1987).

64. H.I. Kantor, C.M. Michael, H. Shore and H.W. Ludvigson, Administration of estrogens to older women, a psychometric evaluation, <u>Am. J. Obstet. Gynecol.</u> 101:58 (1968).

65. C.H. Michael, H.I. Kantor and H. Shore, Further psychometric evaluation of older women-the effect of estrogen administration, <u>J. Gerontol.</u> 25:337 (1970).

66. H. Fillit, H. Weinreb, I. Cholst, V. Luine, B. McEwen, R. Amador and J. Zabriskie, Observations in a preliminary open trial of estradiol therapy for senile dementia-Alzheimer's type, <u>Psychoneuronedocrinol.</u> 11:337 (1986).

67. B.W. Hackman and D. Galbraith, Replacement therapy with piperazine oestrone sulfate ("Harmogen") and its effect on memory, <u>Current Medical Research and Opinion</u> 4:303 (1976).

68. M. Raskind, Biological parameters in the differential diagnosis of dementia and depression, <u>in</u>: "Biology and Treatment of Dementia in the Elderly," C.A. Shamoian, Ed., American Psychiatric Press, Washington, D.C. (1983).

69. V. Chan-Palay, Y.S. Allen, W. Lang, V. Haesler and J.M. Polak, II. Cortical neurons immunoreactive with antisera against neuropeptide Y are altered in Alzheimer's-type dementia, <u>J. Comp. Neurol.</u> 238:391 (1985).

70. P. Davies, R. Katzman and R.D. Terry, Reduced somatostatin-like immunoreactivity in cerebral cortex from cases of Alzheimer's disease and Alzheimer's senile dementia, <u>Nature</u> 288:279 (1980).

IMMUNOLOGIC APPROACH TO THERAPY IN ALZHEIMER'S DISEASE

Vijendra K. Singh and Reed P. Warren

Department of Biology and DCHP
Utah State University
Logan, Utah 84322-6800, USA

INTRODUCTION

Alzheimer's disease (AD) is a progresssive neurodegenerative disorder of aging characterized clinically by the loss of memory (especially of recent events), intellect and cognitive functions. The etiology and the pathogenesis of AD is unknown, and there is no effective treatment available. However, some good hypotheses are presently being investigated (see ref. #1-3). These include speculations that AD is caused by: (a) an infectious agent, perhaps a virus; (b) abnormal function of immune system or immunoincompetence; (c) genetic predisposition as in 'familial' AD; (d) disturbance of brain biochemistry (neurotransmitters, neuropeptides and/or neurotropic factors); and (e) exposure to toxic substances like aluminum. Current immune studies have shown abnormalities of both cell-mediated and humoral immunity, supporting an immune hypothesis in the pathogenesis of AD or at least in a subset of immune origin (4-6), especially since clinical as well as genetic heterogeneity (7) exists among patients presented with this disease. One possible immune mechanism may involve autoimmunity perhaps secondary to a virus infection (i.e. a humoral immune response to body's own constituents, specifically brain antigens in the case of AD). Relevant ot this hypothesis is a recent observation which showed a temporal link of a unconventional virus infection in AD; this was shown based upon the transmissibility of Creutzfeldt-Jacob disease (CJD)-like histopathology in the hamsters inoculated intracerebrally with buffy coat cells (white blood cells) of the blood from AD patients (8). This paper describes the rationale for the development of therapy with immunomodulating agents.

INTERRELATIONSHIP BETWEEN CENTRAL NERVOUS SYSTEM AND IMMUNE SYSTEM

As summarized in Table 1, there exists a reciprocal structural and functional reltionship between the central nervous system (CNS) and immune system. This observation led us to hypothesize that the white blood cells can be used to study various neuropsychiatric diseases (6). Blalock and Smith (9) previously suggested that the immune system represents body's "mobile brain", and the term "immunotransmitter" synonymously to "neurotransmitter" was coined to refer to the soluble products of the immune system cells (10). Several antigenic proteins of the CNS have been localized on the immune cells, and neuropeptides like endorphins and corticotropins are natural products of both brain cells and immune cells. The high-affinity binding receptor sites for several neurotransmitters (acetylcholine, serotonin, dopamine, histamine) and neuropeptides (substance P, somatostatin, endorphins, corticotropin-

Table 1. Interactiveness between CNS and immune system*

A. Structural Similarities:

1. Thy-1 antigen, a membrane glycoprotein of sequence homology with IgG, is present on both lymphoid and CNS cells.
2. MRC OX-2 antigen is a glycoprotein of sequence homology with the light chain of Ig molecule and is distributed on thymocytes, dendritic cells, some B cells and nerve cells of the CNS.
3. Human T cell antigens are expressed on both glial cells (oligodendrocytes) and neurons (Purkinje cells).
4. Natural killer (NK) cells and myelin sheath share an antigen which is marked by the monoclonal antibody anti-Leu-7.
5. Monocyte monoclonal antibody (OKM1) stains cells in the white matter of the brain; Fc receptors and Ia antigens are found on B lymphocytes and monocytes as well as on astrocytes and microglia in the brain.
6. Various ion-channels (Na^+, K^+ and Ca^{++}) are found on neurons and lymphocytes.
7. Receptor entities for neurotransmitters and neuropeptides are localized on both brain and immune cells.
8. Interleukin-1 receptors are present on brain cells and the helper T cell antigen CD4 is detected on brain astrocytes.
9. Receptor binding sites for CRF neurohormone are localized on white blood cells and brain cells.

B. Functional Relationship:

1. Interferon exposure induces the expression of Ia and MHC-restricted antigens by normal brain cells; it also modifies electrophysiological responses.
2. Brain lesions modify immune responses directly or indirectly via neuroendocrine sysytem.
3. Immune responses invoke firing of CNS noradrenergic cells.
4. Both monocytes and astrocytes present 'antigen' to T cells; both these cell types produce interleukin-1 cytokine which has a trophic effect on astroglial cells. Interleukin-2, a helper T cell factor, induces proliferation of CNS oligodendroglial cells.
5. Both neurons and lymphocytes synthesize endorphin- and corticotropin-like neuropeptides.
6. Neuropeptides like substance P, *beta*-endorphin and somatostatin modulate immune functions.
7. Recombinant interleukin-1 induces the synthesis and secretion of CRF neurohormone by hypothalamic cells.
8. CRF neurohormone stimulates lymphocyte proliferation and interleukin-2-receptor expression by T cells.

*Note: For detailed references, see citation number (6) and (16).

releasing factor or (CRF) have been found on the membranes of blood lymphocytes. In addition, the receptor sites for immune cell products, e.g. interleukin-1, have been identified on CNS cells.

In terms of functions, both CNS and immune system cells have the property of 'memory'. The astrocytes present antigens to T cells just like monocytes do, and the interleukins (IL-1 or IL-2) act as supplementary growth factors for neuronal cultures. Likewise, several neuropeptides modify the function of immune cells, e.g. IL-1 stimulates the secretion of CRF by hypothalamic cells in the brain. We recently reported that CRF, in turn, stimulates lymphocyte proliferation and the IL-2-receptor expression on T cells (11). These findings, thus, provide a basis for a complete circuit between CNS and immune system, and accordingly, it was suggested that certain neuropsychiatric disorders can

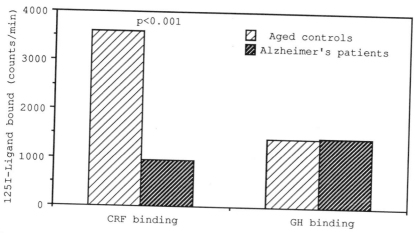

<u>Figure 1</u>. Binding of ^{125}I-CRF and ^{125}I-growth hormone (GH) to blood mononuclear cells of AD patients and non-AD controls. The details of the binding experiments were the same as described elsewhere (12).

be studied by the use of blood lymphocytes (6), in addition to brain biopsies or autopsies. Four different sets of experiments now support this hypothesis: (a) the lymphocyte receptor binding for neurohormone CRF, but not growth hormone (Fig.1), is markedly reduced in about 80% of AD patients compared to non-AD controls (12);(b) the acetylcholinesterase activity of blood lymphocytes was is lower in AD patients than the aged controls (13); the mitogen-induced uptake of calcium by blood lymphocytes is decreased in AD patients (14); and (d) the membrane fluidity of blood platelets is reduced in AD patients (15). Thus, the use of blood lymphocytes to discern nerve cell dysfucntion is a feasible approach for the studies of neuropsychiatric disorders.

IMMUNOPATHOLOGICAL CONSIDERATIONS IN ALZHEIMER'S DISEASE

Several lines of investigations suggest the importance of studying immune parameters in AD (16). These are: (a) AD is a disease of loss of memory function, a property shared by both central nervous system (CNS) and immune system, and the two systems display remarkable structural-functional relationships with each other, and the immune cells can be used to resolve alterations of counterpart brain cells in AD; (b) AD is a disease of the aging, and there is a general decline of function of immune cells with aging accompanied by an increased incidence of diseases, especially autoimmune diseases; (c) amyloidosis or the accumulation of unusually large amounts of amyloid occurs in the brain of AD patients, and amyloid is presumably of immune origin because of its immunoreactivity with antibodies to immunoglobulin light chains; (d) Down's Syndrome (DS), a high-risk factor in AD, has been considered as an appropriate model of both primary immunodeficiency and accelerated aging in humans, and we recently found depressed immune function in patients with both AD and DS (5); (e) immune-mediated mechanisms have been associated with other diseases of the nervous system (e.g. multiple sclerosis, myasthenia gravis, autism, and schizophrenia), and patients with some of these disorders respond to immunotherapy; and (f) abberrations of both cell-mediated as well as humoral immunity have been found in AD patients (see below). Each one of these considerations is sufficiently important so as to implicate immunologic mechanisms in the pathophysiology of AD.

An immune hypothesis involving autoimmunity in the pathological processes of AD has long been suggested, although very little is known about the mechanism of tissue damage. Conceivably, circulating autoantibodies may have direct cytotoxic effect or the tissue damage may be mediated by immune complexes or immune activation of T cells may generate CD8+-suppressor/cytotoxic cells. It's noteworthy, however, that the cytotoxic/suppressor (CD8+) T cells were recently localized in the brain tissue of AD patients (17) which may be indicative of a cell-mediated immune response in the disease. Abnormal neuropathology in AD is certainly capable of disseminating brain antigens which can be recognized by patients' own immune system, generating circulating autoantibodies. Brain autoantibodies have been detected in many patients with AD (4,18,19). Whether these autoantibodies are cytotoxic, especially to brain cells, is not known. However, the isotype of brain autoantibody in AD is mainly of IgG3 subclass (19,20), which most effectively activates classic pathway, but not alternate pathway, of complement system and thus it may be involved in cell cytotoxicity. Once the C1 complement system is activated, immune complexes via Fc portion of the immunoglobulin molecule bind to complement receptors (C3 or C3b) on various cells causing cellular destruction in the target organ. Moreover, elevated levels of immune complexes containing IgG antibody are generally seen in autoimmune diseases, and upon deposition in tissue, they can cause tissue damage in a complement-dependent mechanism (21)

IMMUNOLOGIC DYSFUNCTION IN ALZHEIMER'S DISEASE

Abnormal function of one or another immune parameters has been demonstrated in AD patients. In terms of cell-mediated immunity (T cell function), the lymphocyte proliferation in response to stimulation with T cell mitogens (phytohemagglutinin, concanavalin A, pokeweed mitogen and anti-CD3) was severely depressed in many patients with AD (5). The T cell stimulation by non-T cells (B cells and monocytes) in the autologous-mixed leucocyte reaction was also abnormal in a subset of patients. The deficient function of T cells was furthermore found by the reduced activity of CD8+ suppressor T cells (22), and by depressed responsiveness to Con A-stimulated lymphocyte blastogenesis and BCG vaccine-induced delayed-type hypersensitivity (23). Our unpublished data showed that the ratio of helper/suppressor T cells was increased in many patients as reflected by an increase in the proportion of helper T cells in 10 of 16 cases but decrease of suppressor T cells in 6 of 16 cases. All of these data point to a basic defect of immunoregulatory T cells in AD patients.

Impairement of humoral immunity has also been found in a subset of AD. Inconsistent results have been reported with regards to the serum concentration of immunoglobulins (IgM, IgG and IgA): IgG and IgA normal but decreased IgM (24) or IgG and IgA increased but IgM normal (25). This discrepancy is apparently related to the clinical diagnosis of the disease since patients either had presenile dementia (24) or dementia was due to reasons other than AD, e.g. cerebral artherosclerosis (25). Recent analysis of serum IgG isotypes showed that the distribution of IgG1, IgG2 and IgG4 was normal, but the level of IgG3 isotype was significantly elevated in about 45% of AD patients (20) and this isotype was related to brain autoantibodies detected in AD serum (4, 20).

Circulating autoantibodies to neural tissue antigens have been detected in a subset of AD patients (4, 18, 19). Unlike AD patients, the patients with Down's syndrome did not have brain antibodies, and in this respect, the Down's syndrome differed from AD (4). There is now evidence that in some patients, the brain autoantibody is mainly due to IgG3 isotype directed against cholinergic neurons (18,19). Autoantibodies to other neural antigens, e.g. neuron-axon filament proteins (16,26), pituitary cells (27) and neurofibrillary tangles (28) have also been reported.

The generation of circulating tissue-specific antibodies is generally considered as an indication of an autoimmune phenomenon in a given disease, e.g. brain autoantibodies in AD and antibodies to myelin basic protein in MS. Consistent with this idea is a recent report showing the presence of leucocyte antigen positive cells and suppressor /cytotoxic T cells in the brain tissue of AD patients but not of healthy subjects (17). This finding may be interpreted as an indication of lymphocytic infiltrate or sensitization of brain antigens.

IMMUNOTHERAPEUTIC IMPLICATIONS IN ALZHEIMER'S DISEASE

The clinical as well as the genetic heterogeneity (7) amongst the subjects with AD suggests that this disease is a syndrome of subsets with different etiologies, one of which is immunologic in origin (or an immune subset). This concept is advocated to suggest that different therapeutic modalities will be necessary in the hopes of developing any form of successful treatment for patients with AD. Thus, the therapy based on neurotransmitter or neurotrophic factor deficiency may identify a neurochemical subset; therapy based on an immunologic deficit or dysfunction may define an immune subset; and other forms of therapy may necessitate yet other unknown subsets. Hence, it is not unreasonable to think that more than one type of agents should be developed for the improvement of cognitive deficits seen in AD patients.

The development of an immunotherapeutic approach for the treatment of patients will depend upon the nature of the immune deficit, appropriate immunomodulating agent, and responsiveness to therapy with these agents. These requisites would imply that within the immune subsets, there may be several sub-categories: one immune subset with the deficiency of cell-mediated immunity (T cell function), another one with the impairement of humoral immunity (or an autoimmune subset), another one with lymphocyte deficiencies of biochemical and/or molecular factors, still another one based on the deficiency of a neuroendocrine-immune circuity (Fig. 2), e.g. CRF lymphocyte receptor deficiency (12).

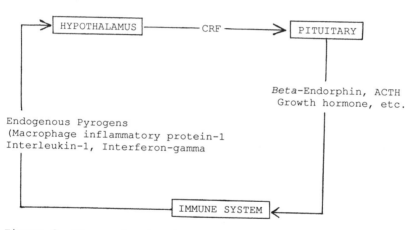

Figure 2. Neuroendocrine-immune circuity involving CRF and endogenous pyrogens

The present situation of treatment for AD resembles, in many respects, another neurological disease, multiple sclerosis (MS), for which, nearly 150 'therapies' have been advocated during the last fifty years (29) yet there is no successful treatment available today. A point of interest, however, is the fact that current approaches to therapy for MS are based on the thinking that the disease is the net outcome of a virus infection and/or autoimmunization against some component of the myelin sheath, although the etiology of MS still remains a big mystery. Likewise in AD, the etiology and the pathogenesis is not known, there are preliminary indications of a viral infection and/or autosensitization against some brain antigen, pointing to the possibility of treatment of AD patients with immunomodulating or immunosuppressive or antiviral agents. Recently, therapy with Transfer Factor (TF) was shown to produce some benefits of secondary symptoms (30), but these results are difficult to evaluate due to the 'open-label' nature and the lack of neuropsychiatric assessment in the study. However, the TF therapy should be discouraged since the white blood cells from the so-called healthy relatives of AD patients (whose white blood cells would normally be used as the source of TF) have been shown to transmit CJD-like disease in the experimental animals (8) . In addition, the biochemical nature of TF is not known (what if it is a unknown viral constituent?), TF therapy is of unproven validity, and it produces no positive results in patients with at least two other CNS diseases, MS (31) and autism (32).

In AD patients, the depression of cell-mediated immunity or immunoincompetence may be potentiated with agents such as recombinant interleukins, interferons, thymic hormones, isoprinosine, etc. The immunosuppressants like cyclosporin A may be tested for patients in the autoimmune subset having autoantibodies to brain tissue antigens. Cyclosporine was recently shown to produce some benefits in patients with amyotrophic lateral sclerosis (33) which may also involve autoimmune factors. These immunoactive compounds, not only restore the deficient function of immune cells, may indeed act directly on the CNS cells, thereby improving the CNS function also, e.g. interleukin-1 stimulates hypothalamic cells for the synthesis and secretion of CRF (34) . Additionally, agents with neurotrophic activity, e.g. NGF, may be active in restoring the function of immune cells. Thus, the immunomodulating agents could possibly stimulate the function of 'atrophied' neurons in vivo, which led us to conclude that the importance of immunotherapy should not be precluded from our current thinking about the therapeutic modalities in Alzheimer's disease.

REFERENCES

1. Glenner, G.G. (1985) On causative theories in Alzheimer's disease. Human Pathol. 16: 433-435.
2. Wisniewski, H.M., Merz, G.S. and Carp, R.I. (1985) Current hypothesis of the etiology and pathogenesis of senile dementia of the Alzheimer's type. Interdiscipl. Topics Geront. 19: 45-53.
3. Khachaturian, Z.S . (1986) Aluminum toxicity among other views on the etiology of Alzheimer's disease. Neurobiol. Aging 7: 537-539.
4. Singh, V.K. and Fudenberg, H.H. (1986) Detection of brain autoantibodies in the serum of patients with Alzheimer's disease but not Down's syndrome. Immunol. Lett. 12: 277-280.
5. Singh, V.K., Fudenberg, H.H. and Brown, F.R. (III) (1987) Immunologic dysfunction: simultaneous study of Alzheimer's and Down's patients. Mech. Ageing Develop. 37: 257-264.
6. Singh, V.K. and Fudenberg, H.H. (1986) Can blood immunocytes be used to study neuropsychiatric disorders? J. Clin. Psychiatr. 47: 592-595.
7. Schellenberg, G.D., Bird, T.D., Wijsman, E.M., Moore, D.K., Boehnke, M., Bryant, E.M., Lamp, T.H., Nochlin, D., Sumi, S.M., Deeb, S.S., Beyreuther, K. and Martin, G.M. (1988) Absence of linkage of chromosome 21q21 markers to familial Alzheimer' s disease. Science 241: 1506-1510.
8. Manuelidis, E.E., de Figuiredo, J.M., Kim, J.H., Fritch, W.W. and Manuelidis, L. (1988) Transmission studies from blood of Alzheimer's disease patients and relatives. Proc. Natl. Acad.Sci., USA. 85: 4898- 4901.
9. Blalock J.E. and Smith, E.M. (1985) The immune system: our mobile brain? Immunol. Today 6: 115-117.
10. Hall, N.R., McGilliS, J.P., Spangelo, B.L. and Goldstein, A.L. (1985)Evidence that thymosins and other biologic response modifiers can function as neuroactive immunotransmitters. J. Immunol. 135: 806s-811s.
11. Singh, V.K. (1989) Stimulatory effect of corticotropin-releasing factor on human lymphocyte proliferation and interleukin-2-receptor expression. J. Neuroimmunol. (in press).
12. Singh, V.K. and Fudenberg, H.H. (1988) Binding of [125I] corticotropin releasing factor to blood immunocytes and its reduction in Alzheimer's disease. Immunol. Lett. 18: 5-8.

13. Bartha, E., Szelenji, K., Szilagji, K., Venter, V., Thu Ha, N.T., Paldi-Harris, P. and Hollan, S. (1987) Altered lymphocyte acetylcholinesterase in patients with senile dementia. <u>Neurosci. Lett</u>. 79: 190-194.

14. Gibson, G.E., Nielson, P., Sherman, K.A. and Blass, J.P. (1987) Diminished mitogen-induced calcium uptake by lymphocytes from Alzheimer's patients. <u>Biol. Psychiatr</u>. 22: 1079-1086.

15. Zubenko, G.S., Wusylko, M., Cohen, B.M., Boller, F. and Teply, I. (1987) Family study of platelet membrane fluidity in Alzheimer's disease. <u>Science</u> 238: 539-542.

16. Singh, V.K. and Fudenberg, H.H. (1988) Implications of immunomodulant therapy in Alzheimer's disease. <u>Progress Drug Res</u>. 32: 21-42.

17. Itagaki, S., McGeer, P.L. and Akiyama, H. (1988) Presence of T-cytotoxic suppressor and leukocyte common antigen positive cells in Alzheimer's disease brain tissue. <u>Neurosci. Lett</u>. 91:259-264.

18. Fillit, H., Luine, V.N., Reisberg, B., Amador, R., McEwen, B. and Zabriskie, J.B. (1985) Studies of the specificity of antibrain antibodies in Alzheimer's disease. In: <u>Senile Dementia of the Alzheimer's type</u> (eds: Hutton, J.T. and Kenney, A.D.), Alan R. Liss Publ.,N.Y., pp.307-318.

19. Mcrae-Degueurce, A., Booj, S., Haglid, K., Rosengren, L., Karlsson, J.E., Karlsson, I., Wallin, A., Svennerholm, L., Gottfries, C.G. and Dahlstrom, A. (1987) Antibodies in the CSF of some Alzheimer's patients recognize cholinergic neurons in the rodent central nervous system. <u>Proc. Natl. Acad. Sci</u>., USA. 84: 9214-9218.

20. Singh, V.K. and Fudenberg, H.H.(1989) Increase of immunoglobulin G3 subclass is related to brain autoantibody in Alzheimer's disease but not in Down's syndrome. <u>Autoimmunity</u> (in press).

21. Williams, R.C. (1981) Immune complexes in Human diseases. <u>Ann. Rev. Med</u>. 32: 13-28.

22. Skias, D., Bania, M., Reder, A.T., Luchins, D. and Antel, J.P. (1985) Senile dementia of Alzheimer's type (SDAT): reduced T8+ cell-mediated suppressor activity. <u>Neurology</u> 35: 1635-1638.

23. Torack, R.M. (1986) T-lymphocyte function in Alzheimer's disease. <u>Neurosci. Lett</u>. 71: 365-369.

24. Tavolato, B. and Argentiero, V. (1980) Immunological indices in presenile Alzheimer's disease. <u>J. Neurolog. Sci</u>. 46: 325-331.

25. Cohen, D. and Eisdorfer, C. (1980) Serum immunoglobulins and cognitive status in the elderly: I. a population study. <u>Brit. J. Psychiatr</u>. 136: 33-39.

26. Toh, B.H., Gibbs, C.J., Gajdusek, D.C., Goudsmit, J. and Dahl, D. (1985) The 200- and 150- kDa neurofilament proteins react with IgG autoantibodies from patients with kuru, Creutzfeldt-Jacob disease, and other neurological diseases. <u>Proc. Natl. Acad. Sci</u>. USA. 82: 3485-3489.

27. Pouplard, A. and Emile, J. (1985) New immunological findings in senile dementia. <u>Interdiscipl.Topics Geront</u>. 19: 62-71.

28. Gaskin, F., Kingsley, B.S. and Fu, S.M. (1987) Autoantibodies to neurofibrillary tangles and brain tissue in Alzheimer's disease. <u>J. Exp. Med</u>. 165: 245-250.

29. Waksman, B.H. (1987) A multiple sclerosis therapy. <u>Nature</u> 328: 664-665.

30. Fudenberg, H.H. (1987) Immunodiagnosis and immunotherapy of patients with Alzheimer's syndrome. Paper presented to the IPSEN Foundation, Angers, France.

31. Van Haver, H., Lissoir, F., Droissart, C., Ketelaer, P., Van Hees, J., Theys, P., Verliet, G., Claeys, H., Gautama, K., Vermylen, C. and Carton, H. (1986) Transfer factor therapy in multiple sclerosis: A three- year prospective double-blind clinical trial. <u>Neurology</u> 36: 1399-1402.

32. Stubbs, E.G., Budden, S.S., Burger, D.R. and Vandenbark, A.A. (1980) Transfer factor immunotherapy of an autistic child with congenital cytomegalovirus. <u>J. Aut. Develop. Dis</u>. 10: 451-458.

33. Appel, S.H., Stewart, S.S., Appel, V., Harati, Y., Mietlowski, W., Weiss, N. and Belendiuk, G.W. (1988) A double-blind study of the effectiveness of cyclosporine in amyotrophic lateral sclerosis. Arch. Neurol. 45: 381-386.
34. Sapolsky R., Rivier, C., Yamamoto, G., Plotsky, P. and Vale, W. (1987) Interleukin-1 stimulates the secretion of hypothalamic corticotropin-releasing factor. Science 238: 522-524.

THE INFLUENCES OF ACTH 4-9 ANALOG UPON AVOIDANCE LEARNING IN

NORMAL AND BRAIN DAMAGED RATS

W. F. McDaniel, M. S. Schmidt, F. I. Chirino Barcelo and
B. K. Davis

Department of Psychology
Georgia College
Milledgeville, GA   31061

INTRODUCTION

The potential benefits of exogenous administration of the
adrenocorticotropic hormone (ACTH) and some of its fragments following
nervous system damage has been examined sporadically over the past 40 years.
Early research (e.g., 1) reported that administration of ACTH resulted in
limited functional recovery in some animals after spinal cord damage, and
these beneficial effects seemed to be associated with administration shortly
after the injury. Strand and Kung (2) found that ACTH accelerated the rate
of nerve regeneration following nerve crush in adrenalectomized animals and
concluded that ACTH stimulated an increase in protein and RNA synthesis in
spinal motor neurons. Strand and Smith (3) have hypothesized that this
enhanced protein synthesis results in increased synthesis and/or delivery of
neurotransmitters or neurotrophic substances to sprouting axons. Similarly,
it has been reported (4,5) that ACTH 1-39 facilitates functional
reorganization of motor units and hastens functional recovery following
either peroneal or sciatic nerve crush. Bijlsma and colleagues (6)
concluded that the 4-10 amino acid sequence of ACTH was responsible for the
hormone's beneficial action on peripheral nerve regeneration and accelerated
recovery of a foot-flick response. In a test of this hypothesis, these
researchers repeated their earlier methodology, again using animals with
crushed sciatic nerves, and found that treatment with ACTH 4-10 resulted in
a striking increase in the number of myelinated axons throughout the
regeneration process. Treatment with the 11-24 fragment of ACTH produced no
beneficial effects. This observation has been replicated recently (7) with
both fiber density and regeneration rate facilitated by ACTH 4-10 following
sciatic nerve crush. Since the 4-10 (and 4-9) sequence of the hormone fails
to exert an endocrine effect upon the adrenal cortex (8), it has been
concluded that the facilitated nerve regeneration is independent of the
corticotropic (or peripheral) influences of the hormone (6).

Investigations of systemically administered fragments of ACTH following
brain injury have been few. Using the entire hormone, Bush, Lovely and
Pagano (9) found that administration of 16 I.U. to rats with bilateral
amygdalectomies one hour before shuttle-box avoidance training reversed the
acquisition impairment associated with this lesion. Isaacson and Poplawsky
(10) have reported that administration of 1 μg of an analog of ACTH 4-9 for

four consecutive days immediately following bilateral septal lesions reduces the amount of hyperemotionality and hastens the rate of declining hyperemotionality seen with repeated testing. Since behavioral testing began two weeks after the surgeries, it is possible that the accelerated recovery produced by the 4-9 analog was mediated by a facilitation of neuronal sprouting in non-injured brain tissue. Interestingly, administration of neither 1 nor 10 μg of ACTH 4-10 was beneficial (11). More recently, Veldhuis, Nyakas, and DeWied (12) have found that chronic administration (8 injections total) of either the analog ACTH 4-9 (10 or 50 μg, subcutaneously, beginning on the third day after surgery) or alpha-MSH (same doses) attenuated or reversed a cognitive learning impairment associated with bilateral parafascicular thalamic nucleus injury. That is, the ability to learn a T-maze reversal task was significantly facilitated by the 10 μg dose of either neuropeptide, but still inferior to the sham-operated controls; however, 50 μg doses resulted in acquisition rates that were parallel to those observed in normal rats. Motor dysfunctions that result from the lesion were not altered.

Age-related neural and behavioral changes can also be affected by administration of the ACTH 4-9 analog. For example, administration of 12 μg of the peptide per day via an osmotic mini-pump restored the number of hippocampal corticosterone receptors, which declines markedly with age, to a level seen in young adult rats (13). Also, declines in social interactions (14) observed in senescent rats have been reported to be reversed. Further, Walker and Sandman (15) have reported that administration of the ACTH 4-9 analog to mentally retarded adults improved performance on several neuropsychological test measures (e.g., the Halstead-Reitan, Benton Visual Recognition Test). These investigators concluded that the improved performance reflected facilitated attentional processes, previously thought to be irreversible, in the retarded. The fragment of interest here, or related (i.e. centrally active) pro-opiomelanocortin fragments have also been reported to reverse amnesias induced by circadian rhythm disruption (16), CO_2 exposure (17), as well as ECS and protein synthesis inhibitors (8). Most researchers have concluded that ACTH-mediated effects upon learning and memory result from limbic system arousal and resultant increases in attention and facilitation of memory retrieval (see 8, 18 and 19 for reviews), although habituation and selective attention may be diminished.

The purpose of this research effort was to examine the potential benefits upon learning after brain injury of immediate postsurgical administration of ACTH 4-9 analog as compared to administration concomitant with acquisition. Lesions located in the medial frontal (MF) and posterior parietal (PP) neocortices result in a constellation of behavioral deficits in instrumental tasks (20-25). Both areas are the recipients of cholinergic afferents from the nucleus basalis (26), a region whose atrophy has been implicated in the memorial and cognitive declines that accompany Alzheimer's disease (27), and significant numbers of neurons in these regions atrophy several months following nucleus basalis lesions (28). The effects of the two administration regimes above on acquisition and extinction of a two-way shuttle avoidance response was the principle task used. It was hypothesized that chronic administration of the peptide immediately following an injury would facilitate postoperative acquisition of the two-way avoidance response. Furthermore it was predicted that administration concomitant with learning would either have no influence upon learning rates or possibly retard learning as we have recently reported (21) for acquisition of the spatial alternation strategy. Detectable levels of ACTH 4-9 analog have been found in the brain following subcutaneous administration (29), and the ACTH 4-9 analog has been described as exerting a 1000-fold greater effect upon measures of learning and memory than ACTH 4-10 (30).

222

GENERAL METHODS

Subjects

A total of 98 male and female adult rats (90–180 days; derived from the Long-Evans strain) were used. All animals were bred in this laboratory, had been housed individually in standard rodent cages since approximately 50 days of age, and had been entrained to a reversed light-dark cycle since birth (onset 8:00 pm, offset 8:00 am). Both food and water were available ad libitum.

Surgery and Histology

All animals were weighed prior to surgery and administered Nembutal (sodium pentobarbital: 50 mg/kg for females and 55 mg/kg for males). After the animal was completely anesthetized, signaled by absence of a tail-pinch reflex, the scalp was shaved and scrubbed with a Povidone-iodine solution (10% USP). The animal was mounted in a Kopf stereotaxic instrument and, using sterile surgical instruments, a midline incision was made exposing the dorsal cranium. Animals designated for sham injuries had their wounds stapled with wound clips at this point and Mycitracin triple antibiotic applied liberally to the wound. Landmarks used to guide cranial trephining and achieve access to the cortical regions under investigation here have been reported previously (21). For animals receiving ablations, the following measurements are used to guide placement of the initial trephine hole (2.5 mm): PP lesions, 3 mm posterior to bregma and 1.5 mm lateral to the sagittal sulcus; MF lesions 3.5 mm anterior to bregma and 1 mm lateral to the sagittal sulcus. In all cases, microrongeurs were also used to create a cranial opening in the shape of the underlying cortical region. The lesions were made by gentle aspiration using a 1.5 mm glass pipette and a dissecting microscope for visual guidance. After closing the wound as described above, a 1 cm incision was placed in the animal's back 2 cm caudal to the neck for the animals in Experiments 2 and 3. Those animals designated for postsurgical ACTH 4-9 analog or saline treatment had mini-pumps installed at this time. Wound clips were used to close the incisions and the animals were kept warm until recovery from anesthesia was apparent. In Experiments 1 and 2, behavioral testing was conducted with the trainers blind to an animal's surgical and drug condition.

At the end of behavioral testing, the animals with lesions were overdosed with Nembutal and perfused through the heart with 0.85% saline followed by 10% formalin (50 cc each). The brains were removed and stored first in formalin. After photographing the brains from the dorsal perspective, they were transferred to a 10% formalin-30% sucrose solution and stored in a refrigerator. The brains were blocked to include the lesion and thalamus, and sectioned through the coronal plane at 40 μm in a cryostat. Every tenth section was mounted on a slide and stained with standard cresyl-violet acetate procedures. The stained sections were used to reconstruct the lesion and resulting pattern of retrograde degeneration. The photographs were used to confirm regional lesion location.

ACTH 4-9 Administration

In Experiments 1, ACTH 4-9 analog was delivered via subcutaneous injection on alternate days (i.e., 3 per week). Each injection contained 25 μg of the peptide dissolved in a volume of 0.30 ml bacteriostatic saline. Control animals received an equivalent volume of the solvent. This single dose of ACTH 4-9 and injection routine was selected because of the results reported by Velduis et al. (12). In their study 10 μg facilitated acquisition and 50 μg completely reversed a learning deficit associated with parafascicular thalamic nucleus lesions. Our peptide level is intermediate between these doses. In Experiments 2 and 3, 12.5 ug of ACTH 4-9 was delivered each 24 hours by an Alzet model 2002 osmotic mini-pump. Each pump has a reservoir of 0.2 ml and administers its contents at a constant rate of 0.5 ul/hr. The pump has a nominal pumping life of 14 days and a constant release rate is obtained 4 hr after placement. The company literature shows that the contents of the pump are fully exhausted after 16 days. The dosage of 12.5 ug per day was obtained by dissolving 5 mg ACTH 4-9 in 2.4 ml bacteriostatic saline. For drug control animals, a pump that was filled with bacteriostatic saline was installed. It should be mentioned that the subcutaneous route of administration does produce detectable levels of the neuropeptide in the brain (29), and previous reports that the 4-9 analog exerts a 1000-fold greater effect upon passive avoidance behavior than the unaltered 4-10 sequence of the neuropeptide (30) relates to its greater metabolic stability (29).

Equipment and Behavioral Procedures

A Lafayette automated shuttle apparatus (model 85251SS) was used in Experiments 1 through 3. A compound CS (conditioned stimulus) consisting of an auditory tone (2800 Hz, 100 db measured in the center of a chamber) onset and guillotine door opening preceded onset of a 0.4 mA footshock by 3 sec in Experiments 1 and 2. Because of the results of Experiment 2, a third avoidance study was conducted using a CS of 10 sec duration, but all other parameters were identical to those used in Experiments 1 and 2. In all three experiments, the animal could terminate footshock, which had a maximal duration of 20 trials per day, 5 days per week. In Experiment 1, all rats were trained 25 sessions. In Experiments 2 and 3, training was terminated and extinction was begun after an animal attained a learning criterion of 70% avoidances or better in two sessions. Animals were trained a maximum of 40 sessions in Experiment 2 and 35 sessions in Experiment 3.

Designs and Specifics for the Experiments

Experiment 1. Thirty-six female rats were randomly assigned to one of six factorial conditions that had equal ns. After extensive handling, the animals were given either sham, MF, or pp lesions. Following a 28 day post-operative recovery period, one-half of the animals in each lesion group were injected on alternate days with either ACTH 4-9 analog or saline. Within a range of 2 to 6 hours after the injections, the animals were trained in the automated shuttle apparatus. Training concomitant with exposure to ACTH 4-9 analog continued for 5 weeks (25 sessions) for all animals regardless of performance.

Experiment 2. Twenty-four male and female rats were assigned randomly to one of four factorial groups matched on the basis of gender. These animals were prepared with either MF or sham lesions and administered either ACTH 4-9 analog or saline through an osmotic mini-pump. After a 28 day recovery period, acquisition of the two-way avoidance task was assessed to a ceiling of two sessions of 70% avoidances or for a maximum of 8 weeks.

Experiment 3. This experiment repeated the methodology of Experiment 2 with one exception. The latency between CS onset and US (unconditioned change was to reduce the vigilance required for accurate performance of the two-way avoidance task. Acquisition training continued to the ceiling used in Experiment 2 or to a ceiling of 35 sessions.

RESULTS

Histology

At this time careful histological analysis has been achieved only on
the animals in Experiments 1 and 2. The nature of the MF and PP lesions and
the thalamic retrograde degeneration that accompanied the lesions conformed
to that describe in our previous research efforts (e.g. 21,22), and
representative lesions are shown from the dorsal view in Fig. 1.
Microscopic evaluation of the sectioned brains showed that the MF lesions
extended from the frontal pole to the genu of the corpus callosum. Most

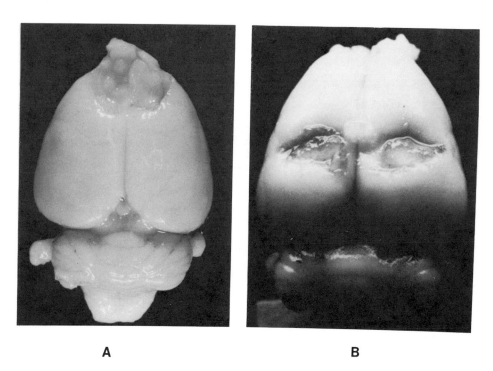

A   **B**

Fig. 1. Photographs of the MF (A) and PP (B) lesions in representative cases
taken from the dorsal view.

often the tissue along the medial walls of the sagittal sulcus, including
the cingulate cortex, was spared. It is probably due to the small size of
the lesions that retrograde degeneration was not detected in the mediodorsal
thalamic nucleus. PP lesions removed area 7, portions of area 39, and
frequently extended rostral into somatosensory cortex. The underlying
corpus callosum was damaged in most cases, and gliosis was evident in the
posterior and lateral thalamic nuclei. Degeneration was frequently observed
in the ventral thalamic nuclei when lesions included somatosensory cortex.

Behavior

The principle dependent measure for each avoidance learning study was the proportion avoidance made in each block of 100 trials. An analysis of variance (ANOVA) for a completely randomized factorial design was used to examine this data. When post-hoc multiple comparisons tests were warranted, the Fisher's least significant difference test was used. The number of training sessions required to achieve an acquisition criterion of two days of 0.70 or more avoidances and an extinction criterion of 0.15 avoidances were assessed in Experiments 2 and 3. In each avoidance experiment, an ANOVA on the proportion avoidances made on day 1 of training showed that the groups were equivalent (i.e., equally naive) at the initiation of training.

TABLE 1

ANOVA RESULTS FOR EXPERIMENT 1

Block	Significant Effects ($p<.05$)	$\underline{F}$	$\underline{df}$	$\underline{P}$	Conclusion from Fisher's LSD ($p<.05$)
1	Main Effect for Lesion	8.31	2,30	.002	MFs retarded relative to Shams and PPs
2	Main Effect for Lesion	8.04	2,30	.002	Same as Block 1
3	Main Effect for Lesion	3.99	2,30	.028	MFs retarded relative to Shams only. PPs intermediate.
4	Main Effect for Lesion	3.34	2,30	.048	Same as Block 3
5	Main Effect for Lesion	4.55	2,30	.018	Same as Block 3

Experiment 1. As can be seen in Fig.2 and Table 1, one consistent observation accrued from this study. Animals with MF injuries were deficient in learning the shuttle-box avoidance habit relative to sham operated controls. They were also inferior to rats with PP injuries during the first two blocks of sessions. The rats with PP injuries were never found to differ significantly from the sham group and they were more proficient learners than the animals with MF lesions during the early stages of training, that is blocks 1 and 2. No other differences (i.e., the main effect for ACTH 4-9 analog and the interaction of lesion by peptide) achieved significance.

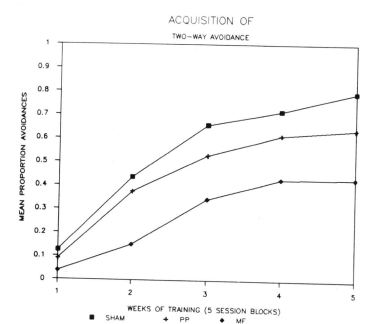

Fig. 2. Mean proportion avoidance across blocks of 100 trials for each brain lesion group.

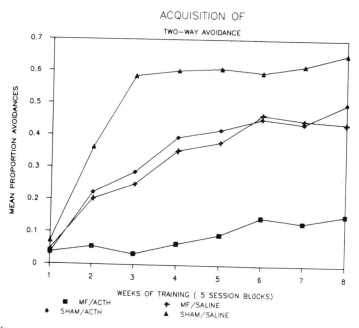

Fig. 3. Mean proportion avoidances across blocks of 100 trials for each factorial group.

Experiment 2. An ANOVA on the number of training sessions to criterion or a ceiling of 40 sessions produced significant main effects for the lesion [$\underline{F}(1,20)$ = 5.98, $\underline{p}$ = .023] and ACTH 4-9 analog [$\underline{f}(1,20)$ = 4.63, $\underline{p}$ = .042] conditions. That is, pooled across ACTH 4-9 doses, the sham animals learned the task more rapidly than the animals with MF injuries. Also, pooled across lesions, the animals exposed to 12.5 μg of ACTH 4-9 analog for a two week period four weeks prior to the initiation of training learned the avoidance task at a <u>retarded</u> rate. The interaction was not significant. Fig. 3 shows the learning curves for all four groups and Table 2 presents the results of ANOVAs for 2 X 2 factorial designs for each block of 100 trials. Exposure to ACTH 4-9 analog impaired learning in both the sham and MF injured groups relative to saline. As can be seen, the learning curves for sham animals administered ACTH 4-9 and MF injured animals administered saline show substantial overlap. Contrary to our predictions, the behavior of rats with MF lesions that were exposed to ACTH 4-9 analog failed to benefit from the extensive instrumental conditioning (800 trials) offered. The number of sessions to extinction was assessed for those animals that attained criterion (8 of 12 shams and 4 of 12 MF injured rats) with the $\underline{t}$ test. No differences were detected between the lesion groups. A $\underline{t}$ test comparing extinction sessions for animals exposed to ACTH 4-9 ($\underline{n}$ = 4) and those exposed to saline ($\underline{n}$ = 8) was also nonsignificant.

Experiment 3. This experiment repeated all conditions of Experiment 2 with one exception, the CS was of 10 sec duration rather than 3 sec. No significant differences resulted from analyses of sessions to criterion, sessions to extinction, or the proportion avoidances per block of 100 trials. Fig. 4 shows the learning curves for each factorial group so that they might be contrasted with the results of Experiment 2 shown in Fig. 3.

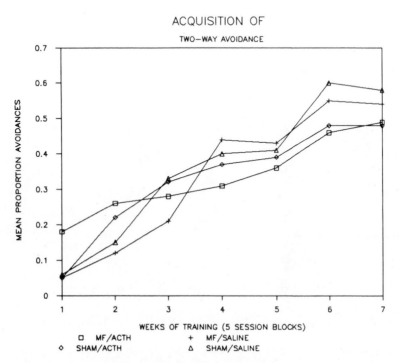

Fig. 4. Mean proportion avoidances across blocks of 100 training trials.

TABLE 2

ANOVA RESULTS FOR EXPERIMENT 2

Block		Significant Effects ($p<.05$)	F	df	P	Conclusion from Fisher's LSD ($p<.05$)
1		None				
2		None (but lesion and drug main effects yield Fs with $p<.10$)				
3	a.	Main Effect for Lesion	9.82	1,20	.005	MFs retarded relative to Shams.
	b.	Main Effect for ACTH 4-9	7.43	1,20	.013	ACTH 4-9 exposure produces inferior performance.
4	a.	Main Effect for Lesion	8.34	1,20	.009	Same as Block 3
	b.	Main Effect for ACTH 4-9	6.11	1,20	.021	
5	a.	Main Effect for Lesion	8.40	1,20	.009	Same as Block 3
	b.	Main Effect for ACTH 4-9	6.24	1,20	.020	
6		None (but same as Block 2, Fs with $p<.10$)				
7	a.	Main Effect for Lesion	5.24	1,20	.031	Same as Block 3
	b.	Main Effect for ACTH 4-9	5.68	1,20	.026	
8	a.	Main Effect for Lesion	7.88	1,20	.011	Same as Block 3
	b.	Main Effect for ACTH 4-9	4.85	1,20	.038	

DISCUSSION

The results of these experiments contradict several studies in which it has been reported that treatment with the 4-9 (or 4-10) analog sequence of the adrenocorticotrophic hormone restores behavioral functions that are compromised by neural injury (10,12). Treatment on alternate days with 25 μg of the peptide contemporaneous with two-way active avoidance training was found to neither facilitate nor retard learning. Injuries located within the medial frontal cortex, but not the posterior parietal cortex, impaired

acquisition. Chronic administration of 12.5 ug ACTH 4-9 analog per day
for 14 days immediately following medial frontal or sham neural injuries
was found to retard acquisition relative to saline even though training
was initiated 14 days after the contents of the osmotic mini-pump had
been exhausted. This result corroborates the findings of a recent
experiment conducted in this laboratory in which spatial alternation
learning was impaired by continuous exposure to 1 ug of ACTH 4-9 analog
per day, infused via an osmotic mini-pump, in rats with medial frontal,
posterior parietal, and sham injuries. In that study, the peptide was
administered simultaneous with training (21).

However, we are not the first to present data showing that
behavioral functions might be disturbed rather than enhanced by
administration of this neuropeptide fragment. Although not reported by
the authors, there is evidence that ACTH 4-9 analog disturbed learning
in the senescent rats (26 mos) studied by Rigter et al. (13). In their
experiment, chronic exposure to ACTH 4-9 analog (12 ug per day) fail to
improve learning in these rats relative to senescent rats treated with
saline, but it impaired learning of an 18 arm spatial task that is
anlogous to the radial arm maze. Our analysis of their data (see p.
394, Table 1) revealed that the senescent rats required more time to
find the correct goal box than the old rats exposed to saline, t(16) =
3.19, p < .01. In all three experiments that have demonstrated an
impairment of learning in animals receiving the ACTH 4- 9 analog the
peptide was delivered chronically via an osmotic pump. In the
experiments showing either a faciliation of learning or no effect of the
peptide upon behavior that have been reported here and elsewhere.
Chronic exposure to ACTH-like peptides may suppress the release of
hypothalamic releaseng hormones (e.g., corticotropin releasing hormone)
via the well-known negative feedback systems of the
hypothalamic-pituitary axis, thereby altering the synthesis of
pro-opiomelanocortins and, hence, a host of pituitary hormones for a
relatively long period. Acute administration may offer neurons in these
regions an opportunity to recover from the suppression induced by
exogenous administration of the peptide following its metabolism. It is
concluded tentatively, pending a planned test of the hypotheses, that
the mechanism of delivery, as well as the dose administered is a crucial
factor in interpretation of the behavioral results of ACTH 4-9 analog
administration.

In the third experiment reported here it was found that extending
the duration of the auditory CS form 3 sec (Wxperiments 1 and 2) to 10
sec reversed thelearning deficiences that were observed in rats with MF
lesions, as well as the learning impairment induced by post-surgical
chronic treatment with 12.5 ug ACTH 4-9 analog daily. This result is of
special relevance to an interpretation of the nature of the learning
dysfunction associated with both the MF lesion and ACTH 4-9 analog. It
appears that both impairments emerge in paradigms that require
exceptional vigilance (i.e., responding during the brief 3 sec CS as was
true for Experiments 1 and 2). Concerning the behavioral influences of
centrallly active ACTH fragments in both humans (31) and animals (32),
several authors have concluded that the peptide facilitates memory
retrieval by stimulation limbic structures and thereby enhancing general
attentional (or arousal) processes. However, this disinhibitory
influence might be accomplished at the cost of impaired habituation and
selective attention. Such an impairment might be expected to impede
learning in behavioral pardigms that demand sustained vigilance and 30hr
working memory. A study to examine the influence of ACTH 4-9 upon rates
of habituation of the startle response is underway in this laboratory.

Passingham et al. (33) have recently argued that the medial tissue occupying the dorsal convexity of the frontal cortex in rat (i.e., the tissue removed in creating our MF lesions) is both homologous and analogous to primate premotor cortex rather than prefrontal cortex. Removal of this tissue might be expected to disturb the rapid execution of locomotor responses required to escape or avoid an aversive stimulus. However, providing a longer period for executing such motor responses might mask the motoric disability. Interestingly, we observed no obvious motor dysfunctions in our animals. Finally, the shuttle-box avoidance learning curves for the MF damaged rats studied here are nearly identical to the curves for rats prepared with nucleus basalis lesions (34). On the basis of this behavioral similarity and the fact that the MF cortex is a principle recipient of cholinergic axons from the nucleus basalis (26,28), it might be suggested that this lesion offers the behavioral neuroscientist a model for the investigation of factors that might be of value in the treatment of declines in learning and memory functions that accompany the neuropathology of Alzheimer's type as well as neocortical brain damage.

Although centrally active ACTH-like peptides have been shown to augment several indices of nerve repair in the peripheral nervous system and to improve some behavioral functions following central nervous system injury, the beneficial influences of these compounds may be limited. At this time we conclude that facilitated functional recovery following treatment with ACTH-like fragments may not generalize to lesions of the frontal and parietal neocortices, to tasks like those discussed here, and to paradigms involving continuous chronic peptide delivery routines. Further research will be necessary to examine the multiple factors contributing to the positive and negative influences of the analog of ACTH 4-9 upon the recovery of behavioral functions following brain injury.

Acknowledgements

This research was made possible by two Georgia College Faculty Research Grants to the first author. We wish to acknowledge the assistance of Mr. Tim Vacula in the preparation of photographs. Some of the interpretations of our data grew out of discussions with Ms. Pam Prosser.

REFERENCES

1. McMasters, R. E. (1962) Regeneration of the spinal cord in the rat. Effects of piromen and ACTH upon the regenerative capacity. J. Comp. Neurol. 119: 113-125.
2. Strand, F. L., & Kung, T. T. (1980) ACTH accelerates recovery of neuromuscular function following crushing of peripheral nerve. Peptides 1: 135-138.
3. Strand, F. L., & Smith, C. M. (1980) LPH, ACTH, MSH, and motor systems. Pharmacol. Ther. 11: 509-533.
4. Saint-Come, C., Acker, G. R., & Strand, F. L. (1982) Peptide influences on the development and regeneration of motor performance. Peptides 3: 439-449.
5. Bijlsma, W. A., Jennekens, F. G. I., Schotman, P., & Gispen, W. H. (1981) Effects of corticotrophin (ACTH) on recovery of sensorimotor function in the rat: Structure-activity study. Eur. J. Pharmac. 76: 73-79.
6. Bijlsma, W. A., Jennekens, F. G. I., Schotman, P., & Gispen, W. H. (1983) Stimulation by ACTH 4-10 of nerve fiber regeneration following sciatic nerve crush. Muscle Nerve 6: 102-110.

7. Girlanda, P., Muglia, U., Vita, G., Dattola, R., Santoro, M., Toscano, A., Venuto, C., Roberto, M. L., Baradello, A., Romano, M., & Messina, C. (1988) Effect of ACTH 4-10 on nerve fiber regeneration afte sciatic nerve crush in rabbits: an electrophysiological and morphological study. Exp. Neurol. 99: 454-460.

8. DeWied, D. (1980) Hormonal influences on motivation, learning, memory, and psychosis. In D. T. Krieger and J. C. Hughes (eds.), Neuroendocrinology, Sutherland, MA: Sinauer Associates, Inc., 194-204.

9. Bush, D. F., Lovely, R. H., & Pagano, R. R. (1973) Injection of ACTH induces recovery from shuttle-box avoidance deficits in rats with amygdaloid lesions. J. Comp. Physiol. Psychol. 83: 168-172.

10. Isaacson, R. L., & Poplawsky, A. (1983) An ACTH 4-9 analog (ORG 2766) speeds recovery from septal hyperemotionality in the rat. Behav. Neural Biol. 39: 52-59.

11. Isaacson, R. L., & Poplawsky, A. (1985) ACTH 4-10 produces a transient decrease in septal hyperemotionality. Behav. Neural Biol. 43: 109-113.

12. Veldhuis, H. D., Nyakas, C., & DeWied, D. (1985) Neuropeptides and functional recovery after brain damage. In B. E. Will, P. Schmitt, & J. C. Dalrymple-Alford (eds.), Brain Plasticity, Learning, and Memory, New York: Plenum Press, 473-480.

13. Rigter, H., Veldhuis, H. D., & deKloet, E. R. (1984) Spatial learning and the hippocampal corticosterone receptor system of old rats: effect of the ACTH 4-9 analogue ORG 2766. Brain Res. 309: 393-398.

14. Spruijt, B. M., Rombouts, L., & Gispen, W. H. (1987) Effects of ACTH (4-9) on behavioral plasticity in aging animals. New Trends in Aging Research (Abstract Book), Italian Study Group on Brain Aging, International Symposium, April 12-15, Sirmione, Italy, 28.

15. Walker, B. B., & Sandman, C. A. (1979) Influences of an analog of the neuropeptide ACTH 4-9 on mentally retarded adults. Am. J. Ment. Defic. 83: 346-352.

16. Fekete, M., Van Ree, J. M., & DeWied, D. (1986) The ACTH-(4-9) analog ORG 2766 and desglycinamide 9-(Arg8)-vasopressin reverse the retrograde amnesia induced by disrupting circadian rhythms in rats. Peptides 7: 563-568.

17. Rigter, H. H., Van Riezen, H., & DeWied, D. (1974) The effect of ACTH- and vasopressin analogues on CO2-induced retrograde amnesia in rats. Physiol. Behav. 13: 381-388.

18. de Wied, D., & van Ree, J. M. (1982) Neuropeptides, mental performance and aging. Life Sci. 31: 709-719.

19. Krieger, D. T. (1983) Brain peptides: what, where, and why? Science 22: 975-985.

20. McDaniel, W. F. (1985) Functions of the posterior neocortex of the rat. IRCS J. Med. Sci. 13: 286-289.

21. McDaniel, W. F., Davall, E. J., & Walker, P. E. ACTH 4-9 analog can retard spatial alternation learning in brain damaged and normal rats. Behav. Neural Biol. (in press).

22. McDaniel, W. F., & Wall, T. T. (1988) Visuospatial functions in the rat following injuries to striate, peristriate, and parietal neocortical sites. Psychobiol. 16: 251-260.

23. Kolb, B. (1984) Functions of the frontal cortex of the rat: a comparative review. Brain Res. Rev. 8: 65-98.

24. Kolb, B., Sutherland, R. J., & Whishaw, I. Q. (1983) A comparison of th contributions of the frontal and parietal association cortex to spatial localization in rats. Behav. Neurosci. 97: 13-27.

25. Kolb, B., & Walkey, J. (1987) Behavioural and anatomical studies of the posterior parietal cortex in the rat. Behav. Brain Res. 23: 127-145.

26. Johnston, M.V., McKinney, M. & Coyle, J.T. (1981) Neocortical cholinergic innervation: a description of extrinsic and intrinsic components in the rat. Exp. Brain Res. 43: 159-172.

27. Bartus, R.T., Dean, R. L., Beer, B. & Lippa, A.S. (1982) The cholinergic hypothesis of geriatric memory dysfunction. Science 217: 408-416.

28. Arendash, G.W., Millard, W.J., Dunn, A.J., & Meyer, E.M. (1987) Long-term neuropathological and neurochemical effects of nucleus basalis lesions in the rat. Science 238: 952-956.

29. Verhoef, J., & Witter, A. (1976) In vivo fate of a behaviorally active ACTH 4-9 analog in rats after systemic administration. Pharmacol. Biochem. Behav. 4: 583-590.

30. Fekete, M., & DeWied, D. (1982) Potency and duration of action of the ACTH 4-9 analog (ORG 2766) as compared to ACTH 4-10 on active and passive avoidance behavior of rats. Pharmacol. Biochem. Behav. 16: 387-392.

31. Born, J., Fehm, H.L., & Voigt, K.H. (1986) ACTH and attention in humans: a review. Neuropsychobiol. 15: 165-186.

32. Van Wimersma Greidanus, T.B., Bohus, B., Kovacs, G.L., Versteeg, D.H.G., Burbach, J.P.H., & DeWied, D. (1983) Sites of behavioral and neurochemical action of ACTH-like peptides and neurohypophyseal hormones. Neurosci. Biobehav. Rev. 7: 453-463.

33. Passingham, R.E., Meyers, C., Rawlins, N., Lightfoot, V., & Fearn, S., (1988) Premotor cortex in the rat. Behav. Neurosci. 102: 101-109.

34. Arendash, G.W., Strong, P.N., & Mouton, P.R. (1985) Intracerebral transplantation of cholinergic neurons in a new animal model for Alzheimer's disease. In: Senile Dementia of the Alzheimer Type (eds: Hutton, J.T. and Kenney, A.D.), Alan R. Liss, Inc., New York, 351-376.

TRANSNEURONAL NEUROCHEMICAL AND NEUROPATHOLOGICAL CHANGES INDUCED BY NUCLEUS BASALIS LESIONS: A POSSIBLE DEGENERATIVE MECHANISM IN ALZHEIMER'S DISEASE

Gary W. Arendash[1], Gregory J. Sengstock[1], Gerry Shaw[3], and William J. Millard[4]

[1]Department of Biology, University of South Florida, Tampa, FL 33620; [2] Department of Neuroscience, [3] Department of Pharmacodynamics, University of Florida, Gainesville, FL 32610

INTRODUCTION

A considerable body of evidence indicates that neurons within a number of CNS systems may atrophy or degenerate following a loss of their afferents (1). This transneuronal atrophy or degeneration secondary to deafferentation is commonly referred to as "anterograde transneuronal degeneration." Perhaps the best example of this phenomenon is the atrophy/degeneration of neurons within the lateral geniculate nucleus following interruption of their afferent input from the optic nerve (2). Such transneuronal changes may occur very slowly, often taking months or years to manifest themselves. Although the mechanism(s) responsible for atrophy or degeneration of neurons which have suffered no direct injury are basically unknown, a likely mechanism involves loss of a neurotransmitter and/or neurotrophic factor(s) formerly released onto these neurons by eliminated afferent nerve terminals.

Since senile dementia of the Alzheimer's type (SDAT) is characterized by a degeneration of neurons within several neurotransmitter systems originating subcortically, it is important to consider the possibility that widespread transneuronal changes may be occurring in the Alzheimer's-diseased brain as a result of these degenerated/dysfunctional neurons. Along this line, a consistent observation in SDAT brains is a degeneration or atrophy of cholinergic neurons that originate in the subcortical nucleus basalis and provide the primary cholinergic innervation to the neocortex (3-5). The characteristic cholinergic hypofunction in neocortex of SDAT brains (6-8) probably reflects this loss of nucleus basalis cholinergic neurons. Furthermore, a relationship exists between loss of nucleus basalis neurons, the occurrence of cortical pathology, and the degree of cognitive impairment in SDAT patients (5).

Although the aforementioned findings indicate an important role for nucleus basalis cholinergic neurons in the pathogenesis of SDAT, these neurons should not be perceived in isolation from the neurons they innervate directly or indirectly. Indeed, of the four other forebrain areas most severely affected pathologically in SDAT, two (the neocortex and amygdala) are innervated directly by nucleus basalis cholinergic neurons and the remaining two (the entorhinal cortex and hippocampus) are indirectly innervated by these cholinergic neurons. Thus, the areas of most profound SDAT pathology and synaptically linked directly or indirectly to the nucleus basalis.

This relationship may provide the anatomical substrate for anterograde transneuronal changes in these four brain areas resulting from an initial degeneration of nucleus basalis cholinergic neurons. In this context, we have recently obtained data from rats suggestive that the death of nucleus basalis cholinergic neurons initiates a cascade of transneuronal events within the neocortex, amygdala, entorhinal cortex, and hippocampus (9). These data involve excitotoxic lesioning of the rat nucleus basalis to eliminate, and thus mimic to some extent, the loss of similar cholinergic neurons in SDAT-diseased brains. Certainly, a host of studies have shown that such lesions result in reduced presynaptic cholinergic markers in neocortex (10-16), as seen in SDAT. Furthermore, nucleus basalis lesioned-rats have been shown to be deficient in learning and memory abilities (8, 10-16), as are SDAT patients. Prior to our recent report (9), however, the long-term effects of these lesions were largely unknown. The present chapter extends this earlier report by indicating more comprehensively the extensive neuronal losses and atrophy, neurofibrillary changes, and neuropeptide changes that can be observed in the rat forebrain long-term after nucleus basalis lesions done in "young adult" rats. Since the loss of nucleus basalis cholinergic neurons may not occur until later in the life of SDAT patients, lesioning the nucleus basalis of "aged" rats may provide a more realistic appraisal of the impact that degeneration of nucleus basalis cholinergic neurons may be having in SDAT patients. Thus, initial results of nucleus basalis lesioning in "aged" rats will also be presented.

Our data from both young and aged nucleus basalis legioned rats indicate that, in addition to cognitive deficits, a variety of transneuronal neurochemical and neuropathological changes occur gradually throughout the forebrain over many months. Because similar transneuronal changes may be occurring in the pathogenesis of SDAT, it is important to fully characterize these transneuronal changes in rats. In that manner, a partial animal model for SDAT (based on an initial cholinergic dysfunction) may be established from which various treatment or preventive strategies for SDAT could be tested.

NUCLEUS BASALIS LESIONING IN YOUNG ADULT RATS: NEUROPATHOLOGICAL CHANGES

The neurotoxin ibotenic acid (5 ug/1 ul PBS) was infused either unilaterally or bilaterally into the nucleus basalis of 2 month old adult male Sprague-Dawley rats as previously described (9,14). We have found this lesioning protocol to be effective in eliminating most (i.e. 80-95%) acetylcholinesterase-positive cell bodies within the nucleus basalis and to provide a marked, essentially permanent cholinergic hypofunction in neocortex (9,14,17). Moreover, animals with bilateral lesions are learning/memory deficient in a variety of cognitive tasks including passive avoidance, 1-way and 2-way active avoidance, and Lashley III spatial maze (see chapter by Strong et al. in this volume).

As indicated earlier, lesion-induced neuropathological changes occur in the same four forebrain areas most affected by SDAT: the neocortex, amygdala, entorhinal cortex, and hippocampus. Neuropathology within these areas is considered below for animals sacrificed between 3 and 22 months after lesioning. It is important to state that the entire forebrain appears histologically unaffected for a number of months following nucleus basalis lesions, with an obvious exception being the ibotenic acid infusion sites in the ventromedial globus pallidus; at those sites, neuronal losses and a restricted gliosis are routinely seen as a direct result of excitotoxin infusion.

The neocortex appears to be the first forebrain region affected "indirectly" by nucleus basalis lesions. In fronto-parietal cortex, significant neuronal losses were first evident at about 5 months following unilateral lesions and became progressively more severe (often 30% or higher) at time points thereafter (Table 1). The sizable neuronal losses seen in layers II, III-V, and VI at 10 and 14 months after bilateral lesions were similar to those seen 14 months following unilateral lesions (Fig. 1). Moreover, many surviving neurons in fronto-parietal cortex were clearly atrophied as a result of lesioning (Fig. 1).

Also beginning 5-10 months post-lesioning, considerable numbers of neurons within the fronto-parietal cortex were seen to stain very intensely for silver impregnation, particularly the pyramidal cells in cortical layers III and V (Fig. 2); such heavily silver-embedded neurons were generally atrophic as well. This enhanced silver staining after lesions appears to be due, in large part, to an elevated neuronal content of neurofilamentous protein since we have obtained preliminary data showing that neocortical neurons exhibit increased monoclonal antibody staining for several neurofilamentous proteins long-term after nucleus basalis lesions (Fig. 3). Consistent with aforementioned silver staining results, nucleus basalis lesions induced pyramidal cells in cortical layers III and V to stain very intensely for neurofibrillary proteins and to do so in higher number than pyramidal cells in control cortical tissues (Fig. 3). Such lesion-induced increases in monoclonal antibody staining are most obvious in unilaterally-lesioned animals. We have thus far obtained no evidence, however, that the enhanced content of neurofilamentous protein within these cortical neurons is due to induction of abnormal, paired helical filament formation by nucleus basalis lesioning. Rather, the intracellular distribution of monoclonal antibody staining for several neurofilamentous proteins suggests a neurofilament distribution consistent with a lesion-induced enhancement of normal neurofilamentous protein in affected cortical neurons.

For the basolateral nucleus of the amygdala, which normally receives cholinergic afferents from the nucleus basalis (18), unilateral lesions did not result in ipsilateral neuronal losses at 14 months post-lesioning. Rather, a marked 36% decrease in mean neuronal areas was observed ipsilaterally within this amygdaloid nucleus (Fig. 4). Similarly, no neuronal loss was ever seen in layers 2 and 3 of entorhinal cortex through 14 months after nucleus basalis lesioning. Rather, a significant neuronal atrophy within entorhinal cortex layer 2 was present by 5 months following unilateral lesions; this entorhinal atrophy was more severe by 14 months post-lesioning (Fig. 5). Though less consistently observed, neuronal loss and/or atrophy were also evident in CA1 and CA3 regions of the dorsal hippocampus by 14 months post-lesioning (9). Particularly in the basolateral nucleus of the amygdala and layers 2-3 of entorhinal cortex, silver impregnation staining revealed large numbers of intensely stained, atrophic neurons long-term after nucleus basalis lesions (9). Though similar in nature to the heavily silver-embedded neurons found in neocortex following lesions, this markedly enhanced silver staining in amygdala and entorhinal cortex appears to require more time to develop after lesions, typically 10 months or longer.

In summary, nucleus basalis lesions induce neuropathological changes in the four forebrain regions most devastated by SDAT: the neocortex, amygdala, entorhinal cortex, and hippocampus. Within these brain regions long-term after lesions, substantial neuronal losses and/or atrophy are present, as well as increased neurofibrillary staining. Furthermore, a slow development of these neuropathological changes occurs following lesions since at least 5 months appear to be required before any neuropathological effects are seen in young adults. The fact that nucleus basalis lesions can induce pathology in four other forebrain regions affected by SDAT suggests that the nucleus basalis may be a primary lesion site in SDAT. However, this is not to the exclusion of other possible primary lesion sites (i.e. neocortex, entorhinal cortex, locus ceruleus), for which considerable evidence also exists.

Table 1.   Effects of Nucleus Basalis Lesions on Neuronal Densities in Neocortex

% CHANGE IN NEURONAL DENSITIES vs CONTROLS

FRONTAL CORTEX	Layer II	Layers III-V	Layer VI
3 Months after Unilateral Lesions	+3	+5	+10
5 Months after Unilateral Lesions	-14*	-10	-6
14 Months after Unilateral Lesions	-21*	-19*	-15*
10 Months after Bilateral Lesions	-25*	-29*	-24*
14 Months after Bilateral Lesions	-22*	-21*	-27*
PARIETAL CORTEX	Layer II	Layers III-V	Layer VI
3 Months after Unilateral Lesions	-2	-7	-2
5 Months after Unilateral Lesions	-19*	-15	-16
14 Months after Unilateral Lesions	-28*	-31*	-24*
10 Months after Bilateral Lesions	-22*	-27*	-20*
14 Months after Bilateral Lesions	-24*	-27*	-20*

Neuronal densities for each animal were determined from five representative brain sections utilizing standard manual counting procedures. Three to five animals comprised each lesion and control group. * = "p" value less than .05 or greater level of significance.

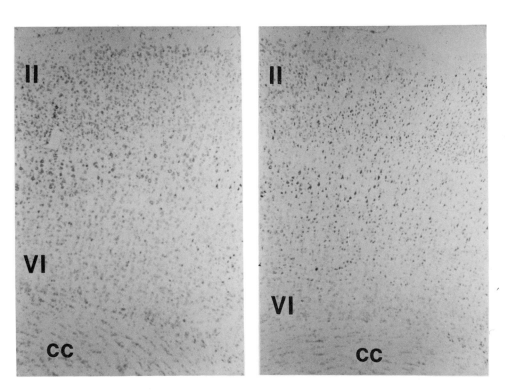

Fig. 1.   Thionin-stained parietal cortex on the control (left) and lesioned (right) side of an animal given a unilateral nucleus basalis lesion 14 months before sacrifice. x63. Note cell losses/atrophy in most cortical layers on lesioned side compared to control side. Both photomicrographs were taken from the same coronal brain section. CC, corpus callosum; II and VI, layers II and VI of parietal cortex.

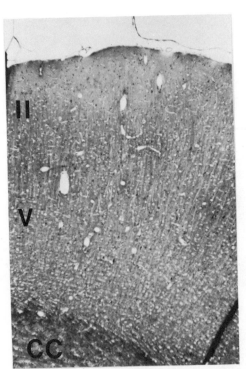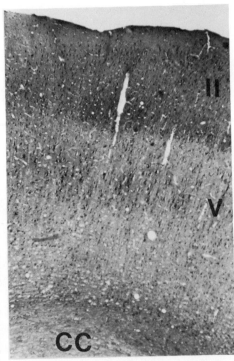

Fig. 2.   Silver-stained parietal cortex immediately adjacent to the thionin-stained brain
section shown in Fig. 1. Animal received a unilateral nucleus basalis lesion on
the right side at 14 months prior to sacrifice. x63. Note the large number of
heavily silver-embedded neurons throughout cortical layers II-VI on the lesioned
(right) side compared to their virtual absence on the control (left) side. This
lesion-induced intense staining for silver impregnation is most prominent in the
pyramidal cells of cortical layer V. Both photomicrographs were taken from
the same coronal brain section. CC, corpus callosum; II and V, layers II and
V of parietal cortex.

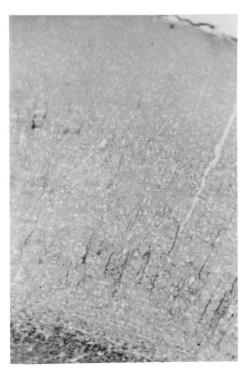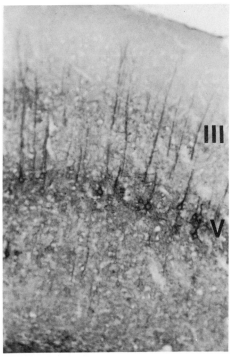

Fig. 3.   Monoclonal antibody staining for neurofilamentous protein in parietal cortex of an animal given a unilateral nucleus basalis lesion 21.5 months before sacrifice. Sternberger antibody SM1-32 was utilized in conjunction with PAP staining procedures. In contrast to the general lack of staining on the control (left) side, an intense staining of pyramidal cells is evident in cortical layer V on the lesioned (right) side, as is a less intense staining in cortical layer III. Both photomicrographs were taken from the same coronal brain section. x100.

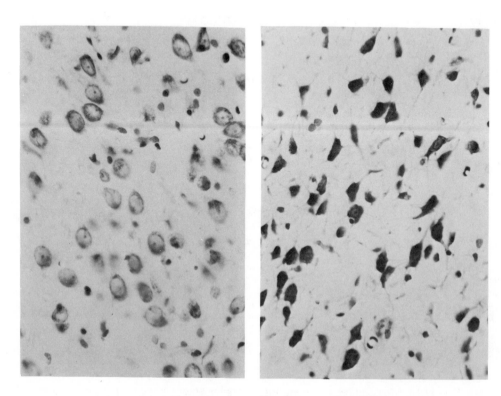

Fig. 4.   Thionin-stained neurons within the basolateral nucleus of the amygdala at 14
months following unilateral nucleus basalis lesioning. Neurons on the lesioned
(right) side are atrophied and stain more intensely for thionin compared to
those on the control (left) side of the brain.   x400.   Both photomicrographs
were taken from the same coronal brain section.

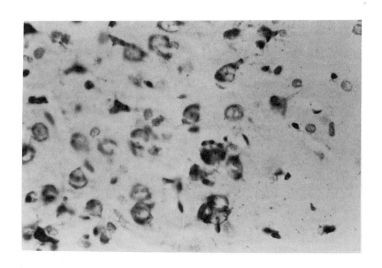

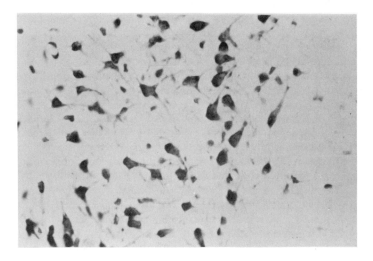

Fig. 5.   Layer 2 of entorhinal cortex stained with thionin at 14 months after unilateral nucleus basalis lesioning. Note the marked atrophy of entorhinal neurons on the lesioned side (lower photo) compared to the control side (upper photo) of the brain. x400. Both photomicrographs were taken from the same coronal brain section.

What possible mechanism(s) could account for the neuropathology seen long-term following nucleus basalis lesioning? We have hypothesized (9) that the lesion-induced cell loss/atrophy in neocortex and amygdala are due to loss of a necessary, stimulatory influence on neurons within these regions provided by direct cholinergic projections from the nucleus basalis (18). In this context, nucleus basalis lesions have been shown to reduce total electrical activity in the neocortex (19) and the iontophoretic application of acetylcholine has long been known to excite cortical neurons (20, 21). Alternatively, since most cholinergic terminals in neocortex have been shown to contain vasoactive intestinal polypeptide (VIP; 22), a lesion-induced loss of this neuroactive peptide's possible neuronotrophic action on neocortical cells could be responsible for at least some of the neuropathology observed. Thus, we hypothesize that cortical/amygdaloid neurons, denied some critical excitatory or neuronotrophic input from cholinergic neurons after nucleus basalis lesioning, become dysfunctional and eventually die or atrophy through the process of anterograde transneuronal degeneration. Since nucleus basalis cholinergic neurons do not project directly to either the entorhinal cortex or hippocampus, the degenerative changes we have observed in these two forebrain areas may reflect subsequent "secondary" transneuronal effects occurring in response to altered or dysfunctional neocortical input to entorhinal cortex which, in turn, causes dysfunctional entorhinal input to the hippocampus via the perforant pathway. A transneuronal cascade of neuropathological events may, therefore, transpire long-term following nucleus basalis lesioning. It is important to note that the entorhinal cortex and its perforant pathway become degenerative in SDAT (23), thus effectively dissociating two brain regions important for memory - the neocortex and hippocampus.

NUCLEUS BASALIS LESIONING IN YOUNG ADULT RATS: NEUROCHEMICAL CHANGES

Although mounting data indicate the involvement of multiple transmitter systems in SDAT, a cholinergic deficit clearly characterizes most SDAT brains (6,24) and, in that context, is the only neurotransmitter deficit that has been consistently linked to the cognitive dysfunctions of SDAT (25,26). Specifically, decreases in cortical cholinergic markers such as CAT activity (25,27,28), acetylcholine synthesis (29), and high affinity choline transport (7) have been found in SDAT brains. This cortical cholinergic hypofunction of presynaptic markers is thought to be due, in large part, to a dysfunction/degeneration of nucleus basalis cholinergic neurons. A similar cortical cholinergic hypofunction can be induced in rats through nucleus basalis lesioning (9-17). Along this line, we have given young adult rats either unilateral or bilateral ibotenic acid infusions into their nucleus basalis and assayed the frontal cortex for cholinergic markers at 2.5, 5, 10, 14, and 19 months later. Irrespective of whether unilateral or bilateral lesions were done, cortical CAT activity was always substantially reduced at these post-lesion time points. Compared to controls, mean lesion group decreases of 35-55% in cortical CAT activity were usually observed. Moreover, high affinity choline transport and acetylcholine synthesis in frontal cortex were reduced by 27-52% at 10 and 14 months following bilateral nucleus basalis lesions (9,17). Thus, our lesioning procedure induces a substantial and essentially permanent cholinergic hypofunction in neocortex.

Recently, we found that lesions of the rat nucleus basalis produce not only this long-term cholinergic hypofunction in neocortex, but surprising changes in neocortical content of the neuropeptides somatostatin, neuropeptide Y (NPY), and corticotropin-releasing hormone (CRH) as well; all three of these neuropeptides are reduced in the neocortex of SDAT brains (30-34). These lesion affects on cortical peptide content involve a complicated transneuronal mechanism that depends on the time post-lesioning and whether the lesions are unilateral or bilateral. For example, significant decreases of 17% and 24% in cortical somatostatin content were seen at 2.5 and 10 months following unilateral lesions, but not at 1 month post-lesion. By 14 months following unilateral lesions, somatostatin content (though still reduced) was not significantly different compared to control values. In sharp contrast, bilateral lesions resulted in a dramatic 107% increase in cortical somatostatin levels at 10 months after lesioning; similarly robust increases were observed at 14 and 19 months post-lesioning as well. Whatever the intriguing transneuronal mechanism responsible for this peptide elevation, it apparently becomes manifested between 5 and 10 months post-lesioning since bilateral lesions have no effect on cortical somatostatin content at either 2.5 or 5 months after lesioning.

NPY and CRH content in neocortex were affected by unilateral and bilateral nucleus basalis lesions similar to somatostatin levels. Thus, unilateral lesions did not affect neocortical NPY content at 1 month post-lesioning, but did induce a substantial 39% reduction in cortical NPY levels by 2.5 months following lesions. Bilateral lesions resulted in elevations of at least 240% in this peptide at 10, 14, and 19 months after lesions. Although unilateral lesions had no effect on cortical CRH levels through 14 months post-lesioning, bilateral lesions elevated this peptide by at least 152% at 10, 14, and 19 months following lesions - an effect similar to that seen for somatostatin and NPY. It is interesting to note that the parallel changes in cortical somatostatin and NPY that we observe after nucleus basalis lesions are consistent with several studies showing neuronal partial co-localization of these neuropeptides in the rat, as well as human neocortex (35,36). We have in fact found a significant correlation between the elevations in cortical somatostatin and NPY following bilateral lesions.

The above data clearly indicate that: 1) unilateral nucleus basalis lesions can significantly decrease cortical somatostatin and NPY levels by 2.5 months following lesions; and 2) bilateral lesions result in dramatically elevated cortical content of all three neuropeptides (somatostatin, NPY, and CRH) by 10 months after lesions. These results suggest that a functional relationship exists between nucleus basalis neurons projecting to the neocortex and certain neuropeptide systems intrinsic to the neocortex. While it seems likely that these neuropeptide changes are due (at least in part) to the destruction of nucleus basalis cholinergic neurons, it is also possible that other nucleus basalis transmitter systems are directly or indirectly involved. Nonetheless, our data support the notion that the dysfunctional and/or degenerative changes occuring in such neuropeptide-containing neurons of SDAT brains may be secondary to a dysfunction or loss of nucleus basalis cholinergic neurons.

Of the many cerebral cortical neuropeptides measured post-mortem in SDAT victims, somatostatin and CRH are the most commonly found to be reduced (30,31,33,34). Cortical NPY content has also been reported to be reduced in some autopsied brains of SDAT patients (32), but not in others (37). These reported reductions in cortical neuropeptide concentrations from autopsied patients should be interpreted with caution since: 1) the potassium-induced release of somatostatin from biopsied cortical tissue of SDAT patients is normal (38); and 2) the least reliable measurement of a given neurotransmitter's activity is its concentration. Keeping these points in mind, the decreased cortical content of somatostatin and NPY that we see at time points between 2.5 and 14 months after unilateral nucleus basalis lesioning is similar to the reductions in these two peptides reported for autopsied SDAT brains (30-32). A loss of excitatory cholinergic input to cortical neuropeptide-containing cells could be involved in such decreases. In fact, the decreases in cortical somatostatin and NPY content following unilateral lesions may be greater and more consistent over time than the data indicate, since neuropeptide levels in contralateral (control) cortices were generally suppressed in comparison to cortical levels from bilateral sham-lesioned control animals. This suggests that unilateral lesions may be affecting neuropeptide content in both ipsilateral and contralateral cortex, perhaps thru cortico-cortical connections. It is most likely that unilateral lesion-induced changes in neuropeptide levels take several months to occur through transneuronal mechanisms since we found no neuropeptide decreases at 1 month after lesions. This is consistent with a report by McKinney et al. (39) in which no effect on cortical somatostatin content was found several weeks after unilateral lesioning.

The marked elevations in cortical somatostatin, NPY and CRH content by 10 months after bilateral lesions are in sharp contrast to the decreased cortical content of somatostatin and NPY following unilateral lesions. Increased neuropeptide concentrations after bilateral lesions could result from: 1) decreased neuropeptide release; 2) decreased neuropeptide processing/transport; and/or 3) increased neuropeptide synthesis. Regarding a possible increase in neuropeptide synthesis, it is known that both somatostatin and NPY are encoded by genes whose transcription is increased by cyclic AMP (40). Since cyclic AMP accumulation can be inhibited by activation of brain muscarinic receptors (41), it is possible that a loss of nucleus basalis cholinergic neurons may gradually increase cortical neuropeptide content by disinhibiting cyclic AMP accumulation. The possibility that these changes in neuropeptide levels may reflect changes in gene-transcription is discussed elsewhere in this volume (Poulakos et al.).

An alternate, non-synthetic explanation for elevated cortical peptide levels following bilateral nucleus basalis lesions involves decreased peptide release following loss of excitatory cholinergic innervation. Supportive of this mechanism are studies showing that acetylcholine is a powerful releaser of somatostatin in rat cortex, as well as a potent secretagogue of NPY in the adrenal medulla (42). Although the involvement of nucleus basalis cholinergic neurons in lesion-induced neuropeptide elevations remains to be determined, a loss of cortical cholinergic innervation from nucleus basalis may eventually lead to an accumulation of neuropeptides in neocortex through this mechanism.

The delay of 5-10 months required for elevating cortical neuropeptide concentrations following bilateral lesions presumably involves a slow transneuronal mechanism. As indicated in the previous section describing lesion-induced neuropathology, a variety of neuropathological changes are seen in the forebrain no sooner than 5 months post-lesioniong. These changes include neuronal losses/atrophy and neurofibrillary changes in the frontoparietal cortex, amygdala, entorhinal cortex, and hippocampus. The slow development of such neuropathological changes also suggests a transneuronal mechanism. Indeed, transneuronal neuropathological and neurochemical changes caused by nucleus basalis lesioning may be intimately related. For example, the probable lesion-induced loss of cortico-cortical neurons through a transneuronal mechanism may account for the exactly opposite effects of unilateral and bilateral nucleus basalis lesions on cortical neuropeptide content. Since these cortico-cortical neurons are believed to use glutamate as their transmitter (43) their loss after lesioning could result in decreased excitatory input to neuropeptide-containing neurons contralateral to such lesions.

From our neuropeptide results, it is apparent that some functional relationship exists between nucleus basalis neurons projecting to the neocortex (perhaps cholinergic) and several neuropeptide systems intrinsic to the neocortex. Elucidating the molecular basis of this relationship in the nucleus basalis lesioned rat could be important for an understanding of cholinergic/peptidergic interactions in the SDAT-diseased brain.

NUCLEUS BASALIS LESIONING IN AGED RATS: NEUROCHEMICAL, NEUROPATHOLOGICAL, AND BEHAVIORAL CHANGES

The aged rodent would appear to have substantial limitations as an animal model for SDAT. Firstly, a cholinergic hypofunction does not seem to develop spontaneously in the aging rat brain since most cholinergic markers remain unaffected - only acetylcholine release is consistently reduced (44,45). Thus, it is not surprising that no substantial loss of nucleus basalis cholinergic neurons occurs during brain aging in rats or mice; rather, an age-related atrophy of these neurons has been reported to occur (46,47). Secondly, despite several reports of neuronal losses in the aging rodent brain (48-50), others have shown little evidence for such age-related losses in senescent rodents (51-52). Thirdly, the major neuropathological markers for SDAT - neurofibrillary tangles and neuritic plaques - appear to be absent in the aging rat brain. Nonetheless, aged rats and mice have been reported to be impaired in a variety of learning and memory tasks (53-61) and, in that context, are similar to SDAT patients. Since cholinergic function in aged rodents is not generally reduced, however, a direct involvement of cholinergic transmission in these cognitive deficits is questionable. In view of the aforementioned limitations, the intact aged rat does not seem to sufficiently mimic most of the neurochemical and neuropathological aspects of SDAT, making it a largely inappropriate choice for evaluating various treatment or preventive strategies relevant to the disease.

As outlined earlier in this chapter, nucleus basalis lesioning in young (2 month old) adult rats can induce certain characteristics reflective of SDAT including: 1) a permanent cortical cholinergic hypofunction; 2) cortical neuropeptide dysfunctions; 3) learning/memory deficits; and 4) neuropathological changes in the same forebrain regions affected by SDAT. If, however, the rationale for nucleus basalis cholinergic neurons is SDAT, it would seem more appropriate to destroy the rat's analogous cholinergic neurons much later in the aging process. In this manner, the probable loss or dysfunction of these cholinergic neurons later in the life of SDAT patients could be simulated and the impact of this neuronal loss more closely approximated in terms of neuropathological, neurochemical, and cognitive effects. For these reasons, we have begun investigating the impact of nucleus basalis lesioning in aged rats and report below some of our findings.

Aged Sprague Dawley male rats (20-21 months of age) were given unilateral or bilateral nucleus basalis infusions of ibotenic acid and sacrificed 2.5 or 5 months later. A histological examination of subcortical tissues revealed well-circumscribed lesions especially effective in eliminating neurons in the caudal 75% of the nucleus basalis. Consistent with these histological findings were marked decreases of 41-45% in frontal cortex CAT activity after either unilateral or bilateral lesions. Despite this cortical cholinergic hypofunction, neocortical concentrations of somatostatin and NPY were unaffected at both 2.5 and 5 months post-lesioning. For bilaterally-lesioned aged animals, the lack of effect on peptide levels is the same result seen in young bilaterally-lesioned rats at similar post-lesion time points. As was also the case at 2.5 months after bilateral lesions in young rats, a significant reduction in mRNA encoding for neuropeptide Y was seen for aged, bilaterally-lesioned rats. It is interesting to note that 2.5 months following unilateral lesions in young adult animals, neocortical levels of both somatostatin and NPY were significantly reduced - yet similar unilateral lesions in aged rats had no such effect. With this exception, then, lesions in young and aged rats had similar effects on cortical neuropeptides at 2.5 and 5 months post-lesioning.

What cognitive effects do nucleus basalis lesions have when done in aged rats and how do these effects compare to those we have previously characterized in younger animals after lesioning? To address these questions, we have tested aged, lesioned animals on three tests of learning/memory ability: passive avoidance, 2-way active avoidance, and Lashley III spatial maze. In passive avoidance testing, aged rats that were sham-lesioned showed excellent memory retention at 1 or 2.5 months after surgery; in fact, their retention was no different from that of young sham-lesioned adults. By contrast, aged animals given bilateral lesions were markedly deficient in memory retention at 1 or 2.5 months after lesioniong. Bilateral lesioning was necessary to obtain this memory dysfunction since aged animals receiving only unilateral lesions showed excellent memory retention, comparable to that of sham-lesioned control animals. Thus, bilateral nucleus basalis lesioning was able to induce a memory retention deficit in aged rats that would not have otherwise been present.

This ability of lesioning to induce cognitive deficits in aged animals was further revealed during 2-way active avoidance testing. Aged, sham-lesioned animals learned to acquire this avoidance behavior at a rate similar to that of young, sham-lesioned rats. However, aged rats given bilateral nucleus basalis lesions showed an acquisitional deficit so severe that the memory (retention) phase of active avoidance testing could not be performed (i.e. lesioned animals did not even learn this task well enough to have their memory of it tested). Despite the deleterious effects of nucleus basalis lesioning in aged rats on passive and active avoidance performance, no effect of lesioning was observed during Lashley III spatial maze learning. This may be due, at least in part, to a deleterious effect of aging itself on learning of this task since sham-lesioned aged animals performed it at a generally lower level than sham-lesioned young animals.

In summary to this point, nucleus basalis lesions in aged rats can provide a marked cortical cholinergic hypofunction, as well as learning/memory deficits in avoidance tasks. Although the involvement of nucleus basalis cholinergic neurons in these cognitive deficits is implicit, further study is obviously required to more succinctly define any relationship that may exist.

Some of the most intriguing data we have thus far obtained from aged, nucleus basalis lesioned rats involves neuropathology seen 5 months following unilateral lesions. Although only three aged, nucleus basalis-lesioned animals are involved in these preliminary results, we find a remarkably accelerated and accentuated loss of neurons in the neocortex and entorhinal cortex compared to young lesioned rats. For example, neuronal loss in parietal cortex layers III-V was 15% (not significant) at 5 months after lesioning in young animals, but was 26% (highly significant) in aged animals after the same post-lesion time interval. This more dramatic cortical cell loss at 5 months after unilateral lesioning in aged rats was also seen in frontal cortex. In fact, the 23% cell loss in frontal cortex layer II was at least as great as that seen in this same area at 14 months after unilateral or bilateral lesions in young adults. These enhanced neuronal losses in fronto-parietal cortex after lesioning in aged rats suggest that aged cortical neurons are less plastic in their ability to survive a loss of nucleus basalis innervation, perhaps cholinergic in nature.

An even more marked effect of nucleus basalis lesioning in aged rats was seen in the entorhinal cortex. As indicated in an earlier section of this chapter, lesions in young adults never resulted in cell losses within layers II and III of entorhinal cortex through 14 months post-lesions. At five months after unilateral lesioning in aged animals, however, highly significant neuronal losses of 38% and 21% were evident in layers II and III, respectively, of entorhinal cortex. These substantial neuronal losses in entorhinal cortex after lesions in aged, but not young, rats presents the intriguing possibility that the cascade of transsynaptic degenerative events we hypothesize to occur after nucleus basalis lesions (9) is actually accelerated and accentuated in the aged rat. In this context, enhanced neocortical cell losses in the aged, lesioned rat could result in a dysfunctional/degenerative neocortical input to entorhinal cortex much sooner, thus causing degenerative events to occur in entorhinal cortex faster and to a greater extent. Parenthetically, it should be mentioned that neuronal counts in neocortex and entorhinal cortex involved manual counting procedures; an image analysis determination of neuronal counts from these same tissues could result in different quantitative decreases after lesioning.

Neuropathology induced by nucleus basalis lesions in aged rats extended beyond cortical neuronal losses to also include effects on dendritic branching of cortical pyramidal cells. These results are detailed in the chapter by Mervis et al. within this volume. They involve rapid Golgi impregnation of brain sections from aged rats given unilateral lesions and sacrificed 5 months later. In brief, results show that nucleus basalis lesions induce a significant increase in the amount of dendritic branching of ipsilateral pyramidal cells in neocortex relative to controls in the contralateral hemisphere or sham-lesioned controls. Moreover, there is a significant increase in the radius of dendritic domains for pyramidal neurons ipsilateral to lesioning. Such dendritic expansion could be related to the neuronal loss in neocortex that we also find present by 5 months after lesioning. Along this line, lesion-induced increases in dendritic domain may be an expression of compensatory dendritic hypertrophy, whereby the dendritic branching of surviving pyramidal cells extends into regions formerly occupied by neighboring neurons. There is evidence that a similar process of compensatory dendritic hypertrophy may be occuring in SDAT-diseased brains as well. Furthermore, the data suggest that cortical neurons in aged rats retain a surprising degree of neuronal plasticity through their expression of dendritic growth.

In general, then, it appears that the aged, nucleus basalis lesioned rat is characterized by many of the same neurochemical, behavioral, and neuropathological changes that occur after lesioning in young animals. Both models provide a long-term cholinergic hypofunction and reduced NPY mRNA levels in neocortex, but no effect on cortical neuropeptide levels through 5 months post-lesioning. Both models induce memory retention deficits in passive avoidance testing and learning (acquisitional) dysfunctions in active avoidance testing. Both models are characterized by neuronal loss or atrophy in neocortex and entorhinal cortex, although more profound neuronal losses appear to occur in the aged, lesioned rat within a shorter time interval. A continued characterization of each model - neuropathologically, neurochemically, and behaviorally - must be done to determine which, if either, is a better model for SDAT based on an initial cholinergic hypofunction.

SUMMARY AND CONCLUSIONS

SDAT is a late-developing disease, insidious in onset and progressing over a number of years. A major purpose of this chapter was to suggest that transneuronal degeneration may play a fundamental role in the pathogenesis of this disease, possibly due to an initial loss of basal forebrain cholinergic neurons. The neuroanatomical substrate for such transneuronal degeneration is provided by the fact that the other forebrain areas most affected neuropathologically in SDAT (neocortex, amygdala, entorhinal cortex, and hippocampus) are directly or indirectly innervated by cholinergic neurons originating in the nucleus basalis. In this context, we present data indicative that nucleus basalis lesions in the rat can induce various neuropathological and neurochemical changes within these same four forebrain regions, apparently through transneuronal mechanisms because of the long time course involved. These lesion-induced changes include: 1) neuronal losses and/or atrophy; 2) enhanced neurofibrillary content; and 3) changes in cortical concentrations of the neuropeptides somatostatin, NPY, and CRH. A number of months are required to observe such changes in the rat, which again suggests that anterograde transneuronal mechanisms are involved.

A host of previous studies (including our own) have indicated that nucleus basalis lesions, performed in "young" adult rats, induce a cortical cholinergic hypofunction and cognitive dysfunctions - two characteristics of SDAT. Clearly, the intent of these lesions was to mimic the spontaneous degeneration/dysfunction of nucleus basalis cholinergic neurons in SDAT. However, since it is most likely that the loss or dysfunction of such cholinergic neurons occurs later in the life of SDAT patients, we further suggested in this chapter that a more appropriate rat model may involve destruction of the analogous cholinergic neurons in "aged" rats. Aging may affect neurons in ways that alter their response to lesions caused by disease or experimental manipulations. Thus, lesioning the nucleus basalis in aged rats should theoretically provide a more realistic approximation of the impact that a degeneration of nucleus basalis cholinergic neurons is having in SDAT patients. In that context, we presented our initial data from aged, nucleus basalis lesioned rats showing that such lesions induce a marked cortical cholinergic hypofunction and cognitive deficits, as is seen after similar lesions in young adults. However, neuropathological changes in neocortex and entorhinal cortex of aged, lesioned rats appeared to be accelerated and accentuated when compared to the time-course of similar changes in young, lesioned rats. This suggests that the aged brain is less plastic in its ability to survive a loss of nucleus basalis neurons and, further, presents the interesting possibility that transsynaptic degenerative events induced by nucleus basalis lesioning in the aged brain are accelerated. The aged, nucleus basalis-legioned rat would, therefore, appear to deserve intensive further characterization to succinctly define its similarities to SDAT.

As with most animal models for human diseases, certain limitations exist regarding the nucleus basalis-lesioned rat as a model for SDAT based on an initial cholinergic hypofunction. First and foremost, excitotoxic lesions of the nucleus basalis region are non-specific; that is, they induce the death of not only cortically-projecting cholinergic neurons, but also noncholinergic and noncortical-projecting neurons in the nucleus basalis as well. Secondly, excitotoxic infusions cannot be limited to the nucleus basalis; rather, they usually involve much of the adjacent globus pallidus as well. For these reasons, some of the neuropathological, behavioral, and neurochemical effects of nucleus basalis lesions are probably due to this unavoidable destruction of noncholinergic neurons in and around the nucleus basalis. Although a relatively specific cholinotoxin - AF64A - has been developed, we recently found that rats recover from the cortical cholinergic hypofunction induced by cortical infusions of AF64A (62, 63). Unfortunately, this precludes its use to study slowly-developing transneuronal changes involving cortical cholinergic hypofunction. A final limitation of the nucleus basalis lesioned rat that should be mentioned is the fact that it initially compromises only one transmitter system known to be affected in SDAT - the nucleus basalis cholinergic system. Yet considerable evidence supports a possible involvement of non-cholinergic systems in the pathogenesis of SDAT as well, especially ascending monoaminergic systems from the brain stem (64,65). Along the same line, it is likely that several primary lesion sites, in addition to the nucleus basalis, contribute to the pathogenesis of SDAT. Nucleus basalis lesions are thus limited in addressing only one of several possible primary lesion sites in SDAT.

Despite the aforementioned limitations of the nucleus basalis-lesioned rat model, it would appear to be most useful for studying a variety of slow transneuronal pathological and neurochemical changes during long-term neocortical hypofunction. Given the slowly developing nature of SDAT, it is quite possible that similar transneuronal events are spontaneously occurring in the SDAT-diseased brain; transneuronal events that could be directly contributory to the neuropathology and cognitive impairments typical of SDAT patients. Thus, an elucidation of the transneuronal mechanisms responsible for the neuropathological and neurochemical effects of long-term nucleus basalis lesioning may provide considerable new insight into the pathogenesis of SDAT. In this context, we have hypothesized that some of the transneuronal changes seen in neocortex following nucleus basalis lesions may be due to loss of a necessary stimulatory influence, such as acetylcholine and/or vasoactive intestinal polypeptide (VIP) - both of which are present within cholinergic terminals in neocortex. Acetylcholine is known to be an excitatory neurotransmitter in the brain and VIP may have neuronotrophic actions necessary for neuronal survival (66,67).

Of course, a major reason for developing the nucleus basalis rat model, aside from its use in studying a variety of slowly-developing transneuronal events pertinent to the aging brain, is its potential use in testing various treatment or preventive strategies relevant to SDAT. Can the lesion-induced neuronal losses in neocortex be prevented by some therapeutic agent? Can the lesion-induced changes in cortical somatostatin, NPY, or CRH levels be normalized through pharmacological treatment? An obvious choice in attempting to prevent or treat such lesion-induced changes would be the use of cholinomimetic agents, although a variety of more generalized agents (i.e. growth factors, neuronotrophic substances) could conceivably be tested for their therapeutic value through the use of this animal model.

REFERENCES

1. Cowan, W.M. (1970) Anterograde and retrograde transneuronal degeneration in the central and peripheral nervous system. In: Contemporary Research Methods in Neuroanatomy (eds: Nauta, W. and Ebbesson, S.) Springer-Verlag, New York, pp. 217-236.
2. Kupfer, C. (1965) The distribution of cell size in the lateral geniculate nucleus of man following transneuronal cell atrophy. J Neuropath. Exp. Neuro!. 24: 653-661. 3. Nagai, T. McGeer, P., Peng, J., McGeer, E. and Dolman, C. (1983) Choline acetyltransferase immunohistochemistry in brains of Alzheimer's disease patients and controls. Neurosci. Lett. 36: 195-199.
4. Pearson, R., So&oniew, M., Cuello, A., Powell, T., Eckenstein, F., Esiri, M. and Wilcock, G. (1983) Persistence of cholinergic neurons in the basal nucleus in a brain with senile dementia of the Alzheimer's type demonstrated by immunohistochemical staining for choline acetyltransferase. Brain Res. 289: 375-379.
5. Arendt., T., Bigl, V., Tennstedt, A. and Arendt, A. (1985) Neuronal lossin different parts of the nucleus basalis is related to neuritic plaque formation in cortical t rget areas in Alzheimer's disease. Neuroscience 14: 1-14.
6. Bartus, R., Dean, R., Beer, B. and Lippa, A. (1982) The cholinergic hypothesis of geriatric memory dysfunction. Science 217: 408-417.
7. Rylett, R., Ball, M and Colhoun, H. (1983) Evidence for high affinity choline transport in synaptosomes prepared from hippocampal and neocortex of patients with Alzheimer's disease. Brain Res. 289: 169-175.
8. Collerton, D. (1986) Cholinergic function and intellectual decline in Alzheimer's disease. Neuroscience 19: 1-28.
9. Arendash, G., Millard, W., Dunn, A. and Meyer, E. (1987) Long-term neuropathological and neurochemical effects of nucleus basalis lesions in the rat. Science 238: 952-956.
10. Wenk, G., Cribbs, B. and McCall, L. (1984) Nucleus basalis magnocellularis: optimal coordinates for selective reduction of choline acetyltransferase in frortal neocortex by ibotenic acid injections. Exp. Brain Res. 56: 335-340.
11. Flicker, C., Dean, L., Watkins, D., Fisher, S. and Bartus, R. (1983) Behavioral and neurochemical effects following neurotoxic lesions of a major cholinergic input to the cerebral cortex in the rat. Pharmacol. Biochem. Behav. 18: 973-981.
12. Dubois, B., Mayo, W., Agid, Y., LeMoal, M. and Simon, H. (1985) Profound disturbances of spontaneous and learned behaviors following lesion of the nucleus basalis magnocellularis in the rat. Brain Res. 338: 249-258.
13. Hepler, D., Olton, D., Wenk, G. and Coyle, J. (1985) Lesions in nucleus basalis magnocellularis and medial septal area of rats produce qualitatively similar memory impairments. J. Neurosci. 5: 866-873.
14. Arendash, G., Strong, P. and Mouton, P. (1985) Intracerebral transplantation of cholinergic neurons in a new animal model for Alzheimer's disease. In: Senile Dementia of the Alzheimer Type (eds: Hutton, J. and Kenny, A.) Alan R. Liss, Inc., New York, pp. 351-376.

15. Bartus, R., Flicker, C., Dean, R., Pontecorvo, M., Figueiredo, J. and Fisher, S. (1985) Selective memory loss following nucleus basalis lesions: long-term behavioral recovery despite persistent cholinergic deficiencies. Pharm. Biochem. Behav. 23: 125-135.
16. Wenk, G., Hughey, D., Boundy, V. and Kim, A. (1987) Neurotransmitters and memory: role of cholinergic, serotonergic, and noradrenergic systems. Behav. Neurosci. 101:325;332.
17. Arendash, G., Millard, W., Dawson, R., Dunn, A. and Meyer, E. (1989) Different long-term effects of bilateral and unilateral nucleus basalis lesions on rat cerebral cortical neurotransmitter content. Submitted for publication.
18. Mesulam, M. M., Mufson, E., Wainer, B. and Levey, A (1983) Central cholinergic pathways in the rat: an overview based on an alternative nomenclature (Chl-Ch6). Neuroscience 11: 1185-1201.
19. LoConte, G., Casamenti, F., Bigl, V., Milaneschi, E. and Pepeu, G. (1982) Effects of magnocellular forebrain nuclei lesions on acetylcholine output from the cerebral cortex, electrocortigram and behavior. Arch. Ital Biol 120: 176-188.
20. Kryjevic, K, Pumain, R. and Renaud, L (1971) The mechanism of excitation by acetylcholine in the cerebral cortex. J. Physiol. (London) 215: 247-268.
21. Cole, A and Nicoll, R. (1984) Characterization of a slow cholinergic postsynaptic potential recorded in vitro from rat hippocampal pyramidal cells. J. Physiol. (London) 352:173-188.
22. Agoston, D., Borroni, E. and Richardson, P. (1988) Cholinergic surface antigen chol-1 is present in a subclass of VIP containing rat cortical synaptosomes. J. Neurochem. 50: 1659:1662.
23. Hyman, B., Van Hoesen, G., Damasio, A. and Barnes, C. (1984) Alzheimer's disease: cell-specific pathology isolates the hippocampal formation. Science 225: 1168-11270.
24. Coyle, J., Price, D. and DeLong, M. (1983) Alzheimer's disease: a disorder of cortical cholinergic innervation. Science 219: 1184-1190.
25. Neary, D., Snowden, J., Bowen, D., Sims, N., Mann, D., Northen, B., Yates, P. and Davison, A. (1986) Alzheimer's disease: a correlative study. J. Neurol. Neurosurg. Psychiat. 49: 229-237.
26. Perry, E., Blessed, G., Tomlinson, B., Perry, R., Crow, T., Cross, A., Dockray, G., Dimeline, R. and Arregui, A. (1981) Neurochemical activity in human temporal lobe related to aging and Alzheimer-type changes. Neurobiol. Aging 4: 251-256.
27. Bowen, D., Smith, C., White, P. and Davison, A. (1976) Neurotransmitter-related enzymes and indices of hypoxia in senile dementia and other abiotrophies. Brain 99: 459-496.
28. Davies, P. (1979) Neurotransmitter-related enzymes in senile dementia of the Alzheimer type. Brain Res. 171: 319-327.
29. Bowen, D., Sims, M., Benton, J., Curzon, G., Neary, D., Thomas, D. and Davison, A. (1981) Treatment of Alzheimer's disease: a cautionary note. N. Engl. J. Med. 305: 1016-1019
30. Davies, P., Katzman, R. and Terry, R. (1980) Reduced somatostatin-like immunoreactivity in cerebral cortex from cases of Alzheimer's disease and Alzheimer senile dementia. Nature 288: 279-280.
31. Rossor, M., Emson, P., Mountjoy, C. et al. (1980) Reduced amounts of immunoreactive somatostatin in the temporal cortex in senile dementia of Alzheimer type. Neurosci. Lett. 20: 373-377.
32. Beal, M., Mazurek, M., Chattha, G., Svendsen, C., Bird, E. and Martin, J. (1986) Neuropeptide Y immunoreactivity is reduce in cerebral cortex in Alzheimer's disease. Ann. Neurol. 20: 282-288.
33. DeSouza, E. (1988) CRH defects in Alzheimer's and other neurological diseases. Hosp. Practice 23: 59-71.
34. DeSouza, E., Whitehouse, P., Kuhar, M. Price, D. and Vale, W. (1986) Reciprocal changes m corticotropin-releasing factor (CRF) - like immunoreactivity and CRF receptors in the cerebral cortex of Alzheimer's disease. Nature 319: 593-595.
35. Chronwall, B., Chase, T. and O'Donohue, T. (1984) Coexistence of neuropeptide Y and somatostatin in rat and human cortical and rat hypothalamus neurons. Neurosci. Lett. 52:213-217.

36. Vincent, S., Johansson, D. and Hokfelt, T. (1982) Neuropeptide coexistence in human cortical neurons. Nature 298: 65-67.
37. Dawbarn, D., Rossor, M., Mountjoy, C., Roth, M. and Emson, P. (1986) Decreased somatostatin immunoreactivity but not neuropeptide Y immunoreactivity in cerebral cortex in senile dementia of Alzheimer type. Neurosci. Lett. 70: 154-159.
38. Francis, P. and Bowen, D. (1985) Relevance of reduced concentrations of somatostatin in Alzheimer's disease. Biochem. Society Transactions 13: 170-171.
39. McKinney, M., Davies, P. and Coyle, J. (1982) Somatostatin is not co-localized in cholinergic neurons innervating the rat cerebral cortex-hippocampal functions. Brain Res. 243: 169-172.
40. Montminy, M. and Bilezikjian, L. (1987) Binding of a nuclear protein to the cyclic AMP response element of the somatostatin gene. Nature 328: 175-178.
41. Olianas, M., Onali, P. Neff, N. and Costa, E. (1983) Adenylate cyclase activity of synaptic membranes from rat striatum: inhibition by muscarinic agonists. Mol. Pharmacol. 23: 393-398.
42. Robbins, R., Sutton, R. and Reichlin, S. (1982) Effects of neurotransmitter and cyclic AMP on somatostatin release from cultured cerebral cortical cells. Brain Res. 234: 377-386.
43. Fagg, G. and Foster, A. (1983) Amino acid neurotransmitters and their pathways in the mammalian central nervous system. Neuroscience 9: 701-719.
44. Meyer, E. St. Onge, E. and Crews, F. (1984) Effects of aging on rat cortical presynaptic cholinergic processes. Neurobioloy of Aging 5: 315-317.
45. Pedata, R. Slavikova, J. Kotas, A. and Pepeu, G. (1983) Acetylcholine release from rat cortical slices during postnatal development and aging. Neurobiology of Aging 4: 31-35.
46. Hornberger, J., Buell, S., Flood, D., NcNeill, T. and Coleman, P. (1985) Stability of numbers but not size of mouse forebrain cholinergic neurons to 53 months. Neurobiology of Aging 6: 269-275.
47. Armstrong, D., Buzaki, G., Chen, K, Ruiz, R., Sheffield, R. and F. Gage (1987) Cholinergic neurotransmission in the aged rat: a behavioral, electrophysiological, and anatomical study. Soc. Neuroscience Abstr. 13: 434.
48. Landfield, P. Rose, G., Sandles, L., Wohlstadter, T. and Lynch, G. (1977) Patterns of astroglial hypertrophy and neuronal degeneration in the hippocampus of aged, memory-deficient rats. Journal of Gerontology 32: 3/12.
49. Sabel, B. and Stein, D. (1981) Extensive loss of subcortical neurons in the aging rat brain. Experimental Neurology 73: 507-516.
50. Peng, M. and Lee, L. (1979) regional differences of neuron loss of rat brain in old age. Gerontology 25: 205-211.
51. Peters, A., Feldman, M. and Vaughan, D. (1983) The effect of aging on the neuronal population within area 17 of adult rat cerebral cortex. Neurobiology of Aging 4: 273-282.
52. Freund, G. (1980) Cholinergic receptor loss in brains of aging mice. Life Sciences 26: 371-375.
53. Gallagher, M. and Pelleymounter, M. (1988) Spatial learning deficits in old rats: a model for memoly decline in the aged. Neurobiology of Aging 9: 549-556.
54. Pontecorvo, M., Clissold, D. and Conti, L (1988) Age-related cognitive impairments as assessed with an automated repeated measures memory task: implications for the possible role of acetylcholine and norepinephrine in memory dysfunction. Neurobiology of Aging 9: 617-625.
55. Barnes, C., Nadel, L. and Honig, W. (1980) Spatial memory deficit in senescent rats. Canadian Journal of Psychology 34: 29-39.
56. Van der Staay, R., Raaijmakers, W., Sakkee, A. and Van Bezooijen, C. (1988) Spatial working and reference memory in senescent rats after thiopental anaesthesia. Neurosci. Res. Comm. 3: 55-61.
57. Ingram, D. (1988) Complex maze learning in rodents as a model of age-relatedmemory impairment. Neurobiology of Aging 9: 475-485.
58. Gold, R., McGaugh, J., Hankins, L. Rose, R. and Vasquez, B. (1981) Age dependent changes in retention in rats. Experim. Aging Res. 8: 53-58.
59. Zornetzer, S. Thompson, R. and Rogers, J. (1982) Rapid forgetting in aged rats. Behavioral and Neural Biology 36: 49-60.

60. Goodrick, C. (1972) Learning by mature-young and aged wistar albino rats as a function of test complexity. J. of Gerontology 27: 353-357.
61. Wallace, J., Krauter, E. and Campbell, B. (1980) Animal models of declining memory in the aged: short-term and spatial memory in the aged rat. J. of Gerontology 35: 355-363.
62. Mouton, P., Meyer, E., Dunn, A., Millard, W. and Arendash, G. (1988) Induction of cortical cholinergic hypofunction and memory retention deficits through intracortical AF64A infusions. Brain Res. 444: 104-118.
63. Mouton, P., Meyer, E. and Arendash, G. (1989) Intracortical AF64A: memory impairments and recovery from cholinergic hypofunction. Pharm. Biochem. Behav. 32: in press.
64. Palmer, A., Wilcock, G., Esiri, M., Francis, P. and Bowen, D. (1987) Monoaminergic innervation of the frontal and temporal lobes in Alzheimer's disease. Brain Res. 401: 231-238.
65. Gottfries, C., Adolfsson, R., Awquilonius, S., Carlsson, A., Eckernas, S., Nordberg, A. Oreland, L, Svennerholm, L., Wilberg, A. and Winblad, B. (1983) Biochemical changes in dementia disorders of Alzheimer type (AD/SDAT). Neurobiology of Aging 3: 261-271.
66. Brenneman, D. Eiden, L. (1986) Vasoactive intestinal peptide and electrical activity influence neuronal survival. Proc. Natl. Acad. Sci. 83: 1159-1162.
67. Brenneman, D., Eiden, L and Siegel, R. (1985) Neurotrophic action of VIP on spinal cord cultures. Peptides 6: 35-39.

PRESYNAPTIC MARKERS OF CHOLINERGIC FUNCTION IN CORTEX

FOLLOWING IBOTENIC ACID LESION OF THE BASAL FOREBRAIN

Martha Downen, Kimi Sugaya, Stephen P. Arneric, and
Ezio Giacobini

Dept. of Pharmacology
Southern Illinois University School of Medicine
Springfield, IL

The large neurons of the magnocellular nucleus of the basal forebrain provide the maior extrinsic cholinergic innervation of the cerebral cortex[1,2,3,4,5]. The cells of origin form a diffusely localized cell group known as the nucleus basalis magnocellularis (NBM) and are found in the region of the ventromedial portion of the globus pallidus, the substantia innominata and the preoptic magnocellular nucleus. These cells send widespread projections to the cerebral cortex and the amygdala. This cell group is of particular interest given the finding that an analogous system in the human, known as the nucleus basalis of Meynert, shows considerable damage in Alzheimer's Disease (AD)[6]. Lesions of the rat NBM provide an animal model that.mimics some of the neurochemical pathology associated with AD.

The effects of basal forebrain lesion on some markers of cholinergic function are well known in the cerebral cortex. Following electrolytic or excitotoxic lesion of the NBM, a dramatic decrease in activity of choline acetyltransferase (ChAT) and aceOtylcholinesterase (AChE) occurs[1,7]. High affinity choline uptake[8] and acetylcholine (ACh) release are significantly decreased[9,10]. Similar deficits in ChAT and AChE are observed in postmortem and bioptic samples from AD brain [11,12,13,14,15]. ACh release is also impaired in postmortem and biopsy samples[16,17] taken from AD brain.

Learning and memory deficits are characteristic of AD and are also produced in NBM lesioned animals[18]. The behavioral deficits that occur following NBM lesion have been characterized extensively (for review see [19]). Deficits in ChAT activity significantly correlate with t-maze deficits following ibotenate-lesion of the NBM[20]

The existence of nicotinic receptors on the presynaptic fibers arising from the basal forebrain projection is not well characterized. However, the number of nicotinic receptors is significantly decreased in the cortex of AD patients[21,22] Meyer et al.[23] reported that presynaptic nicotinic receptor modulation failed to alter release in animals with lesions of the NBM and concluded that nicotinic receptors are not located presynaptically on this projection. Moreover, no change is seen in total nicotinic receptors at one and thirteen weeks after NBM lesion[24,25]. A decrease in cortical muscarinic receptors is seen following NBM lesion[7]. However, a lesion-induced alteration in muscarinic receptor modulation of cortical ACh release is not observed[23, 26]

Lesion effects on cortical ChAT, AChE and somatostatin are observed within one week and may persist for at least six months[27]. However, the persistence of lesion-induced alterations in cholinergic function is controversial. Wenk and Olton[28] report a recovery of ChAT activity that occurs within three months following ibotenic acid lesion of the BF. Atack et al.[24] report a recovery of ChAT activity from 51% depletion at one week following ibotenic acid lesion with only 20% depletion at 13 weeks postlesion. Hohman et al.[29] report an age-related recurrence of lesion-induced ChAT depletions. Arendash et al.[30] find a persistence of lesion-induced ChAT deficits at six months following ibotenic acid lesion and see transsynaptic cortical cell death at this time.

A recovery of release of ACh occurs with time following kainic acid lesion of the NBM. Gardiner et al.[26] report a dramatic decrease (71%) in potassium-evoked ACh release from the frontal and parietal cortices after unilateral kainate lesion of the NBM that shows some recovery toward contralateral values at nine weeks in the parietal cortex but not in the frontal cortex. Lo Conte et al.[9] report a slight but non-significant increase in ACh release from the intact contralateral hemisphere at approximately 23 days following a unilateral electrolytic lesion of the BF region.

As with neurochemical deficits, lesion-induced behavioral deficits tend to show some recovery with time. Behavioral recovery occurs by six months following bilateral ibotenic acid lesion but re$overy is dependent on postlesion training in an unrelated task[31].

In these experiments we sought to determine the subchronic changes in presynaptic cortical cholinergic function following ibotenic acid lesions of the BF. The functional integrity of cholinergic neurons in the fronto-parietal cortex was examined in paired contiguous micropunches to determine the short-term rostral-caudal progression of cortical cholinergic dysfunction. Both ChAT activity and ACh release were assessed concurrently to correlate topographically the functional changes in cortex postlesion. Additionally, we sought to determine whether alpha-BTX binding sites reside on the presynaptic projections from the basal forebrain to the cortex.

METHODS

Animals and Surgery

250 - 350 g male Sprague-Dawley rats were anesthetized with 2.5 % halothane, balance O_2 and mounted in a stereotaxic apparatus (David Kopf). Unilateral lesions of the NBM were performed via injection of ibotenic acid (Sigma) 5 µg/0.5 µl in a vehicle of sterile filtered 100 mM phosphate buffer, pH 7.4. Ibotenic acid was delivered with a graduated microliter pipette with an external tip diameter of 75 microns mounted in a pipette holder[32] at 18°. The ventromedial portion of the globus pallidus was stereotaxically localized using the following coordinates: AP = -5.0 mm from bregma, ML = +/- 2.6 mm, 7.5 mm below dura, incisor bar = - 11 from the intra-aural line33. This approach was used in order to avoid penetration through cortical regions that would

be sampled for release and enzyme activity measurements. The toxin was
delivered over a period of 1 min and the micropipette was left in place
for 3 min following injection; vehicle was injected contralaterally.

Neurochemical Mapping

Animals were sacrificed at different time points following lesion.
The animals were lightly anesthetized with halothane, killed by
decapitation and the brains rapidly harvested. The brains were cut into
two major sections and the ventral portion containing the NBM was frozen
in n-Hexane on dry ice, placed in embedding compound and frozen at -90 ^{0}
C for later histological analysis. The cortex was immediately sliced
into 500 micron sections with a McIlwain tissue chopper. Each of ten
sections ranging from + 2.0 mm bregma to - 3.0 mm bregma were dissected
free and placed on a parafilm covered microscope slide. Three
micropunches (1.6 mm diameter) were taken from each hemisphere (fig. 1).
Sixty punches were taken in total, 44 were frozen on dry ice for later
determination of enzyme activity while 16 punches were immediately used
for measurement of ACh release (fig. 2).

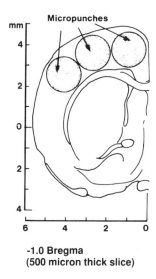

-1.0 Bregma
(500 micron thick slice)

Figure 1. A representative
coronal section indicating the
areas of cerebral cortex sampled
by the micropunch technique to
determine enzyme activities and
ACh release.

Acetylcholine Release

Immediately following dissection, ACh release was determined in
micropunches from the frontal and parietal cortices from each of four of
the areas[33] sampled previously shown to have maximal decreases in ChAT
activity . Release of [^{3}H]-ACh was determined according to the method
of Hadhazy and Szerb[34]. Cortical punches were pre-incubated with [^{3}H]-
choline chloride (NEN) in oxygenated Krebs buffer [mM: 118 NaCl, 4.8

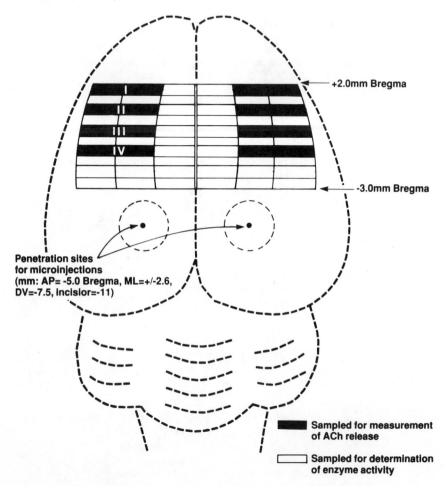

Figure 2. A schematic diagram illustrating regions of the cerebral cortex sampled following unilateral ibotenic acid lesions of the basal forebrain.

KCl, 1.2 NaH_2PO_4, MgSO4, 2.5 $CaCl_2$, 25 $NaHCO_3$, 11 d-glucose, 0.02 choline chloride, 0.1 physostigmine hemisulfate] for 20 min at 37^0 C. Following pre-incubation, the punches were loaded into release chambers constructed from 3 mm filters (Gelman), attached to a 3 cc syringe filled with Krebs solution plus 0.01 mM Hemicholinium-3, and placed in a 37^0C water bath. The tissue was superfused with 250 μl of buffer at five min intervals. Release was elicited at 35 min following exposure to Krebs with 50 mM potassium. Equiosmolar decreases in NaCl were performed to maintain isotonicity. Fractions were collected for an additional 15 min following stimulation. Total [^{3}H]-ACh efflux was determined in an 100 μl aliquot of the release sample plus 5.0 ml Ready value (Beckman). The tissue was resuspended in 200 μl of 100 mM phosphate buffer, pH 7.4 and sonicated (Heat Systems-Ultrasonic inc, Model w225, 30 % duty cycle, o.p. 3). [^{3}H]-ACh was determined in tissue homogenates. Protein was determined in tissue homogenates according to the method of Bradford[35] with bovine serum albumin as standard.

Choline Acetyltransferase activity

ChAT activity was determined according to the method of Fonnum[36]. The tissue punches were resuspended in 100 μl of 10 mM KH_2PO_4, 20 mM EDTA and homogenized using an ultrasonicator (30% power, Microtip, 6 sec). An aliquot was retained for protein determination. Enzyme activity was determined in an aliquot of the homogenate resuspended in 0.2 % BSA and 0.4 % Triton-X 100. [^{3}H]-Acetyl CoA (NEN, 0.05 μCi/0.05 mmol) 0.2 mM final concentration was used as substrate and the reaction mixture consisted of 5.0 mM EDTA, 300 mM NaCl, 0.8 mM choline chloride and 0.1 mM physostigmine sulfate. Following a 40 min incubation at 37^0C, [^{3}H]-ACh synthesized was extracted in 1.0 ml 2-heptanone containing 10 mg tetraphenylboron. Fifteen mls scintillation fluor (Beckman) was added and radioactivity measured in a Beckman LS 5801.

Receptor Autoradiography

Rats were sacrificed by decapitation at various times after ibotenic acid lesion of the NBM for receptor autoradiographic analysis. Following decapitation, the brains were rapidly removed, immersed in n-hexane cooled with dry ice, molded in O.C.T. compound and stored at -90^0C. Cutting was performed at -15^0C with a cryostat microtome. At intervals through each brain, two adjacent coronal sections (20 micron) were taken. Sections were thaw-mounted on acid-cleaned gelatin-coated slides and stored at -90^0 C for at least 24 hr. Slides were pre-incubated in Tris physiological saline buffer (TPB, 10 mM Tris, 1 mM $MgCl_2$, 150 mM NaCl, 3 mM KCl, 3 mM $CaCl_2$, 17 mM glucose, 1 mg/ml BSA, pH 7.4) cfor 30 min and then incubated in TPB which contained 1 nM or 5 nM of ^{125}alpha-bungarotoxin (BTX; Amersham) with or without 1 μM of cold toxin for 2 hr to define total or nonspecific binding. Slides were rinsed in three changes of buffer for 10 min each, dipped into distilled water, and rapidly dried under a stream of compressed air at room temperature and juxtaposed tightly against x-ray film for one week. Films were processed in Kodak D19 developer for five min and fixed for four min with Kodak Rapid Fixer. Computer-assisted image analysis was performed by a video counting and microdensitometry program (BQ IV Software Models, R & M Biometrics, Inc., Nashville, TN) and an IBM AT computer. The analog image data of autoradiographic films seen through a black and white video camera (Dage MTL model 65, Dage-MTI Inc., Michigan City, IN) were converted to digital image data by an AD-converter and stored in the video-RAM board (AT&T Targa M8 Frame Grabber, True Vision, Indianapolis, IN). The optical density was assigned a number, based on an input table with 256 values, from 0 to 255 (8 bit). Background correction which compensates for irregularities in the optical system and subtraction of nonspecific binding from total binding were performed by the computer. The image of the specific binding of ^{125}I-BTX was displayed in black and white on an analog RGB monitor (Nec Multi-Sync II monitor; Nec, Wood Dale, IL) and irregularly shaped regions of interest were defined for measurement of binding of ^{125}I-BTX quantified using ^{125}I microscale standards (Amersham). Interhemispheric differences were compared and statistical significance tested using the Student's t-test.

RESULTS

Confirmation of the lesion site was performed using Nissl staining which verifies loss of cells in the ventromedial portion of the globus pallidus at the level of the anterior commissure (fig. 3).

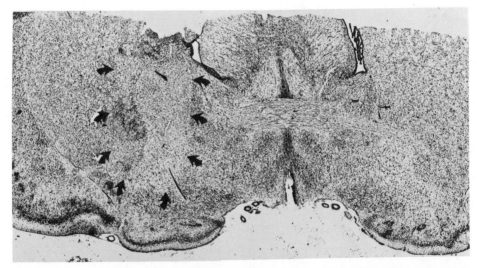

Figure 3. A Nissl stained section illustrating ibotenic acid injection site. Note the loss of cells and glial infiltration in the region of the ventromedial globus pallidus at the level of the anterior commissure.

Baseline release of [3H]-ACh from cortical micropunches was not altered at any time point examined following selective destruction of the cholinergic NBM with ibotenic acid (Data not shown). There was no regional variation in evoked or baseline release at either two or four weeks postlesion in either the intact or lesioned hemisphere. Evoked [3H]-ACh release was significantly depleted at two and four weeks following lesion (figs. 4 and 5).

At six weeks lesion effects on evoked release were regionally selective. Potassium-evoked release was not significantly different in the lesioned versus the unlesioned hemisphere. However, there was a significant regional difference at this time point. Release from the

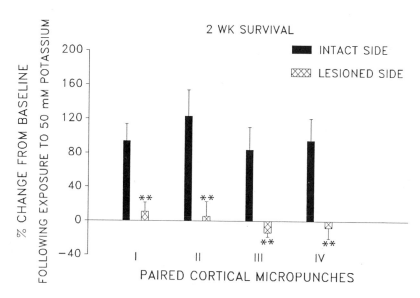

Figure 4. [3H]-ACh release following potassium stimulation in cortical micropunches at 2 weeks following unilateral injection of ibotenic acid into the NBM. ** Indicates significant differences in release from samples from the lesioned and intact hemispheres.

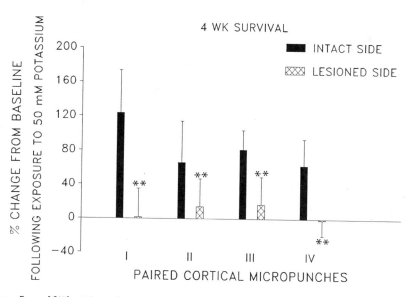

Figure 5. [3H]-ACh release following potassium stimulation of cortical micropunches taken at 4 weeks following unilateral injection of ibotenic acid into the NBM. ** indicates significant difference (p <0.01) in release from lesioned and intact hemispheres.

rostral sections was similar in both hemispheres while there was no potassium-evoked release of [3H]-ACh in the caudal sections from either hemisphere (fig. 6).

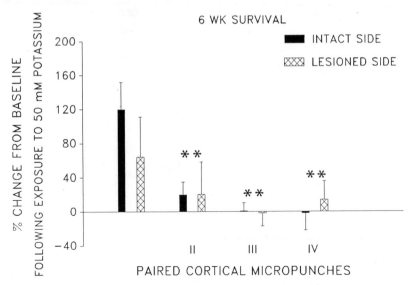

Figure 6. [3H]-ACh release following potassium stimulation in cortical micropunches taken at six weeks following unilateral ibotenic acid injection into the NBM. ** indicates regions II, III, and IV are significantly different from I (p < 0.01).

Depletion of ChAT activity followed, for the most part, a similar pattern as that of release. Lesion effects were expressed as percent difference from the intact contralateral hemisphere. ChAT activity was significantly decreased in the lesioned cortex as compared to the intact hemisphere at all time points measured (p < 0.05). Depletion of ChAT activity at 2 weeks showed a topographical distribution with the most rostral sections showing the greatest depletion. Maximal depletion (71%) was obtained at two weeks in the most frontal micropunches (fig. 7). Enzyme activity was depleted by 48% in the most caudal sections at two weeks following lesion. Enzyme activity remained significantly depleted at 4 and 6 weeks (p <0.05). However, the pattern of enzyme depletion at four and six weeks and differed significantly from that observed at 2 weeks following lesion (fig. 7). A two-way ANOVA with one repeated measure (i. e. regions) revealed a significant time-related lesion effect on enzyme activity (p < 0.05). Percent depletion of ChAT activity at 4 and 6 weeks was less than maximal in the rostral sections with equivalent depletion observed in the caudal punches. Enzyme activity was depleted in the most frontal regions sampled by 38% and 40% at 4 and 6 weeks, respectively. However, the tendency observed for regional differences in % depletion within each of the three time points measured was not significant. It should be noted that in contrast to the effects seen with evoked release of [3H]-ACh at 6 weeks, the caudal regions of the intact side did not show a selective impairment in the ability to synthesize ACh as assessed by ChAT activity.

Alpha-BTX binding in the cerebral cortex was only slightly decreased in cortical regions corresponding to those regions in which ACh release and synthesis were measured when a 1 nM concentration was used to define binding sites (Table 1). Significant decreases in alpha-BTX binding were observed in the most caudal sections taken for autoradiographic analysis (p < 0.05).

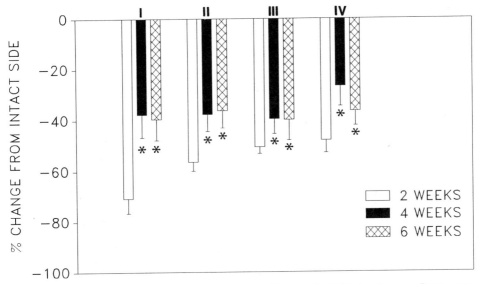

Figure 7. ChAT depletion following unilateral NBM lesion. Data are expressed as % decrease from the contralateral hemisphere. * Indicates significant restoration of enzyme activity at 4 and 6 weeks across regions I - IV as compared to week 2 (p <0.05).

Table I. Alpha-BTX binding in cerebral cortex following unilateral ibotenic acid lesion of the NBM.

mm from bregma		2 WEEKS			4 WEEKS			6 WEEKS		
		LE-SION pCi/g	IN-TACT pCi/g	% DE-CREASE	LE-SION pCi/g	IN-TACT p/Ci/g	% DE-CREASE	LE-SION pCi/g	IN-TACT pCi/g	% DE-CREASE
+2	CCX 1-3	0.279	0.286	2.448	0.316	0.337	6.231	0.284	0.286	0.699
	CCX 4-6	0.456	0.484	5.785	0.616	0.660	6.667	0.500	0.542	7.749
0	CCX 1-3	0.280	0.299	6.355	0.321	0.353	9.065	0.309	0.306	-0.980
	CCX 4-6	0.409	0.462	11.472	0.563	0.605	6.942	0.594	0.592	-0.338
-2	CCX 1-3	0.350	0.355	1.408	0.334	0.392	14.796*	0.283	0.287	1.394
	CCX 4-6	0.451	0.533	15.385*	0.556	0.573	2.967	0.520	0.490	-6.122

* p < 0.05, (CCX 1-3 = cortical layers 1 through 3; CCX 4-6 = cortical layers 4 through 6)

However, a decrease in binding was observed in the cortex in regions corresponding to those areas where deficits in enzyme activity and release were observed with 5 nM ^{125}I-BTX (fig. 8).

2.0

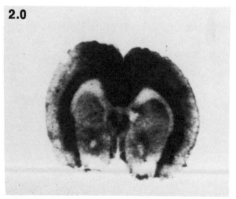

0

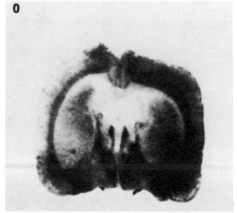

-2.0

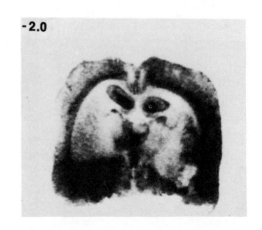

Figure 8. Autoradiograms of alpha-BTX binding following NBM lesion. Sections were taken from regions that correspond with samples neurochemically evaluated (mm from bregma). Note a decrease in binding in the lesioned cortex (left).

DISCUSSION

The lesion effects on [3H]-ACh release observed in this study at 2 and 4 weeks suggest a minimal contribution by cortical interneurons to potassium-evoked ACh release given the finding that release was almost completely abolished in the lesioned hemisphere at these times. However, the NBM lesion only produced a maximum depletion of ChAT activity of 71% with an average depletion of 43% observed. The residual enzyme activity that remains following lesion indicates either a sparing of some of the cells of the NBM projection, the presence of ChAT-containing cortical interneurons, or ChAT-containing endothelial cells. Previous research suggests that approximately 30% of the cholinergic innervation of the cortex is provided by interneurons[1], whereas, approximately 2% of the cortical ChAT activity is associated with microvascular elements[37]. Gardiner et al.[38] did not observe a deficit in cortical ACh release evoked by potassium following excitotoxic lesion of the cortex. However, these authors did observe a significant depletion of cortical ACh release after NBM lesion. In addition, Arneric and co-workers observed modest, 20 - 30%, reductions in the potassium-evoked release of [3H]-ACh from micropunches of cerebral cortex receiving local excitotoxic lesions with ibotenic acid (unpublished observations). Taken together, these findings suggest that cortical interneurons do not contribute substantially to potassium-evoked ACh release.

The downregulation of ACh release observed in the contralateral hemisphere in these experiments is inexplicable at this time. The cholinergic innervation to the cortex from the NBM is primarily considered an ipsilaterally projecting pathway. However, a few reports in the literature point out contralateral effects following unilateral lesions. In a recent publication, recovery of lesion-induced neurochemical and behavioral deficits occurred only in unilaterally lesioned animals while animals receiving bilateral lesions remained deficient in passive avoidance retention, high affinity choline uptake and ChAT activity at six months following lesion[39]. Pearson et al.[40] observed hypertrophy of the contralateral NBM following a unilateral devascularizing lesion of the cortex. Additionally, Atack et al.[24] reported bilateral changes in muscarinic binding sites following unilateral ibotenic acid lesions of the NBM. While these data do not provide evidence for any direct pathway to the contralateral cortex, they do indicate some communication between the NBM and the contralateral hemisphere at least through some indirect pathway.

The changes in alpha-BTX were localized at the deepest layer of the cortex (5 and 6) which are known for a high density of ChAT-immunoreactive fibers[41,3]. The contrasting findings between the 1 nM and 5 nM concentrations of alpha-BTX observed here are puzzling. Perhaps the higher concentration of alpha-BTX labels low-affinity antagonist binding sites which represent a high affinity agonist (i.e. nicotine) binding site. The reduction of alpha-BTX binding sites in the 2 week animal provides evidence for a presynaptic localization of these binding sites. Previous reports have not supported the hypothesis that cortical nicotinic receptors reside presynaptically on the projection from the NBM[23,24,25]. Given the small effect seen here with 1 nM alpha-BTX and the apparently dramatic effect seen at the higher concentration of 5 nM, the existence of presynaptic nicotinic binding sites on the NBM projection remains an area open for further investigation.

The time-related lesion effects on ACh release observed here indicate some recovery in the most rostral regions sampled with an unexpected down-regulation of release in the caudal sections of the contralateral hemisphere. The effects observed on ChAT activity also indicate some regionally selective "recovery" process. A "recovery" toward control values was observed only in the rostral regions sampled. However, ChAT activity in the rostral sections at 6 weeks remained significantly depleted while ACh release returned to normal. Thus, functional presynaptic activity such as release and high affinity choline uptake may provide more sensitive measures with which to assess the persistence of the lesion-induced deficits in cortical cholinergic parameters. Enzyme activity maybe a more crude measure with which to assess these deficiencies and a total "recovery" of enzyme is not necessary in order to regain presynaptic function. Whether the effects observed here are due to a recovery of function, an upregulation of presynaptic function in cells spared from excitotoxic lesion effects or possibly some upregulation of the contribution of cortical interneurons to the evoked release pool can not be inferred from these data.

BIBLIOGRAPHY

1. Johnston, M. V., McKinney, M. & Coyle, J. T. (1981) Neocortical cholinergic innervation: A description of extrinsic and intrinsic components in the rat. Exp. Br. Res. 43: 159 - 172.
2. Mesulam, M.-M., Mufson, E. J., Levey, A. I., and Wainer, B. H. (1983) Cholinergic innervation of cortex by the basal forebrain: Cytochemistry and cortical connections of the septal area, diagonal band nuclei, nucleus basalis (substantia inominata) and hypothalamus in the rhesus monkey. J. Comp. Neurol. 214: 170 - 197.
3. Saper, C. B. (1984) Organization of cerebral cortical afferent systems in the rat. II. Magnocellular basal nucleus. J. Comp. Neurol. 222: 313 - 342.
4. Shute, C. C. D. and Lewis, P. R. (1967) The ascending cholinergic reticular system: Neocortical, olfactory and subcortical projections. Brain 90: 497 - 520.
5. Rye, D. B., Wainer, B. H., Mesulam, M.-M., Mufson, E. J., and Saper, C. B.(1984) Cortical projections arising from the basal forebrain: A study of cholinergic and non-cholinergic components employing combined retrograde tracing and immunohistochemical localization of choline acetyltransferase. Neurosci. 13: 627 - 643.
6. Etienne, P., Robitaille, Y., Wood, P., Gauthier, S., Nair, N. P. V. and Quirion, R. (1986) Nucleus basalis neuronal loss, neuritic plaques and choline acetyltransferase activity in advanced Alzheimer's Disease. Neurosci. 19: 1279 - 1291.
7. Watson, M., Vickroy, T. W., Fibiger, H. C., Roeske, W. R. and Yamamura, H. I. (1985) Effects of bilateral ibotenate-induced lesions of the nucleus basalis magnocellularis upon selective cholinergic biochemical markers in the rat anterior cerebral cortex. Br. Res. 346: 387 - 391.
8. Pedata, F., Lo Conte, G., Sorki, S., Marconini-Pepeu, I., Pepeu, G. (1982) Changes in high-affinity choline uptake in rat cortex following lesions of the magnocellular forebrain nuclei. Br. Res. 233: 359 - 367.
9. Lo Conte, G., Casamenti, F., Bigl, V., Milaneschi, E., and Pepeu, G. (1982) Effect of magnocellular forebrain nuclei lesions on ACh output from the cerebral cortex, electrocorticogram and behavior. Arch.Ital. Biol. 120: 176 - 188.
10. Casamenti, F., Pedata, F., Sorki, S., LoConte, G. and Pepeu, G. (1981) Lesions of the globus pallidus: Changes in cortical ChAT, choline uptake and acetylcholine output in the rat. In: Cholinergic Mechanisms: Phylogenetic and ontogenetic aspects, central and peripheral synapses, clinical significance. (Eds.: G. Pepeu and H. Ladinsky), Plenum Publ. Comp., New York, pp. 685 - 694.
11. Bowen, D. M., Allen, S. J., Benton, J. S., Goodhardt, M. H., Haan, E. A., Palmer, A. M., Sims, N R., Smith, C. C. T., Spillane, J. A., Esiri, M. M., Neary, D., Snowdon, J. S., Wilcock, G. K., and Davison, A. N. (1983) Biochemical assessment of serotonergic and cholinergic dysfunction and cerebral atrophy in Alzheimer's Disease. J. Neurochem 41: 266 - 272.
12. Henke, H. and Lang, W. (1983) Cholinergic enzymes in neocortex, hippocampus and basal forebrain of non-neurological and senile dementia of Alzheimer-type patients. Br. Res. 267: 281 - 291.
13. Nagai, T., McGeer, P. L., Peng, J. H., McGeer, E. G., and Dolman, C. E. (1983) Choline acetyltransferase immunohistochemistry in brains of Alzheimer's disease patients and controls. Neurosci.Letters 36: 195 -199.

14. Perry, R. H., Candy, J. M., Perry, E. K. Irving, D., Blessed, G., Fairbairn, A. F., and Tomlinson, B. E. (1982) Extensive loss of choline acetyltransferase activity is not reflected by neuronal loss in the nucleus of meynert in Alzheimer's disease. Neurosci.Letters 33: 311 - 315.

15. Reisine, T. D., Yamamura, H. I., Bird, E. D., Spokes, E. and Enna, S. J. Pre- and postsynaptic neurochemical alterations in Alzheimer's Disease. Br.Res. 159: 477 - 481.

16. Nilsson, L., Nordberg, A., Hardy, J., Wester, P., and Winblad, B. (1986) Physostigmine restores [^{3}H]-acetylcholine efflux from Alzheimer brain slices to normal level. J. Neural Transm. 67: 275 - 285.

17. Sims, N. R., Bowen, D. M., Allen, S. J., Smith C. C. T., Nearry, D., Thomas, D. J. and Davison, A. N. (1983) Presynaptic cholinergic dysfunction in patients with dementia. J. Neurochem. 40: 503 - 509.

18. Bartus, R. T., Dean, R. L., Pontecorvo, M. J., and Flicker, C.(1985) The cholinergic hypothesis: A historical overview, current perspective, and future directions. Annals N.Y. Acad. Sci. 444: 332 - 358.

19. Wenk, G. and Olton, D. S. (1987) Basal forebrain cholinergic neurons and Alzheimer's Disease. In: Animal Models of Dementia (ED.: Coyle, J. T.), Alan R. Liss, New York, pp. 81 - 101.

20. Salamone, J. D., Beart, P. M., Alpert, J. E. and Iverson, S. D. (1984) Impairment in T-maze reinforced alternation performance following nucleus basalis magnocellularis lesions in rats. Behav. Br. Res. 13: 63 - 70.

21. Giacobini, E., DeSarno, P., McIlhany, M., and Clark, B. (1988) In: Nicotinic Acetylcholine Receptors in the Nervous System. R. Clementi, C. Gotti, and E. Sher (Eds.)Series M, Cell biology, NATO ASI series, vol M.25, P. 367 - 378. Springer Verlag.

22. Whitehouse, P. J., Martino, A. M., Antuono, P. G., Lowenstein, P. K., Coyle, J. T., Price, D. L. & Kellar, K. J. (1986) Nicotinic acetylcholine binding sites in Alzheimer's Disease. Br. Res. 371: 146 - 151.

23 Meyer, E. M., Arendash, G. W., Judkins, J. H., Ying, L., Wade, C. and Kem, W. R. (1987) Effects of nucleus basalis lesion on the muscarinic and nicotinic modulation of [^{3}H]-acetylcholine release _. the rat cerebral cortex. J.Neurochem. 49: 1758 - 1762.

24. Atack, J. R., Wenk, G. L., Wagster, M. V., Kellar, K. J., Whitehouse, P. J., and Rapoport, S. I. (1989) Bilateral changes in neocortical [^{3}H]pirenzepine and [^{3}H]oxotremorine-M binding following unilateral lesions of the rat nucleus basalis magnocellularis: an autoradiographic study. Br. Res. 483: 367 - 372.

25. Wenk, G. L. and Rokaeus, A. (1988) Basal forebrain lesions differentially alter galanin levels and acetylcholinergic receptors in the hippocampus and neocortex. Br. Res. 460: 17 - 21.

26. Gardiner, I. M., deBelleroche, J., Premi, B. K., and Hamilton, M. H. (1987) Effect of lesion of the nucleus basalis of rat on ACh release in cerebral cortex: time course of compensatory events. Br. Res. 407: 263 - 271.

27. Mufson, E. J., Kehr, A. D., Wainer, B. H. and Mesulam, M.-M. (1987) Cortical effects of neurotoxin damage to the nucleus basalis in rats: persistent loss of extrinsic cholinergic input and lack of transsynaptic effect upon the number of somatostatin-containing, cholinesterase-positive and cholinergic cortical neurons. Br. Res. 417: 385 - 388.

28. Wenk, G. L. and Olton, D. S. (1984) Recovery of neocortical choline acetyltransferase activity following ibotenic acid injection into the nucleus basalis of Meynert in rats. Br. Res. 293: 184 - 186.

29. Hohman, C. F., Wenk, G. L., Lowenstein, P., Brown, M. E., and Coyle, J. T. (1987) Age-related recurrence of basal forebrain

lesion- induced cholinergic deficits. Neurosci. Letters 82: 254 - 259.

30. Arendash, G. W. Millard, W. J., Dunn, A. and Meyer, E. M. (1987) Longterm neuropathological and neurochemical effects of nucleus basalis lesions in the rat. Science 238: 952 - 956.

31. Bartus,R. T., Pontecorvo, M. J., Flicker, C., Dean, R. L. and Figueiredo, J. C. (1986) Behavioral recovery following bilateral lesions of the nucleus basalis does not occur spontaneously. Pharm. Biochem. Beh. 24: 1287 - 1292.

32. Amaral, D. G. and Price, J. L. (1983) An air pressure system for the injection of tracer substances into the brain. J.Neurosci. Methods

33. May, A. M. and Arneric, S. P. (1987) Effects of basal forebrain lesions and cholinomimetics on cerebral cortical microvascular perfusion (CCMP) in rat: continuous measurement by laser-doppler flowmetry. Neurosci. Abst. 13: 1034.

34. Hadhazy, P. and Szerb, J. C. (1977) The effect of cholinergic drugs on [^{3}H]-acetylcholine release from slices of rat hippocampus, striatum, and cortex. Br. Res. 123: 311 - 322. 35. Bradford, M. (1976) A rapid and sensitive method for the quantitation of microgram quantities of protein utilizing the principle of protein dye-binding. Anal. Biochem. 72: 248 - 254.

36. Fonnum, F. (1969) Radiochemical microassays for the determination of choline acetyltransferase and acetylcholinesterase activities. Biochem. J. 115: 465 - 472.

37. Arneric, S. P., Honig, M. A., Milner, T. A., Greco, S., Iadecola, C. and Reis, D. J. (1988) Neuronal and endothelial sites of acetylcholine synthesis and release associated with microvessels in rat cerebral cortex: ultrastructural and neurochemical studies. Br. Res. 454: 11-30.

38. El-Defrawy, S. R., Coloma, F., Jhamandas, K., Boegman, R. J., Beninger, R. J. and Wisching, B. A. (1985) Functional and neurochemical cortical cholinergic impairment following neurotoxic lesion of the nucleus basalis magnocellularis in the rat. Neurobio. of Aging 6: 325 - 330.

39. Casamenti, F., DiPatre, P. L., Bartolini, L., and Pepeu, G. (1988) Unilateral and bilateral nucleus basalis lesions: differences in neurochemical and behavioral recovery. Neuroscience 24: 209 - 215.

40. Pearson, R. C. A., Sofroniew, M. V., and Powell, T. P. S. (1987) The cholinergic nuclei of the basal forebrain of the rat: hypertrophy following contralateral cortical damage or section of the corpus callosum. Br. Res. 411: 332 - 340.

41. Eckenstein, F. P., Baughman, R. W. and Quinn, J. (1988) An anatomical study of cholinergic innervation in rat cerebral cortex. Neuroscience 25: 457 - 474.

CHOLINERGIC-NEUROPEPTIDE Y INTERACTIONS IN THE RAT CEREBRAL CORTEX: TOWARDS A MODEL FOR THE TRANS-SYNAPTIC EFFECTS OF CHOLINERGIC TRANSMISSION

Jennifer J. Poulakos[1], Gary W. Arendash[2], William J. Millard[3], Nelida Sjak-Shie[1], and Edwin M. Meyer*[1]

1. Department of Pharmacology and Therapeutics, University of Florida College of Medicine, P.O. Box J-267, J. H. Miller Health Center, Gainesville, FL
2. Departments of Biology and Neurology, University of South Florida College of Medicine, Tampa, FL
3. Department of Pharmacodynamics, University of Florida College of Pharmacy Gainesville, FL

Introduction

Cholinergic neurons projecting from the nucleus basalis to the cerebral cortex are among those consistently rendered dysfunctional during the early stages of Alzheimer's disease (1-3). These cholinergic neurons are implicated in the memory and cognitive disorders associated with the disease, based on pharmacological and pathological studies in humans and animals (4-6). Unfortunately, attempts to improve mental status by increasing brain cholinergic transmission have been only marginally successful because of at least four factors: 1) the multitransmitter basis of this disease, especially in its later stages; 2) our inability to diagnose the disease consistently in its earliest stages; 3) the lack of agents that selectively increase cholinergic transmission in brain pathways affected by Alzheimer's disease; and 4) our lack of understanding about the long-term, trans-synaptic effects of cholinergic transmission that may modify the initial response to cholinergic agents. This chapter focuses on the fourth factor, with an emphasis on developing a neurochemical model for trans-synaptic changes associated with cholinergic transmission. Such a model would be particularly useful for characterizing the functional effects of agents purported to alter cholinergic transmission pre- or postsynaptically, e.g., trophic factors, receptor agonists and antagonists, as well as nootrophic drugs.

The trans-synaptic marker we describe here involves changes in neocortical neuropeptide Y (NPY) synthesis and levels. NPY is a 36 amino acid peptide discovered in 1982 by Tatemoto et al.(7). Although particularly high concentrations are localized in the hypothalamus, where it is functionally associated with the regulation of feeding behavior (8-10), neocortical NPY levels are also rather high, and pharmacological studies suggest that NPY in this region may be associated with memory and cognition (11). NPY-containing neurons in the neocortex are predominantly or exclusively intrinsic in nature, and most appear to contain somatostatin as well (12). However, while Alzheimer's disease consistently reduces the levels of cortical somatostatin (13), its effects on NPY levels are much less consistently observed (14 vs. 15,16). Thus, the differential turnover of these co-localized peptides may be an important clue as to the etiology of the disease.

Our interest in studying the effects of cholinergic transmission on NPY turnover derives from the observation that deafferentation of ascending cholinergic projections to the rat neocortex surprisingly and markedly increases (over 100%) levels of NPY in the parietal cortex after extended time intervals (e.g., 10 or more months)(17,18, Arendash et al., this volume). Further, the recovery of passive avoidance behavior following nucleus basalis lesions appears to correlate temporally with these elevated NPY levels but not with cholinergic recovery (18,19), suggesting that this trans-synaptic response could underlie the apparent recovery of memory-related behaviors in this species.

In this chapter, we describe how changes in cholinergic transmission affect the synthesis of this peptide over shorter intervals, using its precursor mRNA as a marker of synthesis. Since we were particularly interested in developing a model for trans-synaptic effects of cholinergic transmission that would be applicable to age-related disorders such as Alzheimer's disease, we also compared the trans-synaptic effects of cholinergic hypofunction in aged rats to those in young adults.

Effects of cholinergic transmission on neocortical NPY turnover.

In order to study the effects of cholinergic deafferentation in the cerebral cortex, we lesioned the nucleus basalis of rats by twice infusing 5 µg of ibotenic acid in 1 µl phosphate buffered saline unilaterally or bilaterally in 3 month old male Sprague Dawley albino rats as described previously (17,18). These lesions typically reduced nucleus basalis cholinesterase-staining by over 90% and frontal cortex choline acetyltransferase levels by 35-45% in the ipsilateral hemispheres. Residual cholinergic activity was presumably due to intrinsic cholinergic neurons (20).

Unilateral and bilateral lesions had different effects on the parietal cortex levels of NPY measured 2 months post-lesioning (Table 1). Decreased levels were observed after bilateral but not after unilateral lesions. This lesion-induced reduction in NPY levels was the opposite of what was observed much longer (10-14 months post-lesioning(17,18) in bilaterally, but not unilaterally lesioned rats (18). Since the time interval post-lesioning and the laterality of the lesions (uni- versus bilateral) both affect how lesions alter parietal cortex NPY levels, our focus remained on the initial deficits in NPY levels observed within 2 months post-lesioning.

Table 1

Type of Nucleus Basalis Lesion	NPY Concentrations (% control)	pre-proNPY mRNA (% control)
Unilateral	59 ± 7*	NM
Bilateral	104 ± 9	73 ± 8*

*Parietal cortex levels of NPY and its encoding mRNA were assayed 2 months after nucleus basalis lesions as described in the text. Dot blot analyses were performed with the same stringency as in Northern blot described in Figure 1. Each value is the mean ± S.E.M. of 4-5 animals/group. Control NPY concentrations (from appropriate sham-operated hemisphere) for unilaterally and bilaterally lesioned rats were 123 ± 11 pg/mg wet weight and 218 ± 23 pg/mg wet weight, respectively. *p < 0.05 compared to sham-operated control. NM: not measured.*

We next measured the levels of the precursor mRNA encoding for pre-proNPY as a marker of synthetic rate. Animals were lesioned bilaterally with ibotenic acid as described above and assayed for parietal cortex mRNA encoding pre-proNPY 2 months afterwards using a dot blot assay as follows.

Total RNA was extracted by the acid guanidinium-phenol-chloroform method described by Chomczynski and Sacchi (21), quantitated by absorption at 260 nm, and then assessed for purity with $A_{260}:A_{280}$ ratios. The integrity of all samples was assessed on a minigel for the presence of 28S and 18S ribosomal bands and the absence of degradation.

For dot blot analyses, neocortical RNA was filtered under slight vacuum through Nitroplus 2000 nitrocellulose membrane (MSI, Inc., Westboro, MA) held in a Hybri-Dot manifold (Bethesda Research Laboratories). The membrane was baked in a vacuum oven for 2 hrs. at 80° C. Each blot was prehybridized for at least 3 hours at 42° C and then hybridized for 16-24 hours at 42° C with hybridization buffer containing 10^6 cpm/ml of [alpha ^{32}P]dCTP labeled pre-proNPY cDNA. The rat pre-proNPY probe (cDNA), which was generously provided by Dr. Janet Allen, Massachusetts General Hospital (22), was digested from the pGEM vector with the restriction enzyme EcoRI and purified by agarose gel electrophoresis. It was labeled with [^{32}P]dCTP (New England Nuclear) by primer extension, purified on a NACS Prepac column (Bethesda Research Laboratories) and used as a hybridization probe (10^6 cpm/ml hybridization buffer). Membranes were washed repeatedly before exposure to Kodak XAR-5 film at -80° C in the presence of a Dupont Lightning-Plus intensifying screen. Autoradiographs were analysed by scanning laser densitometry. These stringency conditions gave only a single broad band typical of the polyadenylated message under Northern blot analyses (Figure 1).

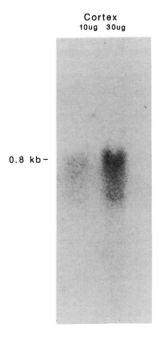

Cortex
10ug 30ug

0.8 kb –

Figure 1. Northern blot of mRNA encoding neuropeptide Y in rat parietal cortex.
Total RNA was isolated from cerebral cortices dissected from 6 month old rats. Northern blot analysis was performed as described in the text, using the probe for the rat cDNA neuropeptide Y gene. To each lane was applied either or μg of total RNA

When mRNA encoding pre-proNPY was assayed in this manner 2 months after bilateral lesions, their levels were decreased by 27% (Table 1), slightly less than the decrease in peptide levels observed at this time interval after unilateral lesioning. These data suggest that a reduction in ascending cholinergic transmission may decrease NPY-synthesis even in bilaterally lesioned animals that show no change in peptide levels themselves. Whether unilateral lesions of the nucleus basalis cause even greater reductions in mRNA encoding pre-proNPY, which would be suggested by the peptide-changes observed above, is under study.

Even shorter term changes in brain cholinergic transmission appear to alter the synthesis of NPY, as shown in Figure 3. Oxotremorine, a full muscarinic agonist with respect to some but not all transduction processes (see chapters by Fisher and by Crews et al., this volume), significantly elevated mRNA encoding for this peptide 4 hr after IP injection (Figure 2). This oxotremorine-induced elevation in NPY-encoding mRNA was blocked by pretreatment with atropine, a non-selective muscarinic antagonist. Atropine alone also tended to increase NPY-encoding mRNA synthesis, but this effect did not reach statistical significance. While any atropine-induced elevation in NPY encoding mRNA would be unexpected based on the foregoing data, it may be due to a blockade of different receptor subtypes than those activated by oxotremorine selectively (M2)(23,24). This hypothesis is supported by the observation that atropine increases pre-proNPY encoding mRNA several fold in primary neuronal cultures from the whole brain of the neonatal rat (Poulakos and Meyer, unpublished observation).

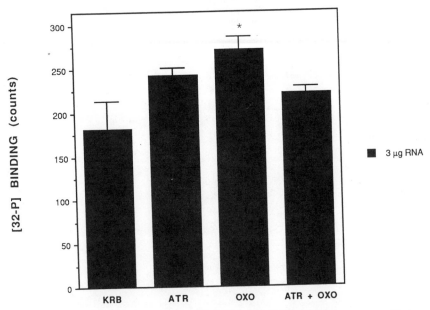

Figure 2. Male Sprague Dawley albino rats were injected with 1 mg/kg of the specified drugs (IP) and decollated 4 hr later. Their parietal cortices were rapidly removed and assayed for mRNA encoding pre-proNPY as described in the text. Each value is the mean ± S.E.M. of 4 animals/group. *p < 0.05 compared to saline injected control value.

With respect to how changes in cholinergic transmission modulate NPY synthesis at the genetic level, is interesting to note that phorbol esters and forskolin, which respectively increase protein kinase C and adenylate cyclase activities, each can increase the synthesis of NPY-encoding mRNA (29,30). These second messenger systems probably act by phosphorylating two different proteins that normally recognize the AP1 site (protein kinase C sensitive) and pallindromic cyclic AMP-sensitive site, each of which can increase gene-transcription when activated. Although the NPY-gene has neither of these sites upstream from the tataa region, it does contain one upstream sequence similar to both of them (30) that may recognize both types of phosphorylated protein. In any case, since muscarinic receptors can modulate both of these second messenger systems (e.g., M1 for PKC activity indirectly; M2 and M4 for adenylate cyclase activity)(31), it is conceivable that changes in cholinergic transmission can regulate not only the release of NPY by standard neurophysiological processes, but the synthesis of the peptide at the genetic level as well.

Another method used to increase cholinergic transmission in selected brain pathways involves the use of trophic factors such as NGF, which act presynaptically on the ACh-neuron. While NGF can enhance choline acetyltransferase activity and other cholinergic markers in the neocortex, hippocampus and other brain regions under a variety of conditions, its effects on cholinergic synaptic transmission remain less well characterized. We therefore investigated whether this trophic factor had trans-synaptic effects on NPY turnover in the rat neocortex.

NGF administered by Alzet osmotic minipumps in the lateral ventricle for two weeks as described previously (25) had no effect on either neocortical choline acetyltransferase activity or levels of mRNA encoding for NPY. Since we found that NGF increased hippocampal choline acetyltransferase activity in partial fimbria-lesioned rats when administered under identical conditions, this peptide-infusion appeared to be sufficient to activate hypofunctional neurons, at least (25). Perhaps lesioning or some other anticholinergic process such as aging is necessary to observe NGF-induced elevations in neocortical cholinergic activity, as suggested elsewhere in this volume (26-28). Of course, ACh-release could be elevated even in the absence of choline acetyltransferase, so it is impossible to conclude whether the lack of an NGF-induced effect on NPY-turnover in the cortex reflects an inability to elevate cholinergic transmission under these conditions or a lack of an effect of ascending cholinergic transmission on NPY-turnover.

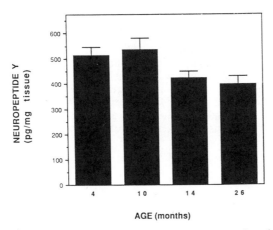

Figure 3. Parietal cortex NPY levels during aging. *Parietal cortices from rats of the specified ages were assayed for NPY by RIA as described in the text. Each value is the mean ± S.E.M. of 5 animals. *p < 0.05 compared to 4 month old animals (one way analysis of variance)*

Effects of aging on cholinergic-NPY interactions.

Aging produces a variety of neurochemical effects in the brain, including the synthesis and turnover of many transmitters. Conceivably, any of these neurochemical changes could underlie the age-related predisposition of certain individuals to neuropathological disorders such as Alzheimer's disease; further, they may render potential pharmacological treatments less effective. Of particular interest to us was the observation that aging decreases neocortical cholinergic transmission by interfering with the depolarization-induced calcium-dependent release process (26,28). This deficit in cholinergic transmission may occur without concomitant deficits in acetylcholine (ACh) synthesis, and appears to reflect changes in the intracellular response to calcium ions. The potential trans-synaptic effects of this cholinergic hypofunction on NPY turnover have not been studied. Indeed, little is known about how aging itself affects NPY turnover. We therefore measured changes in parietal cortex levels of NPY and its encoding mRNA.

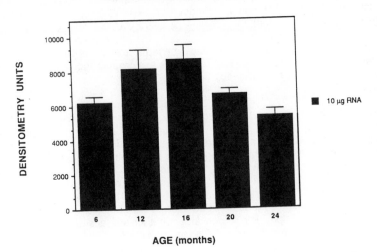

CORTICAL PREPRO NPY mRNA

■ 10 µg RNA

AGE (months)

Figure 4. Parietal cortex levels of mRNA encoding for pre-proNPY during aging
Cerebral cortices from rats of the specified ages were assayed for mRNA encoding
pre-proneuropeptide Y using a dot blot analysis as described in the text.
Each value is the mean ± S.E.M. of 4 animals, except the 20 month time
point (n = 2).

Aging gradually decreased the levels of both NPY and the mRNA encoding for its
precursor to a similar extent (Figures 3 and 4), with the most pronounced changes
observed by 26 months of age. No change was observed in either marker by 12 months of
age. Thus, the decrease in cortical NPY levels occurring with age appeared to be associated
with a decreased rate of synthesis as well. This aging pattern in the NPY system is similar
to that observed for reductions in neocortical ACh release in this rat strain (Table 2) (32).

Table 2

Age (Months)	[^{3}H]ACh Release (dpm/mg protein)	
	5 mM KCl	35 mM KCl
6	7,600 ± 600	11,400 ± 1,000
12	7,200 ± 300	10,700 ± 700
16	7,000 ± 200	10,300 ± 400
20	7,100 ± 400	9,000 ± 400*
24	6,300 ± 200*	8,200 ± 300*
26	6,200 ± 300*	8,000 ± 300*

Legend: Neocortical synaptosomes were prepared from the male Fischer 344
rats of the specified age and loaded with [^{3}H]ACh by incubating with 1 µM
[^{3}H]choline (10 Ci/mmol) for 10 min at 37°C in oxygenated Krebs Ringer
buffer as described previously (32). After washing away residual labelled
choline, the synaptosomes were incubated in Krebs Ringer buffer containing 1
mM calcium chloride, 5 mM KCl, 10 µM eserine, plus or minus 35 mM KCl
added for depolarization. After 2 min at 37°C, this incubation was terminated by
placing the samples on ice and the [^{3}H]ACh released into the medium was
measured and expressed as the mean ± S.E.M. of at least 5 animals/group (each
animal measured in duplicate). *$p < 0.05$ compared to youngest group.

While ACh-release in the presence of a depolarizing concentration of potassium ions gradually decreases from 6 to 26 months of age, no statistically change in ACh-release is observed until after 16 months of age, after which a more pronounced drop occurs.

In order to study how aging affects the neocortical NPY-turnover response to lesion-induced cholinergic deafferentation, male Sprague Dawley albino rats (N=4-5 animals per group) were lesioned bilaterally at 20 months of age as described previously and then assayed 2 months later for parietal cortex levels of NPY and its encoding mRNA. As with the younger animals, these lesions caused a significant reduction in NPY-encoding mRNA (to 66 ± 8% of control values p <0.01 by Student's t-test) without affecting NPY levels themselves. In contrast, we found that rats killed at a similar age (21.5 month, yet lesioned bilaterally at 2 months of age, displayed elevations in cortical NPY levels similar to those reported earlier (240% of sham operated controls) It thus appears that aging per se does not alter the response to nucleus basalis lesions viz neocortical NPY synthesis, while time post-lesioning does.

Summary

These results demonstrate that changes in cholinergic transmission can alter the synthesis and levels of NPY in the parietal cortex. At least some of these changes appear to be attributable to ascending neurons projecting from the nucleus basalis, based on lesion studies. While the cholinergic drugs used in this study could act anywhere in the brain, the observation that oxotremorine and nucleus basalis lesions exert opposite effects on NPY-encoding mRNA levels is at least consistent with the hypothesis that the agonist mimics the actions of endogenous ACh released from the ascending cholinergic neurons.

The trans-synaptic effects of cholinergic transmission with respect to NPY turnover remain correlational and somewhat complex at this point. Why do NPY levels eventually rise only in bilaterally lesioned animals? Why do NPY levels decrease only in unilaterally lesioned animals, even though bilateral lesions reduce NPY synthesis? What is the role of cross-hemispheric communication in the NPY response to cholinergic deafferentation? Will the answers to these and other questions require a better understanding of the synaptic connections among cholinergic, NPY and other types of neurons, or will it be sufficient to measure changes in the synthesis storage and, eventually, release of the NPY as we are attempting presently?.

The present results also demonstrate for the first time that aging alone reduces the trans-synaptic levels of rat parietal cortex NPY as well as the mRNA encoding it. Previous studies have shown aging to reduce the levels of other neuroactive peptides or their encoding mRNAs, so this result is not particularly surprising. Nevertheless, ongoing NPY-synthesis may be important for its continued function in this brain region, and the present evidence suggests that aging may compromise NPY-transmission. Whether the reduced levels of neuropeptide Y are due solely to a decrease in the synthesis of mRNA cannot be ascertained from the present results; indeed, it is conceivable that aging reduces the number of neuropeptidergic neurons without any decrease in the functionality of the individual cells themselves.

Another type of unresolved question pertains to the behavioral correlates of changes in NPY synthesis that are mediated by cholinergic transmission. One intriguing possibility is that even short term changes in cholinergic transmission may have long term effects on NPY levels. This peptide is synthesized primarily in the perikaryon and transported to the nerve terminal where no protein synthesis occurs de novo. Thus, changes in cholinergic transmission in the neocortex would eventually (given time for transcription, translation, post-translational modifications, and axonal transport to occur) result in much later and longer lasting changes in NPY-transmission. Such a long term trans-synaptic response could be a substrate for one or more types of memory-related behavior.

Acknowledgements. The authors wish to thank Corinne Pruysers and Jacob Burks for technical support. This work was funded in part by the Taiho Pharmaceuticals Co.

REFERENCES

1. Coyle, J.T., Price, D.L. and Delong, M.R. (1983) Alzheimer's disease: a disorder of cortical cholineric innervation. Science 219, 1184-1190.
2. Whitehouse, P.J., Price, D.L., Struble, R.G., Clark, A.W., Coyle, J.T. and Delong, M.R. (1982) Alzheimer's disease and senile dementia: loss of neurons in the basal forebrain. Science 215: 1237-1239.
3. Davies, P. (1986) Cholinergic and somatostatin deficits in Alzheimer's disease. In: Treatment Development Strategies for Alzheimer's Disease.(T. Crook, R. Bartus, S. Ferris and S. Gershon, eds.) Mark Powley Associates, CT, p. 385-420.
4. Bartus, R.T., Dean, R.L., Beer, B. and Lippa, A.S. (1982) The cholinergic hypothesis of geriatric memory dysfunction. Science 217, 408-414.
5. Murray, C.L. and Fibiger, H.C. (1985) Learning and memory deficits after lesions of the nucleus basalis magnocellularis: reversal by physostigmine. Neuroscience 14, 1025-1032.
6. Bartus, R.T., Flicker, C., Dean, R.L., Pontecorvo, M., Figueiredo, J.C. and Fisher, S.K. (1985) Selective memory loss folowing nucleus basalis lesions: long term behavioral recovery despite persistent cholinergic deficiencies. Pharmacol. Biochem. Behav. 23, 125-135.
7. Tatemoto, K., Carlquist, M. and Mutt, V. (1982) Neuropeptide Y - a novel brain peptide with structural similarities to peptide YY and pancreatic polypeptide. Nature 296, 659-660.
8. Allen, Y.S., Adrian T.E., Allen, J.M., Tatemoto, K., Crow, T.J., Bloom, S.R. and Polak, J.M. (1983) Neuropeptide Y distribution in the rat brain. Science 221, 877-879.
9. Allen, J.M. and Bloom, S.R (1986) Neuropeptide Y: a putative neurotransmitter. Neurochem. Int. 8, 1-8.
10. Stanley, B.G. and Leibowitz S.F. (1985) Neuropeptide Y injected in the paraventricular hypothalamus: a powerful stimulant of feeding behavior. Proc. Natl. Acad. Sci. 82, 3940-3943.
11. Flood, J.F., Hernandez, E.N. and Morley, J.E. (1987) Modulation of memory processing by neuropeptide Y. Brain Res. 241, 280-290.
12. Chronwall, B., Chase, T. and O'Donohue, T. (1984) Coexistence of neuropeptide Y and somatostatin in rat and human cortical and rat hypothalamus neurons. Neurosci. Lett. 52, 213-217.
13. Beal, M.F., Mazurek, M.F., Chattha, G.K., Svendsen, C.V., Bird, E.D. and Martin, J.B. (1986) Neuropeptide Y immunoreactivity is reducd in the cerebral cortex in Alzheimer's disease. Ann. Neurol. 20, 282-289.
14. Dawbarn, D., Rossor, M., Mountjoy, C., Roth, M. and Emson, P. (1986) Decreased somatostatin immunoreactivity but not neuropeptide Y immunoreactivity in cerebral cortex in senile dementia of Alzheimer type. Neurosci. Lett. 70, 154-159.
15. Davies, P., Katzman, R. and Terry, R. (1980) Reduced somatostatin-like immunoreactivity in cerebral cortex from cases of Alzheimer's disease and Alzheimer senile dementia. Nature 288, 279-280.
16. Chan-Palay, V., Allen, Y.S., Lang, W. Hawsler, U., and Polak, J. M. (1985) J. Comp. Neurol. 238, 391.
17. Arendash, G.W., Millard, W.J., Dunn, A.J. and Meyer, E.M. (1987) Long term neuropathological and neurochemical effects of nucleus basalis lesions in the rat. Science 238, 952-956.
18. Arendash, G.W., Millard, W.J., Dunn, A.J., Dawson, R.J. and Meyer, E.M. (in press) Different long term neurochemical effects of unilateral and bilateral nucleus basalis lesions in the rat. Neurochem. Res., in press.
19. Bartus, R.T., Pontecorvo, M., Flicker, C., Dean, R. and Figueiredo, J. (1986) Behavioral recovery following bilateral lesions of the nucleus basalis does not occur spontaneously. Pharmacol. Biochem. Behav. 24, 1287-1292.
20. Wainer, B.H., Levey, A.I., Mufson, E.J. and Mesulam, M.M. (1984) Cholinergic systems in mammalian brain identified with antibodies against choline acetylcholinesterase. Neurochem. Intern. 6, 163-174.

21. Chomczynski, P. and Sacchi, N. (1987) Single-step method of RNA isolation by acid guanidinium thiocyanate-phenol-chloroform extraction. Anal. Biochem. 162, 156-159

22. Allen, J., Novotny, J., Martin, J. and Heinrich, G. (1987) Molecular structure of mammalian neuropeptide Y: analysis by molecular cloning and computer-aided comparison with crystal structure of avian homologue. Proc.Natl. Acad. Sci. 84, 2532-2536.

23. Barnard, E.A. (1988) Separating receptor subtypes from their shadows. Nature 335, 301-302.

24. Gonzales, R.A. and Crews, F.T. (1984) Characterization of the cholinergic stimulation of phosphoinositide hydrolysis in rat brain slices. J. Neurosci. 4, 3120-3127.

25. Sjak-Shie, N.N., Scott, J., Burks, J., Watson, R. and Meyer,.E.M. (1989) Cholinergic peptide interactions in vivo: molecular to behavioral considerations. ICBR Short Report 9, 119.

26. Hefti, F. (1986) Nerve growth factor in the treatment of Alzheimer's disease. J. Neurosci. 6, 2156-2162.

27. Williams, L.R., Varon, S., Peterson, G.M., Wictorin, K., Fischer, W., Bjorklund, A. and Gage, F.H. (1986) Continuous infusion of nerve growth factor prevents basal forebrain neuronal death after fimbria fornix transection. Proc. Natl. Acad. Sci. USA 83, 9231-9235.

28. Williams, L.R., Jodelis, K.S., Donald, M.R. and Yip, H.K. (1989) Exogenous nerve growth factor stimulates choline acetyltransferase activity in basal forebrain of axotomized and aged rats. In: Novel Approaches for the Treatment of Alzheimer's Disease (E.M. Meyer, J.W. Simpkins and J. Yamamoto, Eds.) Plenum Press, New York, in press.

29. Poulakos, J.J., Shakar, R., Millard, W.J. and Meyer, E.M. (1989) The primary neuro-enriched culture from rat brain as a model for studying cholinergic neuropeptide Y interactions. ICBR Short Report 9, 118.

30. Higuchi, H. and Sabol, S.L. (1987) Rat neuropeptide Y; precursor mRNA: characterization, tissue distribution, and regulation by glucocorticoids, cyclic AMP, calcium and NGF. 17th Society for Neurosciences Abstracts, 176.

31. Fisher, S.K., Klinger, P.D. and Agranoff, B.W. (1983) Muscarinic agonist binding and phospholipid turnover in brain. J. Biol. Chem. 258, 7358-7363.

32. Meyer, E.M. and Judkins, J.H. (in press) Effects of aging on acetylcholine release triggered by different secretagogues in the rat cerebral cortex and striatum. Neurobiol. Aging.

THE EFFECTS OF NUCLEUS BASALIS LESIONS IN THE RAT ON ONE WAY PASSIVE

AND ACTIVE AVOIDANCE, TWO WAY AVOIDANCE, AND LASHLY III MAZE

LEARNING: AN ANIMAL MODEL FOR SDAT

Paschal N. Strong[1] and Gary W. Arendash[2]

[1]Department of Psychology
[2]Department of Biology
University of South Florida
Tampa, FL 33620

The development of a useful animal model for senile dementia of the Alzheimer's type (SDAT) entails a number of considerations. Among them are the following:

1. The choice of an appropriate organism. In choosing a candidate organism the following issues should be addressed.

A. Are there well established neurological homologies between the model's CNS and the human CNS?

B. Is the model organism's behavior well enough studied and described so that pathologies in behavior due to disease or lesions have an adequate research base for comparison to normal behavior?

C. Is the organism's behavior homologous to a wide variety of human behavior?

D. Is it practical and cost efficient to use a given organism?

2. Once the organism has been selected, the choice of the behaviors to be studied must have a rational basis. Although this seems obvious, there are subtle nuances often overlooked. When an investigator decides that one way passive avoidance would be a good test for memory function many questions must be answered, such as:

a. Number of pre-shock trials
b. Number of shock trials
c. Intensity of shock
d. Number of spacing of post shock trials

Variations in these parameters can lead to a wide variety of inter-pretations of findings. Furthermore, analysis of the data is often simplistic (such as only measuring latency of entering the shock chamber in one way passive avoidance) when a more sophisticated description and analysis of behavior would lead to more insights into the behavioral deficit. One of the goals of the research to be reported on in this chapter was to achieve a finer analysis of the avoidance behavior often used in research in Alzheimer's disease using various animal models.

279

3. Another important decision is the use of inter-subject designs as opposed to intra-subject designs. By this we mean using different animals for each behavior investigated (inter-subject) or exposing each animal to a wide variety of tasks (intra-subject). While the former has the appeal of noncontamination of one behavior by previous experiences (use of the so called naive subject) it suffers in generalizing to human behavior since humans, and all higher organisms, have a rich variety of experiences against which pathological changes must be assessed. Furthermore, intra-subject designs are more efficient because more information is obtained per subject. Balanced against the above advantages of the intra-subject design is the necessity of determining the order of behaviors to be investigated or the controlling of them through counterbalancing procedures.

Although some writers such as Lockhart (1) and Beach (2) have questioned the use of the laboratory rat as a good model for human behavior, others, such as Boice (3) support its use. In terms of the above considerations, the rat would appear to be a reasonable first choice in Alzheimer's research. The CNS is well researched and elucidated with clear-cut homologies with the human CNS. Of particular interest are the homologies between the nucleus basalis of Meynert in the human and the nucleus basalis magnocellularis in rats, and of the septal/diagonal band nucleus in both organisms. Furthermore, the massive amount of behavioral research done on the rat supplies a rich behavioral repertoire from which to choose. The rat is a highly adaptable, omnivorous, social and curious organism. Except for higher primates, whose costs and need for specialized housing and test apparatus rules them out for the average researcher, the rat may well be the best model organism for use in this area of research. Also, the life span is long enough to look at natural aging effects and yet short enough to be practical for a researcher to study.

The studies to be presented in this chapter represent an attempt to clarify in finer detail the deficits seen in various types of avoidance behaviors demonstrated in rats with lesions in the nucleus basalis magnocellularis. We will also present some preliminary data on maze learning in these rats.

INTRODUCTION

Autopsies of patients suffering from senile dementia of the Alzheimer's type (SDAT) reveal a profound loss of cortical cholinergic neurons as well as loss of neurons in basal forebrain nuclei such as the nucleus of Meynert (NBM), the medial septal nucleus and the nucleus of the diagonal band of Broca (4,5,6,7).

Destruction of the rat analogue to the NBM, the nucleus basalis magnocellularis, leads to a severe depletion of neurons in the frontal, parietal and occipital cortex, while lesions in the medial septal nucleus and diagonal band of Broca lead to the depletion of cholinergic neurons in the hippocampus, cingulate gyrus, and temporal cortex (8,9,10).

Numerous studies investigating the effects of NBM lesions in rats have employed passive and active avoidance paradigms but, while often showing significant deficits in these behaviors, fail to relate them to each other or to analyze the behavior in detail (11-18). The present study employed one way passive avoidance, one way active avoidance and two way shuttle avoidance because these tasks clearly differentiate frontal cortical damage from hippocampal damage and thus should clarify the role of the NBM from the septal, diagonal band complex. Hippocampal damage will cause rats to be impaired in passive avoidance but not in one way active avoidance (19-21). In the two way shuttle avoidance task, both passive and active avoidance behaviors are present with the passive avoidance behaviors interfering with the acquisition of two way avoidance. Hence, hippocampally lesioned animals show superiority in acquisition of this behavior compared to normal rats while cortically damaged rats are deficient (22-23). Subjects were also tested on Lashly III maze learning which Jackson and Strong (24) have shown to differentiate also between cortical and hippocampal damage.

METHOD

SUBJECTS

Male Sprague-Dawley had surgery performed at between 70 and 90 days of age and were begun on behavioral testing two weeks after surgery. The sham surgery group consisted of 11 rats while the NBM lesion group consisted of 14 subjects.

SURGERY

Bilateral lesions of the NBM using the excitotoxin ibotenic acid was performed under sodium pentobarbital anesthesia using the procedures and coordinates previously described (25,26). Sham control animals had identical procedures performed with the exception that no ibotenic acid was injected.

ONE WAY PASSIVE AVOIDANCE

On day one, the subject was placed in a small, lit compartment. Thirty seconds later a guillotine door was raised exposing a larger, unlit compartment. Figure 1. shows the apparatus used. When the animal entered the unlit compartment, the door was lowered and the subject received a two second, 1 mamp foot shock. The subject was then removed from the shock compartment and placed in a holding cage for sixty seconds. It was then placed back in the lighted compartment and thirty seconds later the door was raised. Time to enter the shock compartment was recorded. Latencies were measured to 0.001 seconds. If the subject did not enter in five minutes, it was removed from the starting compartment and returned to its home cage. Subjects were tested in a similar manner 24, 48, and 168 hours (7 days) later. Subjects never received a shock after trial one. An additional group of seven animals, not used in the remaining experiments, were treated in a similar fashion but received no shock on trial one.

TWO WAY ACTIVE (SHUTTLE) AVOIDANCE

Figure 2. shows the apparatus used in the two way shuttle task. The subject received a moderately loud buzzer (CS) for five seconds followed by 15 seconds of a 1 mamp shock. If the animal moves to the other side of the compartment within the first five seconds, the shock was avoided (CAR). If the animal moved to the other side of the shuttle compartment during the shock, the shock was terminated and recorded as an escape responses. Avoidance and escape latencies were measured to 0.01 seconds. Inter-trial interval was varied from 25-35 seconds to avoid temporal conditioning. A new trial was not begun if the subject was moving towards the other side of the shuttle box. Besides response latencies, the number of spontaneous shuttles between trials was also measured. Subjects were given ten trials a day for thirty days or until they made 80% CARs for two consecutive days.

ONE WAY ACTIVE AVOIDANCE

Figure 3 shows the one way active avoidance chamber. It was made of Plexiglas and was ten inches square and twenty four inches high.

On the floor was a shock grid that delivered a 1 mamp. scrambled shock. An overhead light provided the CS. The CS came on for five seconds followed by 15 seconds of shock. In the center of the chamber was a pole covered with hardware cloth. If the subject jumped on the pole before the five second CS interval, he avoided the shock (CAR). If he jumped up on the pole during the shock, the shock was terminated. Avoidance and escape latencies were measured to .01 seconds as well as failure to escape. Subjects were given ten trials a day for 12 days or until two successive days of 80% or better CARs.

LASHLY III MAZE

Figure 4. shows a diagram of the six unit Lashly maze used in this study ,which was similar to the one used by Jackson and Strong (24). Subjects were reduced to 80% of the base body weight and accommodated to a reward of Fruit Loops. After they were eating the reward reliably they were given three days of accommodation to the startbox, alleys, and goals box. Subjects were run for one trial a day for 25 days or until they attained a criterion of one perfect days-run. Subjects were removed from the apparatus if they failed to leave the startbox in 5 minutes or to complete the maze in 10 minutes.

RESULTS

ONE WAY PASSIVE AVOIDANCE

Figure 5. shows the results for the passive avoidance measure. Analysis of variance indicates that there is a significant difference between the control-group and the lesion-but-no shock-group for every postshock trial except for day seven. The lesion group and noshock group did not differ on any postshock trial. The gradual rise in latency over postshock trials for the non shock group is probably due to the fact that being removed from the apparatus is somewhat traumatic for animals which makes them somewhat reluctant to enter the chamber as trials continue. The behavior of those few control animals that did enter the shock chamber on postshock trials was strikingly different from that of the lesioned animals. The control animals would show significant approach-avoidance behavior, repeatedly putting their head and front paws in the chamber and then drawing back. The lesioned animals showed little of this type of behavior; rather they proceeded into the chamber with little hesitation or vacillation.

TWO WAY ACTIVE (SHUTTLE) AVOIDANCE

Analysis of percent conditioned avoidance responses (CARs) and number of animals reaching criteria revealed that the control group was superior to the lesion group, although this difference just failed to reach significance at the 0.05 level. A more detailed analysis of the two groups behaviors, however, clearly reveals the reason for this. Figure 6. shows the distribution of CAR scores for the two groups at the beginning of the training (days 1-5), in the middle of training (days 16-20) and at the end of training (days 26-30). At the beginning, the two groups show the expected positively skewed, unimodal distribution with most animals showing few CARs. At the middle of training, the control animals are showing a bimodal distribution of CAR scores while the lesion group shows a symmetrical, unimodal distribution. This trend continues to develop and is quite striking at the end of training. Both a Chi Square analysis and the Kolmogorv Smirnov test show that the two groups do not differ during the first five days of conditioning but do have significantly different distributions at the middle and end of conditioning. Examination of individual scores reveals that if a control animal makes more than 50% CARs in a given day, it will almost always reach criterion. One control animal had one day of 60%

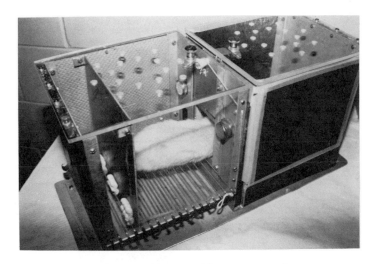

FIG. 1.   Passive avoidance apparatus

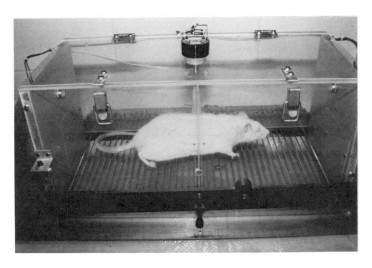

FIG. 2.   Two way shuttle apparatus

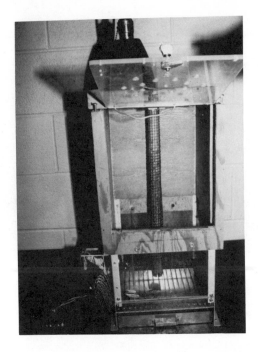

FIG. 3.   One way active avoidance apparatus

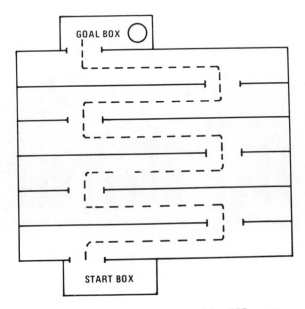

FIG. 4.   Diagram of the Lashly III maze

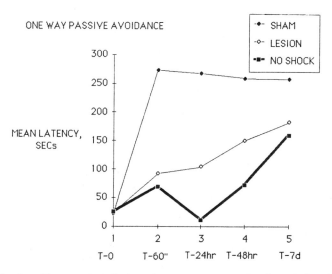

FIG. 5. Mean entry latencies over post shock trials in the passive avoidance task

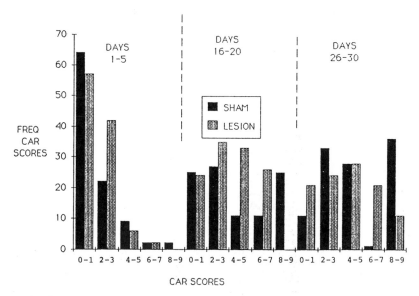

FIG. 6. Distribution of number of CARs during the beginning, middle, and end of 2-way shuttle training

but failed to reach criterion. The lesioned group, on the other hand, had many animals who had many days of 60% or greater CARs who failed to reach criteria. A Fisher's exact test showed this difference to be significant below the 0.01 level.

A bimodal distribution is usually indicative of the presence of two populations and this describes the control group well. They can be characterized as freezers and movers. Freezers quickly adopt a strategy of freezing and quickly jumping to the other side when shock occurs. Movers, on the other hand, show significantly more spontaneous shuttles from side to side between trials and reach the CAR criterion. Figure 7. shows the distribution for both groups for spontaneous shuttles. The four highest individuals in the sham control group reached criteria as did the highest shuttler in the lesion group. The distribution of the sham group supports the contention of two separate populations. The lesion group does not appear to be bimodally distributed in this measure either. It should be emphasized that the high spontaneous shuttlers are not running frantically back and forth, but rather freeze for a period and then cross deliberately to the other side. Their response to the CS is deliberate and clear-cut.

Figure 8. shows the mean escape times for both groups over the course of conditioning. The control group reached an escape latency of 0.35 seconds while the lesion group was almost twice as slow after shock was instigated. The apparatus is so set up that shock and the timer do not stop until the animal crosses to other side. Considering the finite time that this would take, it is probable that the control group is responding almost to the limit of their reaction times, while the lesion group is responding considerably slower and less efficiently. Thus,the control group "freezers" reduce their shock to a very brief pulse and can be considered to have learned almost as effective a response in the situation as the "avoiders." Lesioned animals, on the other hand, are far less effective in escaping shock and this may suggest both an attentional as well as a learning
deficit.

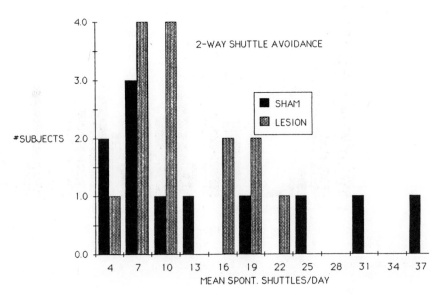

FIG. 7. Frequency distribution of spontaneous shuttles in the 2-way active avoidance task

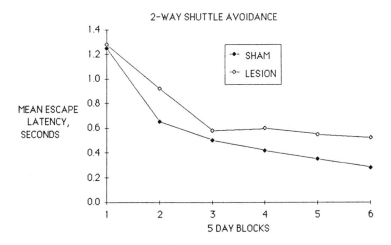

FIG. 8. Mean escape times over 5-day blocks of trials

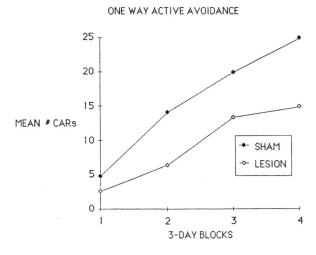

FIG. 9. Mean number of CARs in the one way active avoidance over 3-day blocks

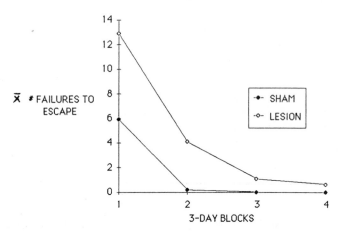

FIG. 10. Mean number of failures to escape over three day blocks during one way active avoidance training

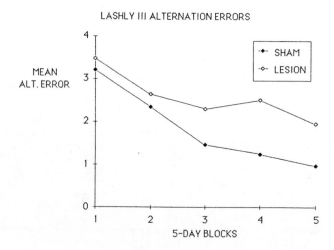

FIG. 11. Mean number of alternation errors over 5-day blocks during Lashly III maze acquisition

ONE WAY ACTIVE AVOIDANCE

Figure 9. shows the mean number of CARs for the two groups.
Analysis of variance indicates a highly significant difference
between the two groups. All control animals reached criteria while
less than half the lesioned animals did so.

As in the two way shuttle avoidance, the two groups escape
behavior also differed significantly. Figure 10 shows the mean
number of failures to make and escape during the shock period. It is
clear that the control group becomes highly efficient at making an
escape response early in training while many of the lesioned animals
continue to fail to escape.

LASHLY III MAZE LEARNING

Two types of errors are scored on the Lashly III maze, door
errors and alternation errors. A door error is scored when the
subject passes a door opening rather than going through it. An
animal can make any number of door errors. An alternation error is
making a turn in the wrong direction after going through a door. An
animal can only make six alternation errors with three being the
chance value. Jackson and Strong (24) have shown that hippocampectomized rats show significantly more door errors than cortical
controls, but no more alternation errors than those due to cortical
damage. Analysis of variance shows no difference between control and
lesioned animals in door errors but a highly significant difference
in alternation errors. Figure 11 shows these results. Inspection of
this figure shows that the lesion group is still operating at chance
levels by the end of training while the control group shows a
significant reduction in alternation errors. Since subjects are
given only one trial a day, the tasks imposes a significant memory
burden on the subject.

DISCUSSION

The use of a standardized assessment battery of behavioral tasks
builds a base of data from which useful comparisons can be made when
a research group runs a number of studies parametrically
investigating an aspect of problems such as SDAT animal model
studies. Our group has now used this battery with the addition of a
radial arm maze a variety of experimental groups such as fetal
transplant studies and normal and lesioned aged rats. Olton (27)
among others has also persuasively argued for such an approach. As
mentioned briefly in the introduction, careful thought must be given
as to the rationale for each test selected. Although a purist
approach would argue for counter balanced designs in order to assess
order effects, the sample size required becomes impractical as the
battery of behavioral measures becomes more numerous. Therefore,
one must use a more rational approach in deciding the order in which
the various measures should be taken. Our experience with the Lashly
III maze clearly illustrates this. In our introduction we indicated
that our Lashly III maze data were preliminary. We found that
testing subjects after they had been subjected to shock in three
different avoidance paradigms caused them to behave in the maze in a
manner that is usually interpreted as highly emotional or fearful.
This was manifested by freezing behavior, defecation, and urination
as well as tentative running. While our results were statistically
significant and fit well into the theoretical thrust of the study,
we now realize that any behavior using appetitive motivation, such
as hunger with food reward, should be run prior to aversive
procedures such as shock. In deciding the order of running the three
avoidance procedures, it seems that the passive avoidance procedure
should be run first since the subject receives only one shock and
thus contamination to the other two procedures should be minimal.
It would be an interesting parametric study to run the three

procedures in a counterbalanced design to see the interaction of the three experiences on each other in normal and lesioned rats but the time and expense of such a study would be great. One study of particular interest would be to see if training in one way active avoidance helped or hindered the two way shuttle learning and changed the ratio of "freezers" to "responders."

In looking at the results of the three avoidance studies, the value of looking at a wide variety of behaviors is well illustrated. Since it takes a lot of time and effort to set up a study, it is a shame not to squeeze as many data from it as possible. Besides, counters, cumulative recorders, timers, photocells, and other objectifying paraphenalia cannot take the place of direct observation of behavior. In the passive avoidance task, the behavior of the sham lesioned animals was qualitatively different from that of the lesioned animals. Even those sham animals that eventually entered the shock compartment clearly manifested their memory of the shock by the approach-avoidance behavior they manifested. This behavior was not evidenced by the lesion group. Furthermore, it seems prudent to study this behavior using more than one postshock trial. The use in our study of an immediate postshock test (the 60" postshock trial) as well as tests at one, two, and seven days later clearly gives a finer grained analysis of the behavior being studied, as does the use of a no-shock control group. In another study (to be submitted) on the effect of fetal tissue transplants in NBM lesioned rats, the only positive effect we found was in the passive avoidance task at the 60" postshock trial, thus showing an effect on immediate memory but not long term memory.

Looking at the 2-way shuttle task, we again see the value of looking at many behaviors. If we had not analyzed the frequency distribution of CARs and escape latencies, our data using just the number of CARs over time and number of animal attaining criterion would have indicated a weak effect. Carefully observing the behavior of our two groups gives insights as to the nature of the NBM deficit and yields strong evidence of lesion effects. This also allows us to see the failure to make escape responses in the one way active avoidance situation in a more integrated fashion. The analysis of the Lashly III maze behavior also indicates the value of a finer grained analysis of behavior. Breaking down the learning process into door and alternation errors has proved to be immensely valuable in gaining insights into the learning process involved. Normal animals running down the runways for the first time almost invariably pause and investigate the door opening. It is a sudden change in the stimulus configuration and elicits the orienting response (OR). Hippo-campectomized animals have a significant deficit in the OR and thus spend many trials running past the door openings. The alternation errors, on the other hand, appear to be more of a cognitive deficit and hippocampectomized animals have no significant difficulty with this aspect of the task while cortically damaged rats do (24).

Since NBM lesioned rats show a partial loss of cholinergic innervation in the frontal, parietal and occipital cortices, while damage to the medial septal and diagonal band nuclei cause loss of cholinergic innervation in the hippocampus, the rationale of the test battery was to select tasks that clearly differentiate between the functions of the two systems as well as having a good homology to the human SDAT condition such as immediate and long term memory, cognitive abilities, and cortical disinhibition. Our results indicate that the above objectives were met. Our lesioned animals did not show behaviors typical of temporal lobe-hippocampus damaged rats, but did show those typical of frontal-parietal cortex damaged rats. Future studies should attempt the same battery on animals with medial septal and diagonal band lesions, as well as animals in which all three systems have been damaged.

REFERENCES

1. Lockard, R.B. (1968) The albino rat: A defensible choice or a bad habit? <u>American Psychologist</u> 23: 734-742.
2. Beach, F.A. (1950). The snark was a boojum. <u>American Psychologist</u> 5: 115-124.
3. Boice, R. (1973) Domestication. <u>Psychological Bulletin</u> 80: 215-230.
4. Rosser, M., Garrett, N., Johnson, A., Mountjoy, C., Ruth, M., and Iverson, I. (1982) A post-mortem study of the cholinergic and GABA systems in senile dementia. <u>Brain</u> 105: 313-330.
5. Bowen, D., Sims, N., Benton, J., Curzon, G., Davison, A., Neary, D., and Thomas, D. (1981) Treatment of Alzheimer's disease: A cautionary Note. <u>New England Journal of Medicine</u> 305: 1016.
6. Whitehouse, P., Price, D., Struble, R., Clark, A., Coyle, J., and Delong, M. (1982) Alzheimer's disease and senile dementia: Loss of neurons in the basal forebrain. <u>Science</u> 215: 1237-1239.
7. Pearson, R., Sofroniew, M., Cuello, A., Powel, T., Eckenstein, F., Esiri, M., and Wilocock, G. (1983) Persistence of cholinergic neurons in the basal nucleus in a brain with senile dementia of the Alzheimer's type demonstrated by immunohistochemistry. <u>Brain Res.</u> 289: 375-379.
8 Johnston, M., McKinney, M., and Coyle, J. (1979) Evidence for a cholinergic projection to neocortex from neurons in basal forebrain. Proceedings of the <u>National Academy of Sciences USA</u> 76: 5392-5396.
9. Lehman, J., Nagy, J., Atmadja, S., and Fibiger, H.C. (1980).The nucleus basalis magnocellularis: The origins of a cholinergic projection to the neocortex of the rat. <u>Neurosciences</u> 5: 1161-1174.
10. Fibiger, H.C. (1982) The organization and some projections of cholinergic neurons of the mammalian forebrain. <u>Brain Research Reviews</u> 4: 327-388.
11. Hepler, D.J., Olton, D.S., Wenk, G.L., and Coyle, J.T. (1985) Lesions ion the nucleus basalis magnocellularis and medial septal area of rats produce qualitatively similar memory impairments. <u>Journal of Neuroscience</u> 5: 866-873.
12. Dunnett, S., Low, W., Iverson, S., Stenevi, U., and Bjorkland, A. (1982) Septal transplants restore maze learning in rats with fimbria-fornix lesions. <u>Brain Research</u> 251: 335-348.
13. Berman, R.F., Crosland, R.D., Jenden, D.J., and Altman, H.J. (1988).Persisting behavioral and neurochemical deficits in rats following lesions of the basal forebrain. <u>Pharmacology Biochemistry and Behavior</u> 29: 581-586.
14. Friedman, E., Lerer, B., and Kuster, J. (1983) Loss of cholinergic neurons in the rat neocortex produces deficits in passive avoidance learning. <u>Pharmacology Biochemistry and Behavior</u> 19: 309-312.
15. Flicker, C., Dean, R.L., Watkins, D.L., Fisher, S.K., and Bartus, R.T. (1983) Behavioral and neurochemical effects following neuro-taxic lesions of a major cholinergic input to the cerebral cortex in the rat. <u>Pharmacology Biochemistry and Behavior</u> 18: 973-981.
16. Lo Conte, G., Bartolini, L., Casamenti, F., Marconcini-Pepeu, I., and Pepeu, G. (1982) Lesions of cholinergic forebrain nuclei: Changes in avoidance behavior and scopolamine actions. <u>Pharmacology Biochemistry and Behavior</u> 17: 933-937.
17. Araki, H., Lichiyama, Y., Kawashima, K., and Aihara, H. (1986) Impairment in memory and changes in neurotransmitters induced by basal forebrain lesions in rats. <u>Japan Journal of Pharmacology</u> 41: 497-504.
18. Miyamoto, M., Shintani, M., Nagaoka, A., and Nagawa, Y. (1985) Lesioning of the rat basal forebrain leads to memory impairments in passive and active avoidance tasks. <u>Brain Research</u> 328: 97-104.

19. Issacson, R.L. and Wicklegrn, W.O. (1962) Hippocampal ablation and passive avoidance. <u>Science</u> 138: 1104-1106.
20. Blanchard, R.J. and Blanchard, D.C. (1972). Effects of hippocampal lesions on the rat's reaction to a cat. <u>Journal of Comparative and Physiological Psychology</u> 78: 77-82.
21. Papsdorf, J.D. and Woodruff, M. (1971) Effects of bilateral hippocampectomies on the rabbit's acquisition of shuttlebox and passive avoidance responses. <u>Journal of Comparative and Physiological Psychology</u> 73: 486-489.
22. Issacson, R.L., Douglas, R.J., and Moore, R.Y. (1961) The effect of radical hippocampal ablation on acquisition of avoidance responses. <u>Journal of Comparative and Physiological Psychology</u> 54: 625-628.
23. Olton, D.C. and Issacson, R.L. (1968) Hippocampal lesions and active avoidance. <u>Physiology and Behavior</u> 3: 719-724.
24. Jackson, W.J. and Strong, P.N. (1969) Differential effect of hippocampal lesions upon sequential tasks and maze learning by the rat. <u>Journal of Comparative and Physiological Psychology</u> 68: 442-450.
25. Arendash, G., Millard, W., Dunn, A., and Meyer, E. (1987). Long term neuropathological and neurochemical effects of nucleus basalis lesions in the rat. <u>Science</u> 238: 952-956.
26. Arendash, G., Strong, P., and Mouton, P. (1985) Intercerebral transplants of cholinergic neurons in a new animal model for Alzheimer's disease. In: <u>Senile Dementia of the Alzheimer's Type</u>, (eds. Hutton, J. and Kenny, A.) Alan R. Liss, Inc. New York, pp 351-376.
27. Olton, D.S. (1983) The use of animal models to evaluate the effects of neurotoxins on cognitive processes. <u>Behavioral Toxicology and Teratology</u> 5: 635-640.

NMDA RECEPTORS, AGING AND ALZHEIMER'S DISEASE

Kevin J. Anderson[1], Daniel T. Monaghan[2] and
James W. Geddes[2]

[1] Departments of Physiological Sciences and Neuroscience,
University of Florida, Gainesville, FL 32610; and [2] Department
of Surgery, University of California, Irvine, CA 92717

Introduction

Much research on the aging of the brain has been devoted in recent years to the possible alterations in specific neurotransmitter systems and the receptors which subserve neural transmission. This emphasis on transmitter systems is the result of the availability of new and specific ligands to probe receptor numbers and function as well as highly sensitive assays to directly measure transmitter content. The possibility that breakdowns in individual transmitter systems may correlate with specific clinical symptoms in aging-related disease has received much support, and indeed is well demonstrated in the dopaminergic dysfunction of Parkinson's disease, and, to a lesser extent, the cholinergic deficits seen in Alzheimer's disease (AD). However, it is not well understood how changes in transmitter systems during the course of "normal" aging affect brain function.

During aging, the organisms response to a number of hormones and neurotransmitters has been shown to be impaired. In most cases, the decline in response is progressive over the lifespan or postmaturity phase. In other systems, many functions are preserved with aging. These differences may be explained by how various tissues, organs or physiological systems differ in the rates at which they age. Alternatively, some systems may show fewer deficits because they possess better adaptive mechanisms to compensate for any losses. Thus, neural plasticity may represent a key variable in determining the outcome of brain aging.

Excitatory Amino Acid Transmitter Systems

Excitatory amino acids (EAA) represent a major neurotransmitter class in the mammalian brain and subserve transmission in the majority of excitatory pathways in the central nervous system. As such, it is important to understand their function, not only in normal synaptic activity but also in development, aging and neuropathology. EAA receptors are not solely involved in mediating normal synaptic transmission within excitatory pathways. Evidence has also implicated EAA receptors in the modification of synaptic connections during development and their participation in certain forms of memory. Moreover, the overactivation of EAA receptors has been implicated as a cause of the neuronal degeneration and cell death in a wide spectrum of neurological disorders (e.g., ischemia, hypoglycemia and stroke) (1,2,3)

EAA receptors have been classified on the basis of the action of a number of agonist compounds. Thus, there appear to be at least 5 classes of receptors corresponding to the agonists N-methyl-D-aspartate (NMDA), kainate (KA), α-amino-3-hydroxy-5-methyl-isoxizole-4-propionate (AMPA), 2-amino-4-phosphonobutyrate (APB) and *Trans*-1-amino-cyclopentyl-1,3-dicarboxylate (ACPD) (4). Of these receptors, the NMDA receptor has received the most attention due to its involvement in various aspects of neuronal plasticity and cell pathology (5).

Excitatory transmission in pathways with NMDA receptors appears distinct from conventional fast-acting transmission such as that found at the neuromuscular junction. NMDA receptors function in a dual receptor system: non-NMDA receptors serve fast-acting responses while NMDA receptors both amplify the synaptic response and permit calcium entry, if there is concurrent postsynaptic depolarization (6).

The pharmacological properties of NMDA receptors have been the subject of intense study in recent years. It now appears that the NMDA receptor is a macromolecular complex which consists of a transmitter binding site, an allosterically regulated ion channel, and an allosteric activating site.

NMDA Receptors and Plasticity Versus Pathology

NMDA receptors appear to be central to mechanisms that control developmental plasticity of neuronal circuits and some forms of learning. In aging and AD, loss of these receptors, or a decline in their functional properties, may contribute to dysfunction in learning and memory.

NMDA receptors play a critical role in the development of sensory systems. The development of most sensory pathways appears to involve at least two staged events; first, fibers are guided to the appropriate target fields and second, their synaptic position is refined in an activity-dependent process. Recent work indicates that the latter step involves the activation of NMDA receptors. In the visual system, for example, chronic blockade of NMDA receptors prevents the formation of retinal-specific columns in the tadpole optic tectum (7). Similarly, NMDA antagonist application prevents the formation of the ocular dominance shift in response to monocular deprivation in the kitten (8).

Previous studies have implicated NMDA receptors as an integral part of the cellular mechanisms that underlie certain forms of learning, such as long-term potentiation (LTP). LTP requires NMDA receptor activation (9) indicating that NMDA receptors may be an important component in the processes involved in learning in the mature CNS. LTP may also be associated with new synapse formation and/or growth (enlargement) of existing synapses (10,11). This suggests, in principle at least, that NMDA-mediated LTP and synaptic plasticity may be related processes that differ in degree but share common mechanisms and endpoints.

In the CNS, NMDA receptors provide a mechanism to enhance the synaptic response and to increase calcium influx. Both of these properties, however, can also lead to excitotoxicity. Several recent investigations have provided evidence that damage to the brain produced by anoxia/ischemia, hypoglycemia, and epilepsy are mediated by the excitatory amino acid receptors, particularly of the NMDA type (12,13,14). As a result of these disorders, excessive amounts of glutamate (up to eightfold) are released into the extracellular space (15) and can be toxic to neurons if the levels remain elevated for periods beyond several minutes (16). Excessive synaptic activation of pathways which use excitatory amino acids can result in neuronal loss with a pattern of cell death identical to that obtained following direct injection of an EAA (17). Several glutamate antagonists, particularly in the NMDA class, offer some protection from seizures and cell loss if applied either immediately before or shortly after insult (18). Thus, plasticity mechanisms that increase the activity of NMDA receptors in aging or disease might render the brain more susceptible to excitotoxic injury.

The functional state of the aged brain probably reflects a balance between age-related losses and compensatory mechanisms. It is becoming increasingly clear that the NMDA receptor plays a pivotal role in maintaining this balance in excitatory pathways. During development, NMDA receptors participate in directing growth so that the most active pathways form the most synapses. In the adult or aged brain NMDA receptors appear to encode particular stimulus patterns in highly adaptive circuits. For example, high frequency stimulation causes a long lasting increase or potentiation (e.g., LTP) in the strength of synaptic transmission. Ironically, however, their overactivation (such as in seizures, stroke or vascular insult) can cause injury to neurons. NMDA receptor activation increases intracellular calcium. Elevated levels of calcium can reach a level that is toxic to neurons. Thus, NMDA receptors are needed for memory but may also cause cell damage.

When one seeks to determine the functional status of the aged brain, the levels of NMDA receptors may prove to provide valuable insights into the process of brain aging. A decreased number of NMDA receptors would indicate that the cellular mechanisms to encode memory is impaired; an increase may indicate a selective vulnerability to excitotoxicity. In view of the critical role of the NMDA receptor in higher brain function, it is essential to understand the properties of this receptor complex in the mature, aged and AD brain. Accordingly, we have examined these receptors in a rodent model of brain aging and in the AD brain.

NMDA Receptors in the Aged Rodent Brain

To examine the fate of NMDA receptors in the aged brain we have utilized an *in vitro* autoradiographic approach in order to study the regional distribution of any aging-related changes. Utilizing this approach one can also quantify the kinetic parameters (e.g., K_D or B_{MAX}) of the receptor in question within a given brain region. NMDA-displaceable L-[^{3}H] glutamate sites are found throughout the brain but predominantly in telencephalic regions (19). The highest levels of binding in the brain are found in the strata oriens and radiatum of hippocampal area CA1. Most of hippocampal area CA3 and the dentate gyrus have moderate levels, whereas the mossy fiber termination zone (stratum lucidum) is quite low in NMDA sites, but rather has a high density of kainate sites. The human hippocampal formation has a similar distribution of NMDA sites; the CA1 region, Sommer's sector, contains the highest density of sites (20).

Among the cortical regions, the highest densities of NMDA receptors are found in the frontal, anterior cingulate and piriform cortices. The entorhinal cortex and subiculum contain a relatively low number of sites for a cortical region, and a sharp zone of demarcation is seen in the transition from perirhinal to entorhinal cortex. In neocortical regions such as the parietal cortex, there is a dense band of sites corresponding to layers I-III and an additional zone in layer IVa. Of non-cortical regions, the highest levels of NMDA sites are found in the nucleus accumbens and caudate/putamen, the dorsolateral septum, and the amygdala.

NMDA Receptors are Lost in Specific Regions of the Aged Brain

When the density of NMDA receptors labelled with L-[3H] glutamate in young-adult (4 month old) Fischer 344 rats was compared with aged (24-26 month old) rats, it was apparent that specific brain regions exhibited a decline in receptor density (Fig. 1). Indeed, quantitative analysis of receptor density confirmed NMDA receptor loss in the aged brain. Brain regions in aged rats that exhibited a greater than 30% decrease in receptor density when compared to young-adults included the lateral striatum, inner (deep) entorhinal cortex and lateral septal nucleus. Regions of brain that were within 10% of controls included the inner parietal cortex and anterior cingulate cortex.

In order to further examine the status of the NMDA receptor complex in the aged brain, [3H] glycine binding was employed to probe the associated allosteric activating site. When compared with L-[3H] glutamate binding, a similar decrease in [3H] glycine binding was seen in the aged brain. Like L-[3H] glutamate labelling, areas that showed the greatest degree of loss included the

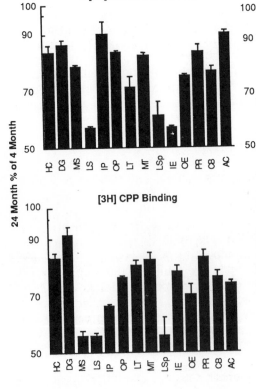

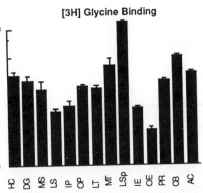

Figure 1. Loss of NMDA receptors in the aged rat brain. NMDA receptor levels in aged rat brain sections are compared with young-adult controls. Three radioligands were used to assess the status of NMDA receptors L-[3H] glutamate, [3H] glycine and [3H] 3((±)-2-carboxypiperazin-4-yl)-propyl-1-phosphonic acid (CPP). Brain regions that were sampled for quantitative analysis were: **HC** = hippocampal area CA1, **DG** = dentate gyrus, **MS** = medial striatum, **LS** = lateral striatum, **IP** = inner parietal cortex, **OP** = outer parietal cortex, **LT** = lateral thalamic nuclei, **MT** = medial thalamic nuclei, **LSp** = lateral septum, **OE** = outer entorhinal cortex, **PR** = perirhinal cortex, **CB** = cerebellar molecular layer, **AC** = anterior cingulate cortex.

striatum, particularly the lateral regions and entorhinal cortex (Fig. 1). However, while the lateral septal nucleus showed a severe decrease in L-[^{3}H] glutamate binding, this decrease was not apparent with [^{3}H] glycine. In addition, the loss of glycine binding sites in aged rats was more profound in the parietal cortex, and outer (superficial) portions of the entorhinal cortex.

Finally, the competitive antagonist [^{3}H] 3 ((±)-2-carboxypiperazin-4-yl)-propyl-1-phosphonic acid (CPP) was used to analyze the density of NMDA receptors in the aged brain. This compound is one of the most potent and selective NMDA antagonists currently available. In the aged brain, a similar decrease in binding to specific brain regions was also seen with [^{3}H]-CPP binding. The regional decrease in CPP binding appeared to fit well with the decrease observed using L-[^{3}H] glutamate.

Since a decrease in ligand binding may represent either a change in affinity or a decrease in the number of receptors, a kinetic analysis of L-[^{3}H] glutamate binding to the NMDA receptor was undertaken. Saturation analysis of L-[^{3}H] glutamate binding showed that within a given brain region that showed a decrease in binding, there was no significant difference in the affinity of the NMDA receptor for L-[^{3}H] glutamate. However, significant decreases were seen in the B_{max} within the most severely affected brain regions, indicating that in the aged brain there was a decrease in the total number of receptors.

One variable that may partially account for an age-related decrease in receptor sites is differential quenching of radioactive emissions due to variations in the amount of total lipid between young and aged rat brain sections. In order to test this possibility, sections of aged and young-adult rat brains were pre-treated with xylene or chloroform to remove lipids from the tissue prior to incubation with L-[^{3}H] glutamate. In autoradiograms from these sections, the decrease in NMDA receptors seen in the aged rat brain were proportionally equivalent between untreated and delipidated slices. This indicates that differential lipid quenching between aged and young-adult rat brain sections does not appear to be a confounding variable in analyzing receptor density.

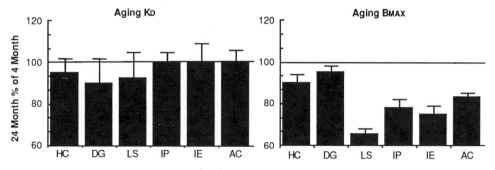

Figure 2. Kinetic analysis of NMDA receptor loss in aging. L-[^{3}H] Glutamate affinity for NMDA receptor is not significantly different between aged and young-adult subjects (left graph). However, aged rats show significant differences in the total number of NMDA receptors in specific brain regions (right graph). Abbreviations: HC= Hippocampal area CA1; DG= Hippocampal Dentate Gyrus; LS= Lateral Striatum; IP= Inner Parietal Cortex; IE= Inner Entorhinal Cortex; AC= Ant. Cingulate Cortex.

In summary, NMDA receptors are lost in specific regions of the senescent rat brain. The reasons for this loss and functional sequelae are as yet, unknown. One possibility is that a decrease in the number of NMDA receptors is due to a general decrease in the number of postsynaptic neurons. While this possibility has not been rigorously tested, our preliminary experiments in rodent and human brains (see below) have indicated that up to 60% of the neurons in area CA1 of the hippocampus can be lost before a significant drop in NMDA receptors is seen.

An alternative possibility is that NMDA receptors are downregulated in brain regions that are vulnerable to excitotoxic damage during aging. It is interesting that NMDA receptors decrease in several specific integrative and highly adaptive brain regions. This would reduce their integrative and storage capacity but it would also protect those areas from toxic damage. It is tempting to speculate that the brain makes a trade-off in order to optimize the potential to preserve the essential circuitry and functions.

NMDA Receptors in AD

An intensive area of recent research has been devoted to determining the state of the NMDA receptor complex in AD. Can the loss of cognitive function seen in the disease be explained by changes in NMDA receptors? The data from AD studies can be illustrated by examining the well-characterized CA1 region of the hippocampal formation. CA1 pyramidal cell dendrites receive a major excitatory input from CA3 pyramidal cells (i.e. Schaffer collaterals). Autoradiographic analysis has shown area CA1 to possess high levels of NMDA receptors while containing low levels of kainic acid receptors. In fact, the highest levels of NMDA receptors in the brain are found in the stratum radiatum and stratum pyramidale. CA1 is particularly vulnerable to the pathology associated with AD and usually contains a high density of neurofibrillary tangles.

It has been reported that NMDA receptors dramatically decrease (80%) in AD (21,22). However, other reports have indicated significantly less decline in the average density of NMDA receptors in AD using NMDA displaceable L-[^{3}H] glutamate binding (20,23). However, this appears to vary from case to case. Upon closer examination, we observed that a marked decline in NMDA receptor density is largest in cases primarily exhibiting very severe neuronal loss in CA1 (20,23). Thus, studies to date suggest that when compared with age-matched controls, NMDA receptor density in AD may be maintained at near normal values as long as neuronal survival is adequate. In correlating cell and receptor density, we estimate that about 60% of the neurons can degenerate before large numbers of receptors are lost. This preservation of receptors may be due to dendritic sprouting of the remaining cells or receptor upregulation. It appears that when the cell loss is severe enough to drop below this critical level, however, major receptor loss is observed. It may be in fact that the density of NMDA sites *per neuron* may increase initially in area CA1 and then decline.

As mentioned above, a decline in hippocampal glutamate receptors of up to 80% has been reported by Young and colleagues (21,22). This observed decrease was attributed to an early loss of NMDA receptors and contrasts our findings that receptor density is maintained in AD, except in the cases exhibiting severe cell loss. Considering the roles of this receptor in higher cognitive function and the extent to which these functions are impacted by AD, it is of extreme importance to determine the status of the NMDA receptor complex in the course of AD. The differences in the findings may be attributable to the severity of the cases examined, differences in experimental methods, or interpretation of the data. Greenamyre et al. (21,22) defined the decrease in NMDA receptors as a loss in high-affinity, quisqualate-insensitive glutamate binding. These studies were also done in the presence of added chloride and calcium. Under similar conditions, we have shown that more than 50% of quisqualate-insensitive, chloride-dependent glutamate binding is also insensitive to NMDA (24,25). This suggests that under the conditions employed by Greenamyre et al (21,22) a substantial amount of the binding measured may not be to the NMDA receptor.

Recent studies have suggested that binding experiments done in the presence of chloride introduce complications associated with transport into both neurons and glia (26,27). Thus, a portion of the reported glutamate receptor loss may actually include the loss of some chloride-dependent glutamate transport sites (28). In light of this, it is interesting that a loss (approximately 20%) of sodium-dependent D-aspartate binding sites has been reported in AD (29). However, if the loss of glutamate sites described by Greenamyre et al., (approximately 80%) represents a loss of chloride-dependent transport sites, then this system may be more heavily impacted than the sodium-dependent system. In addition, since there is a great deal of evidence indicating that astrocytes, both *in vitro* and *in vivo*, possess the ability for sodium-dependent and chloride-dependent transport of glutamate (30,31), the state of EAA metabolism in Alzheimer's disease studies may need to be re-evaluated. A decrease in sodium- or chloride-dependent transport sites in the AD brain may reflect diminished capacity of astrocytes to properly transport EAAs from affected synapses. This, in turn, would suggest that the potential for excitotoxicity is increased in these regions. Clearly, further studies are needed to determine the precise cellular localization of transport binding sites and the status of transport systems in AD in order to evaluate these possibilities.

Other Neurotransmitter Receptors in Aging

Other receptor types appear to be affected during aging with some showing regional variations. The density of dopamine receptors has been examined in the brain of aged rats, monkeys and humans. There appears to be a consistent decrease (25-50%) in striatal D2 dopamine receptors with aging in all species studied (32). However, the fate of D1 dopamine receptors is not as clear. Thus, it has been reported that D1 dopamine receptors increase in the human caudate nucleus and putamen during normal aging, and show modest decreases or no change in the rat striatum (32). Most recently, a study using [3H] SCH 23390 (the most selective D1 antagonist available) has demonstrated a decrease of 37-44% in D1 receptors in the striatum of aged rats (33).

The majority of adrenergic receptor studies in the aged brain have dealt with changes in β-adrenergic receptors. β1 and β2 adrenergic receptors do not appear to undergo an overall decline with age (for review, see ref. 34). Most studies have reported a decrease in the number of receptors with age in the cerebellum where a 30-45% decrease has been observed. More recently, the decrease in cerebellar β-receptors has been shown to be due to a specific decline in β2 receptors, with β1 receptors actually showing an increase in the aged subjects. In other brain regions, changes in β receptors is less clear. Most studies have reported little or no change in β receptors in the cerebral cortex of aged rats, and decreased density in the striatum and brain stem.

Cholinergic muscarinic receptors also show regional changes during senescence. Using [^{3}H] quinuclidinyl benzilate binding Biegon et al. (35) reported that a number of brain regions showed no effect of aging including the hippocampal formation, thalamus and hypothalamus. The neocortical regions and striatum had slight decreases, while the ventral forebrain cholinergic areas demonstrated a 40-60% decrease in the number of receptors. However, Gurwitz et al. (36) using [^{3}H] acetylcholine and [^{3}H]-N-methyl-4-piperidyl benzilate reported that a significant decrease in muscarinic receptors was seen in the cerebral cortex, hippocampus, striatum and olfactory bulb. Moreover, sexual dimorphic variations were reported; aged male rats had a 58% increase in muscarinic receptors in the brainstem while females showed no change with age.

Summary and Conclusion

We have hypothesized that mechanisms exist in the CNS to maintain NMDA receptor density and function in the presence of mild-to-moderate cell loss. This appears to be the case when comparing AD subjects to age-matched controls. A general decline in the density of NMDA receptors does not appear to occur in AD. This indicates that a selective decline of NMDA receptors is not responsible for the loss of cognitive function seen in the disease. However, the cost of maintaining receptor density may be an increased vulnerability to excitotoxic damage. With progressive neuronal loss, maintenance of NMDA receptor density could augment excitotoxic cell death progressing into a cycle where significant functional losses would be eventually realized.

When receptor density is compared between two extremes of the aging spectrum in rodents, highly significant differences in NMDA receptor densities are seen in anatomically discrete brain regions. Furthermore, other studies have demonstrated that a wide variety of receptor systems can decline with age in a number of species including man. What remains to be answered is whether a decline in the density of NMDA receptors, or any other receptor, can be correlated with a functional or behavioral deficit. Perhaps the loss of receptors during senescence is merely a reduction in redundant receptor populations, while function is being maintained at or near normal levels. In light of the involvement of the NMDA receptor in excitotoxic mechanisms, it is also tempting to speculate that a reduction in NMDA receptors during the course of aging represents a protective reaction by the brain to prevent the type of vicious cycle outline above. Further studies will be needed to clarify these issues regarding the aging of the brain.

References

1. Rothman, S.M. and J.W. Olney (1986) Glutamate and the pathology of hypoxic/ischemic brain damage. Ann. Neurol. 19:105-111.
2. Rothman, S.M. and J.W. Olney (1987) Excitotoxicity and the NMDA receptor. TINS 10:299-302.
3. Wieloch, T. (1986) Endogenous excitotoxins as possible mediators of ischemic and hypoglycemic brain damage. Prog. Brain Res. 63:69-85.

4. Monaghan, D.T., Bridges, R.J. and Cotman, C.W. (1989) The excitatory amino acid receptors: their classes, pharmacology, and distinct properties in the function of the central nervous system. Ann. Rev. Pharmacol. Toxicol. 29:365-402.

5. Cotman, C.W. and Iversen, L.L. (1987) Excitatory amino acids in the brain-focus on NMDA receptors. TINS 10:263-264.

6. Ascher, P., and Nowak, L. (1987) Electrophysiological studies of NMDA receptors. TINS 10:284-287.

7. Cline, H.T., Debski, E. and Constantine-Paton, M. (1987) NMDA receptor antagonist desegregates eye specific stripes. Proc. Natl. Acad. Sci. (USA) 84:4342-4345.

8. Kleinschmidt, A., Bear, M.F. and Singer, W. (1987) Blockade of "NMDA" receptors disrupts experience-dependent plasticity of kitten striate cortex. Science 238: 355-358.

9. Collingridge, G.L. and Bliss, T.V.P. (1987) NMDA receptors-their role in long-term potentiation. TINS 10:288-293.

10. Chang, F. and Greenough, W.T. (1984) Transient and enduring morphological correlates of synaptic activity and efficacy change in the rat hippocampal slice. Brain Res. 309:35-46.

11. Lee, K., Schottler, F., Oliver, M., and Lynch, G. (1980) Brief bursts of high frequency stimulation produce two types of structural change in rat hippocampus. J. Neurophysiol. 44:247-258.

12. Wieloch, T. (1985) Neurochemical correlates to selective neuronal vulnerability Prog. Brain Res. 63:69-85.

13. Wieloch, T. (1985) Hypoglycemia-induced neuronal damage prevented by an N-methyl-D-aspartate antagonist. Science 230: 681-682

14. Meldrum, B. (1985) Possible applications of antagonists of excitatory amino acid neurotransmitters. Clin. Sci. 68: 113-122.

15. Beneviste, H., Drejer, J., Schousboe, A., Diemer, N.H. (1984) Elevation of the extracellular concentrations of glutamate and aspartate in rat hippocampus during transient cerebral ischemia monitored by intracerebral microdialysis. J. Neurochem. 43: 1369-74.

16. Rothman, S.M., Olney, J.W. (1986) Glutamate and the pathology of hypoxic/ischemic brain damage. Annal. Neurol. 19: 105-110.

17. Sloviter, R.S. (1983) "Epileptic" brain damage in rats induced by sustained electrical stimulation of the perforant path. I. Acute electrophysiological and light microscopic studies. Brain Res. Bull. 10: 675-697.

18. Rothman, S.R., and Olney, J.W. (1987) Excitotoxicity and the NMDA receptor. TINS 10:299-301.

19. Monaghan, D.T., Cotman, C.W. (1985) Distribution of NMDA-sensitive L-[3H]-glutamate binding sites in rat brain as determined by quantitative autoradiography. J Neurosci 5: 2909-2919.

20. Geddes, J.W., Chang-Chui, H., Cooper, S.M., Lott, I.T., and Cotman, C.W. (1986) Density and distribution of NMDA receptors in the human hippocampus in Alzheimer's disease Brain Res. 399:156-161.

21. Greenamyre, J.T., Penney, J.B., D'Amato, C.J., and Young, A.B. (1987) Dementia of the Alzheimer type: changes in hippocampal L-[3H]glutamate binding. J. Neurochem 48: 543-551.

22. Greenamyre, J.T., Penney, J.B., Young, A.B., D'Amato, C.J., Hicks, C.J., Shoulson, I. (1985) Alterations in L-glutamate binding in Alzheimer's and Huntington's disease. Science 227: 1496-1497.

23. Monaghan, D.T., Geddes, J.W., Yao, D., Chung, C., and Cotman, C.W. (1987) [^{3}H]TCP binding sites in Alzheimer's disease. Neurosci Lett. 73: 197-200

24. Monaghan, D.T., McMillis, M.C., Chamberlin, A.R., and Cotman, C.W. (1983) Synthesis of [^{3}H]-2-amino-4-phosphonobutyric acid and characterization of its binding to rat brain membranes: A selective ligand for the chloride/calcium dependent class of L-glutamate binding sites. Brain Res. 278: 137-144.

25. Monaghan, D.T., Cotman, C.W. (1986) Identification and properties of NMDA receptors in rat brain synaptic plasma membranes. Proc. Natl. Acad. Sci. U.S.A. 83: 7532-36.

26. Bridges, R.J., M. Nieto-Sampedro, M. Kadri and C.W. Cotman (1987) A novel chloride-dependent L-[^{3}H] glutamate binding site in astrocyte membranes, J. Neurochem. 48: 1709-1715.

27. Kessler, M., M. Baudry and G. Lynch (1987) Use of cystine to distinguish glutamate binding from glutamate sequestration. Neurosci. Lett. 81:221-226.

28. Geddes, J.W., Monaghan, D.T., Bridges, R.J., and Cotman, C.W. (1987) Stability of L-glutamate receptors and decrease in a CaCl-dependent [^{3}H]-L-glutamate binding site in Alzheimer's disease. Soc Neurosci Abstr 13:436.

29. Palmer, A.M., A.W. Proctor, G.C. Stratmann and D.M. Bowen (1986) Excitatory amino acid-releasing and cholinergic neurones in Alzheimer's disease. Neurosci. Lett. 66: 199-203.

30. Currie, D.N., and J.S. Kelly (1981) Glial versus neuronal uptake of glutamate J Exp. Biol. 95:181-193.

31. Waniewski, R.A. and D.L. Martin. (1984) Characterization of L-Glutamic acid transport by glioma cells in culture: Evidence for sodium-independent, chloride-dependent high affinity influx. J Neurosci. 4:2237-2246.

32. Morgan, D.G. (1987) The dopamine and serotonin systems during aging in human and rodent brain. A brief review. Prog. Neuro-Psychopharmacol. Biol. Psychiat. 11:153-157.

33. Giorgi, O., Calderini, G., Toffano, G. and Biggio, G. (1987) D-1 dopamine receptors labelled with 3H-SCH 23390: decrease in the striatum of aged rats. Neurobiol. Aging 8:51-54.

34. Scarpace, P.J. and Abrass, I.B. (1988) Alpha- and beta-adrenergic receptor function in the brain during senescence. Neurobiol. Aging 9:53-58.

35. Biegon, A., Duvdevani, R., Greenberger, V. and Segal, M. (1988) Aging and brain cholinergic muscarinic receptors: an autoradiographic study in the rat. J. Neurochem. 51:1381-1385.

36. Gurwitz, D., Egozi, Y., Henis, Y.I., Kloog, Y., and Sokolovsky, M. (1987) Agonist and antagonist binding to rat brain muscarinic receptors: influence of aging. Neurobiol. Aging 8:115-122.

AN EXCITOTOXIC MODEL OF ALZHEIMER'S DISEASE: NMDA LESIONS AND INITIAL

NEURAL GRAFTING RESULTS

D.A. Turner and W.Q. Dong

Department of Neurosurgery
University of Minnesota and Veterans Affairs Medical Center
Minneapolis, MN 55417

SUMMARY

We have developed an animal model of Alzheimer's disease, based on a
critical loss of neurons which are sensitive to the excitotoxic effects of
NMDA glutamate agonists. This model follows an alternative hypothesis for
the etiology of the disease, in assuming a global involvement of cortical
(and subcortical) neurons with NMDA glutamate receptors, as opposed to a
primary subcortical lesion. The initial evaluation of the animal model has
included histological assessment and behavioral testing for cortical memory
function. Treatment with neural grafting has also been performed, to
replace damaged cortical circuitry. The development of animal models of
Alzheimer's disease apart from those with primary cholinergic dysfunction
may be helpful for future understanding of the disease manifestations and
treatment paradigms.

INTRODUCTION

A variety of animal models of Alzheimer's disease have been developed
following a number of hypotheses of the nature of the disease and potential
treatment mechanisms (1,2,3,4,5,6). An initial model was the investigation
of memory deficits and neural grafting in aged animals (7,8,9). Other
models have included ischemic lesions of the hippocampus (10), toxins such
as trimethyltin (11) and the use of pharmacologic cholinergic antagonists
(1). A number of investigators have pursued subcortical models of the
disease, particularly cholinergic destructive models or septal lesions
(12,13,14,15,16,17). These subcortical models have generally assumed the
validity of the cholinergic hypothesis of memory dysfunction (1). However,
attempts to reduce memory impairments in clinical trials using cholinomimetic agents have not been therapeutically successful, possibly because of
the global changes occurring in cortical neurons (2,4,18,19,20,21).

An alternative hypothesis considers the disease in a more global
context of cortical and subcortical dysfunction, particularly involving
changes in the major putative neurotransmitter, glutamate (3,22,23,24,25,26,
27,28,29,30). The initial lesions and manifestations of the human disease
appear to be cortical as well as subcortical, suggesting that a mixed lesion
model of cortical dysfunction may be more applicable to the human disease.
In addition, the primary initial presentation of the disease is often memory

loss and the most severe damage lies in the hippocampus and entorhinal cortex (2,18,21,31). Thus, an alternative animal model of Alzheimer's disease would include bilateral lesions of the hippocampal formation in addition to damage to the subcortical nuclei projecting to the hippocampus.

Two recent clues have helped to solidify this hypothesis of mixed cortical and subcortical damage. The first is the controversial finding that perhaps the N-methyl-D-aspartate (NMDA) class of glutamate receptor may be decreased in number out of proportion to the kainate/quisqualate class in autopsy specimens from patients with Alzheimer's disease (3,18,22,25,29). Findings from autoradiography of human specimens from patients with Alzheimer's disease are also consistent (26) but the technique of separation of glutamate receptor classes remains in dispute. The second clue is the confirmation of the role of an exogenous toxin in the pathogenesis of Guam ALS-Parkinson's-Dementia complex (32). The suspected exogenous toxin, a plant amino acid (L-BMAA), appears to function as an orally active NMDA agonist, and the effects can be blocked by an NMDA antagonist (30).

These two clues point to the global involvement of neurons with post-synaptic receptors for the NMDA class of glutamate receptors (24), which suggests that these neurons appear to be preferentially involved in either the pathogenesis or expression of Alzheimer's disease. The additional finding of severe memory loss with either bilateral restricted CA1 hippocampal damage (31,33) or with the infusion of an NMDA antagonist into the lateral ventricle or hippocampus (34,35) suggests that many of the clinical symptoms in Alzheimer's disease may be attributed to dysfunction of neurons with the NMDA receptor subtype, particularly in the hippocampus.

We have developed an animal model of Alzheimer's disease, which demonstrates combined damage to both the hippocampus and the medial septal nuclei and is directly relevant to the hypothesis of a mixed cortical and subcortical etiology. This model involves a chronic NMDA infusion into the lateral ventricles of rats, since NMDA itself acts as an excitotoxin under these circumstances (36). In correlation with this model, we have performed behavioral testing of spatial memory (37). Additionally, treatment with fetal tissue grafting of hippocampus into the lesioned hippocampus has been performed (38,39,40,41,42,43,44,45). This report will describe the methodology for the induction of the model, histological features and neuropathological areas of involvement, behavioral aspects and initial grafting studies.

METHODS

Experimental Groups and Lesion Induction

The general goal with the experimental groups was to identify the behavioral, anatomical and physiological response to a variety of hippocampal lesions and to subsequent neural grafting. Two main experimental groups and several control groups of Fischer 344 rats were used to differentiate the response of animals with lesions in the hippocampus to neural grafting. The two primary groups included the acute unilateral intraventricular injection of kainic acid (46) and the bilateral chronic intraventricular infusion of NMDA (36). All animals were evaluated by behavioral testing in a serial fashion, as described below. Sham (saline) lesions, animals undergoing lesioning without subsequent grafting and cerebellum grafts were controls for these lesions and grafts.

Kainic acid lesions were created by the stereotaxic injection of the chemical into the posterior lateral ventricle (0.5 μg kainic acid in 0.5 μl of buffer over 30 min; 36,46). The lesion produced by this injection consisted of a dense loss of hippocampal CA3 pyramidal neurons on the side of injection, with a minor loss of CA1 pyramidal cells. The rationale for including this lesion was because of the restricted hippocampal CA3 cell damage. Thus, the integration and synaptic connectivity of the fetal hippocampal grafts may be very different than with the bilateral NMDA infusions.

NMDA lesions were produced by a chronic NMDA infusion, similar to that used for other chronic infusions of chemicals into the cerebral ventricles. An Alzet mini-osmotic pump was connected to an intraventricular cannula, after preloading of NMDA (0.2, 0.5, 0.75 and 1.0 mg total dose, in 210 μl buffer) into the pump (36; Fig. 1). The use of a chronic infusion over two weeks may mimic a slow, long-term cell destruction, similar to the

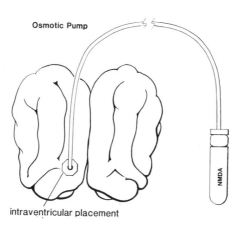

Osmotic Pump

NMDA

intraventricular placement

Fig. 1. NMDA was infused using an osmotic infusion pump. The infusion cannula was placed in the right lateral ventricle, for bilateral effects of the excitotoxin on periventricular regions.

excitotoxic hypothesis concerning the damage associated with neurodegenerative processes (30). In preliminary trials with this technique it was found that the histological pattern of damage showed a moderate cell loss throughout the hippocampus bilaterally, more pronounced on the right (Fig. 6). The end result of the infusion was an animal with moderate bilateral hippocampal damage; the behavioral results will be discussed below in terms of the NMDA dosage.

Behavioral Testing of Spatial Memory

A variety of maze formats have been developed for the purpose of testing hippocampal-related function in rats (7,13,16,31,33,37,42). The Morris water maze, which evaluates place learning, appears to be highly sensitive to hippocampal damage and has been widely used and verified with a substantial number of controls (7,34,37). For these reasons, we chose this test as a standard technique to assess hippocampal-related memory function, before and after lesions and with treatment paradigms. There are also significant internal controls that have been developed within our laboratory for Fischer 344 animals of various ages and with a variety of lesions.

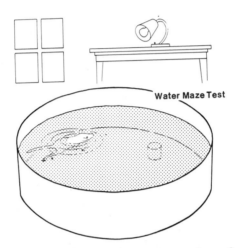

Fig. 2. A diagram of the water maze testing of the rats. The animals were tested for forty trials and the route and time to escape were tracked and logged. The goal of the test was escape onto a platform.

The water maze pool was circular, 150 cm in diameter and 28 cm high (Fig. 2) and the water was darkened with food coloring. The pool was located in a room with several external cues, including a window, a cage and ceiling light. The positive goal of the test was escape from the cold water (approximately 26°C) into the warmer atmosphere. The testing paradigm included the use of both a hidden platform (100 cm^2, just below the water surface) and a visible platform of the same size, with a center pole. The pool was divided into four quadrants and the platform was located at the center of one of the quadrants for the testing of acquisition during a series of trials. The entry point into the water was randomized to any of four points around the circumference of the pool. The behavioral testing was performed on five consecutive days, with a total of eight trials each day. The rats swam until they either found the platform or reached a maximum swim time of 60 s, with 30 s spent on the platform between two trials. Escape latency was measured with a stopwatch and the animal's

trajectory was recorded on diagrams of the pool. The mean escape times were
calculated from all forty trials (7).

Neural Grafting

The procedures for preparation and grafting of fetal hippocampal and
cerebellar tissue were similar to those described by Bjorklund et al. (38),
Ransom et al. (47) and Sunde & Zimmer (44). The timing of the graft
placement into the lesioned host was planned to have the grafts placed
within approximately two to four weeks after the completion of the NMDA
infusion or kainic acid injection. This planned timing allowed a stable
period after the completion of the infusion, during which the behavioral
testing could be performed. Fig. 3 shows a diagram of the technique.

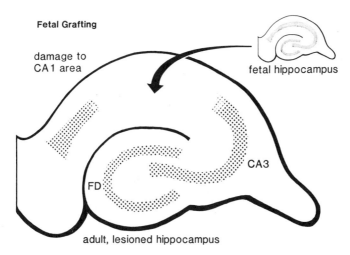

Fig. 3. The neural grafting protocol involved the technique
        of chunk grafting into the lateral ventricle, to
        replace circuitry in the lesioned area of the CA1
        region of the hippocampus.

The 18-19 day rat feti were taken from timed pregnant Fischer 344 rats.
The feti were removed from the uterine horns and placed into a sterile petri
dish containing nutrient tissue medium, kept on ice (47). The brain and
then either the hippocampus or cerebellum was dissected free under
magnification, through a posterior approach. Cerebellar tissue was easier
to separate from the CNS than the hippocampus and was used as control
tissue. The volume of tissue transplanted into each hippocampus was 7-12
μl, drawn up through a metal needle using a micropipet device, and then
stereotactically placed. After finishing the grafting procedure on five
animals (about 2.5 hr), the remainder of the fetal tissue was incubated

using tissue culture, in order to determine both survival of the grafting tissue and the sterility of the procedure.

One of the goals of the graft evaluation was to perform intracellular recording of the neural grafts and adjacent hippocampus, using slices of the hippocampus (10,41,48,49). For this reason, the fetal grafts were placed as separate tissue chunks, adjacent to the CA1 area of the hippocampus (coordinates P 4.0, RL 5.0, D 5.0). These chunks were placed within the ventricle using a metal cannula with a tight fitting plunger,to ensure tissue placement. The cannula was withdrawn over the plunger after the graft was in place. In addition, the lateral ventricle in rats provided a suitable bed for the maintenance of the neural graft (38).

Animals were followed at three month intervals after the grafting with water maze testing, to assess for any changes in either the acquisition or

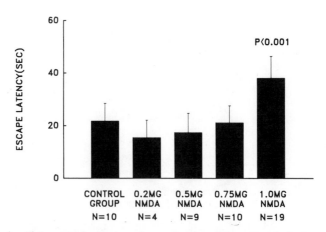

Fig. 4. This graph shows the relationship of total dosage of NMDA to the behavioral effects, as tested with the water maze protocol. Animals with the 1.0 mg dose were significantly impaired.

retention of spatial memory. At various point these animals were sacrificed for either histology or for physiological recording from the grafts.

RESULTS

Behavioral Assessment and Excitotoxin Dosage

NMDA has been suggested as a useful agent for the production of localized,

axon-sparing lesions, mediated presumably through an excitotoxic action,
similar to kainic acid (36). The reported acute intraventricular dose of
NMDA for a localized CA1 region lesion was 1.36 μM, equivalent to 0.2 mg
NMDA. This amount of NMDA was chosen as a starting dose for the chronic
infusion over two weeks. However, this dosage did not lead to permanent
memory deficit, as evaluated by the Morris water maze test. Thus, the
dosages were gradually increased from a total of 0.2 mg, to 0.5, 0.75 and
1.0 mg total dose. The effects of varying dosage on permanent spatial
memory deficit (for the acquisition of escape from new platform locations)
is presented in Fig. 4. The only group with a statistical difference in
memory acquisition, compared to controls, was the 1.0 mg total dose group.
The NMDA did not produce any acute toxic effects at this dose, though the
animals tended to lose weight and to be less well groomed over the period of

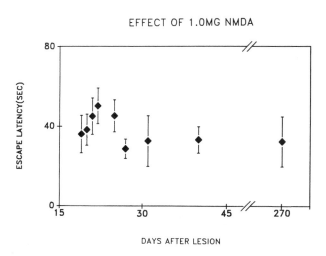

Fig. 5. Stability of NMDA Lesion, as demonstrated by the
behavioral evaluation as a function of time after
the infusion. The lesion may be progressive early
but then appears to be stable to nine months.

observation. In contrast, the kainic acid treated animals did not demonstrate any behavioral deficit, probably due to the restricted hippocampal
damage (36,46).

We evaluated the stability of the lesion effects with the behavioral
testing for the 1.0 mg NMDA group. Different groups of lesioned animals
were tested, beginning at 19 days after completion of the pump infusion
through nine months afterwards (Fig. 5). The only trend in the behavioral
results was that the behavioral impairment effects tended to increase
gradually, and that there was a slight elevation of the escape time in the
animals tested between days 25 and 27 after the completion of the infusion.

The additional long term evaluation shown in Fig. 5 also indicates that the behavioral effects of the NMDA lesion were stable with time, with a trend towards worsening in the behavioral assessment rather than recovery.

Histological Evaluation

The neurotoxic effects of the NMDA infusion were concentrated in the CA1 region of the hippocampus, particularly on the side of the intraventric-

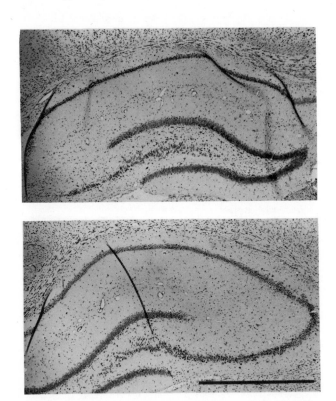

Fig. 6. The NMDA hippocampal lesion mainly involved the CA1 area of the hippocampus, shown on the right in the upper photograph and on the left in the lower illustration. The scale is 1 mm.

ular cannula (Fig. 6). Additional areas of damage included the dentate gyrus, predominantly on the side of the cannula and the medial septal area. In these areas, both pyknotic cells and tissue loss were noted, as early as 30 days after the completion of the infusion of the NMDA. The localization of the lesion was similar to that of increased density of postsynaptic NMDA receptors in the periventricular regions in the rodent CNS (50,51). In some animals there were also additional areas of cell loss in the lateral neocortex, particularly the entorhinal cortex. The areas of damage with the NMDA infusion resembled the topography of regions with high density of NMDA receptors using autoradiography of glutamate receptor subtypes. Thus, the NMDA exhibited some selectivity in terms of the pattern of cell damage.

In contrast, the kainic acid lesions demonstrated only CA3 field damage, ipsilateral to the intraventricular injection (36,46). Both the NMDA and kainic acid cell loss patterns appeared to be histologically stable with time, up to nine months.

Neural Grafting Observations

The grafting procedure involved the bilateral placement of chunk grafts of fetal hippocampus, similar to previous technical descriptions of neural grafting procedures (8,38,39). Because the lateral ventricle offers a cerebrospinal-fluid filled space adjacent to the hippocampal formation, CSF may act as a nutrient medium for the donor graft tissue, prior to vascularization of the tissue. Moreover, since one of the analytic techniques was to evaluate the grafts physiologically in brain slices, fetal hippocampal chunks may be more easily identified on hippocampal slice sections. However, an initial series of grafts did not survive histologically, so a systematic approach to ensure tissue viability was undertaken.

The fetal neural tissue was placed in chilled nutrient media, similar to that used for tissue culture preparations, after dissection from the whole fetus. After placement of grafts into several animals (elapsed time 2.5 hr), the remaining tissue was incubated for culture, with only mild mechanical dissociation. Fig. 7 shows an example of a hippocampal neuron, after 12 days of tissue culture growth, which shows a typical bright soma and extensive dendritic tree (47). Thus, for the majority of the grafting procedures both tissue viability and sterility of the grafted tissue appeared to be excellent.

Though the graft data are preliminary, several animals were sacrificed early, within six weeks of the grafting, to assess graft integration (44). Fig. 8 shows an example of a portion of the hippocampal graft, which was located near the hippocampus. There are numerous surviving neurons within the graft, though the location is not ideal. Fig. 8 is representative of the grafts examined to this point. Thus, both the placement and integrity

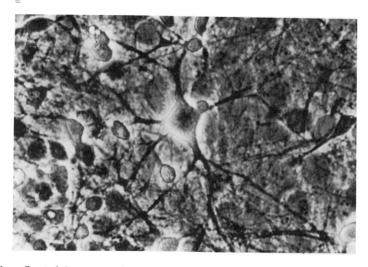

Fig. 7. A hippocampal neuron from tissue culture, which was plated after the remainder of the tissue was used for grafting. Scale shows 50 μm.

of the graft may be improved, through such techniques as attempting to place less volume and adjusting coordinates.

Graft integration will be further assessed with identifying synaptic interconnections physiologically, using an *in vitro* brain slice approach (49). The intracellular recording technique will also be used for Lucifer yellow dye injection, to stain neuron processes. This will allow a very sensitive method to detect graft - host interconnections, by visualizing axon collaterals. Thus, the functional relationship of the fetal hippocampal graft to the host will be assessed by several different methods (39).

DISCUSSION

Characterization of the Excitotoxic Model

The preliminary work with the chronic NMDA infusion model presented here has demonstrated a consistent pattern of behavioral alterations in spatial memory and histological damage to the CA1 area of the hippocampus and medial septum. Because of the slow infusion rate, a higher total dose was required for these effects, as compared to an acute intraventricular infusion (36). However, the slower rate has also resulted in bilateral damage to the hippocampus, and additional areas of involvement, such as the medial septal nucleus. As shown in Fig. 5, the lesion and the behavioral abnormalities also appear to be stable with time. Thus, in spite of the absence of a causal relationship to Alzheimer's disease, this model possesses certain validating properties in terms of the pattern and expression of abnormalities. Long-term survival studies may also show the critical neuropathological features of the disease, such as plaques and tangles (52), which have also been partly reproduced by a cholinergic destruction model (12). In many respects this model is a partial model of the dementia aspect of Guam ALS-Parkinson's-Dementia complex (32).

Since the medial septal nucleus exhibits partial damage, there may be

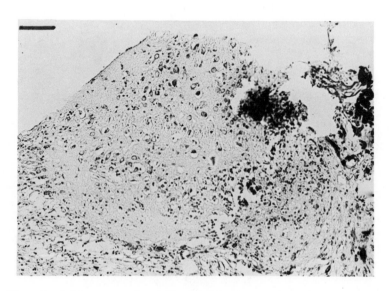

Fig. 8. A hippocampal graft, which shows partial connection to the host hippocampus and multiple surviving neurons. Scale is 100 μm.

at least a cholinergic deficit underlying the spatial memory deficit (7). The characterization of this deficit will require analysis with presynaptic markers for the synthesizing enzyme as well as receptor labelling. If the cholinergic deficit is notable, then fetal septal grafts (rather than hippocampal grafts) may have a role in recovery from the memory deficit, to augment cholinergic function in the hippocampus.

Additional techniques that may help in the characterization of this model include glutamate receptor studies, to confirm primary changes in the NMDA receptor population following the damage or the presence of secondary alterations. In addition to intracellular recording and the physiological assessment of synaptic interconnection between the graft and host (10,39,41), there are other anatomical techniques for evaluating the integration of the graft into the host circuitry (43,45). Additional pharmacological treatment strategies could also be tried with a stable model, such as glutamate enhancement techniques (23). The model could also be extended with an orally-acting excitotoxic agent, such as L-BMAA (32), but which would have primary cortex and hippocampus involvement, rather than spinal cord damage. Thus, there are many directions for further evaluation and extension of this model, particularly if predictive validation could be achieved for treatment paradigms, including neural grafting.

Rationale of the Excitotoxic Model

The cholinergic hypothesis, formulated several years ago (1), pointed to the importance of the cholinergic deficit in the brains of patients with Alzheimer's disease. The learning and memory impairment modeled by an induced cholinergic deficit attracted considerable interest and a number of models are still very important in evaluating this aspect of Alzheimer's disease (4,5,6,12,13,14). However, these models have not proven to be predictive in terms of therapy of patients with Alzheimer's disease, at least with current cholinergic agents (6). Thus, the dissociation between the behavioral response of the animal models to pharmacological manipulation of the cholinergic system and the clinical response may be interpreted in several ways. One way is to examine more closely the spectrum of damage to the cortex and subcortical structures in patients with early Alzheimer's disease, which indicates involvement at both levels, but primarily cortical damage (2,3,18,22,23,25,29,32).

Recently, considerable attention has been directed towards the role of glutaminergic neurotransmission in Alzheimer's disease (18,22,25). The hippocampal formation has been identified as a primary target for Alzheimer's disease, both pathologically and symptomatically, due to the early difficulties with memory in the disease (2,18,31). The current excitotoxic model follows newer hypotheses of primary cortical abnormalities underlying Alzheimer's disease, which may be expressed as alterations in glutamate-mediated synaptic transmission (3,53). The hippocampus may be primarily affected because of the higher density of glutamate receptors, particularly the NMDA class, though the etiology remains unknown. The chronic NMDA infusion of the current model recreates the areas of damage identified from patients, but the etiology remains elusive. Likewise, the memory loss resulting from the hippocampal damage (rather than cholinergic damage alone) may be similar to memory changes noted in patients with the disease. Thus, the NMDA infusion model recreates many of the manifestations reported with early Alzheimer's patients, including the behavioral aspects of memory loss, the pattern of damage in the hippocampus and septum and the loss of neurons with postsynaptic NMDA receptors.

Implications of Loss of Neurons with NMDA Receptors

The function of the NMDA glutamate receptor in the cortex has recently come under considerable scrutiny (22,24,27,35). This receptor possesses special properties, in terms of voltage-sensitivity and calcium influx, which have been implicated in a number of paradigms of learning. There appears to be close association between the high density of NMDA receptors in the CA1 region of the hippocampus (51) and the involvement of these receptors in the spatial learning paradigm in the rat (34). The loss of neurons with NMDA receptors, due to a sensitivity to exogenous toxins (30) thus may have considerable impact on short-term, post-distraction memory (31). Likewise, the pharmacological blockade of NMDA receptors may also impair memory (34,54), creating difficulty in the use of NMDA antagonists for prevention of the excitotoxic damage. Thus, a global loss of neurons with this class of glutamate receptors may have considerable impact on both treatment and symptomatic considerations, as well as plasticity of the CNS.

ACKNOWLEDGEMENTS

This work was supported by grants from the B.S. Turner Foundation, the Veterans Affairs Medical Research Service and the Alzheimer's Disease and Related Disorders Association. We wish to thank Charles Weber and Judy Landry for expert technical assistance. Dr. Dong is a visiting scholar from the Department of Neurobiology, Institute of Acupuncture Research, Shangai Medical University, Shanghai, People's Republic of China.

Address correspondence to: Dennis A. Turner, M.D.
                               Neurosurgery, 112N
                               VA Medical Center
                               54th St. and 48th Ave. S
                               Minneapolis, MN 55417

REFERENCES

1. Bartus, R. T., Dean, R. L., Beer, B. and Lippa, A. S. (1982) The cholinergic hypothesis of geriatric memory dysfunction. Science 217:408-417.

2. Hyman, B. T., Van Hoesen, G. W., Damasio, A. R. and Barnes, C. L. (1984) Alzheimer's disease: Cell-specific pathology isolates the hippocampal formation. Science 225:1168-1170.

3. Maragos, W. F., Greenamyre, J. T., Penney, J. B. and Young, A. B. (1987) Glutamate dysfunction in Alzheimer's disease: An hypothesis. TINS 10:65-68.

4. Perry, E. (1988) Acetylcholine and Alzheimer's disease. British J. Psychiatry 152:737-740.

5. Smith, G. (1988) Animal models of Alzheimer's disease: experimental cholinergic denervation. Brain Res. Rev. 13:103-118.

6. Wilcock, G. K. (1988) Alzheimer's disease - current issues. Quarterly J. Med. Series 66, No. 250, pp 117-124.

7. Gage, F. H. and Bjorklund, A. (1986) Cholinergic septal grafts into the hippocampal formation improve spatial learning and memory in aged rats by an atropine-sensitive mechanism. J. Neuroscience 6:2837-2847.

8. Gage, F. H. and Bjorklund, A. (1986) Neural grafting in the aged rat brain. Annual Review of Physiology 48:447-459.

9.   Gage, F. H., Bjorklund, A., Stenevi, U., Dunnett, S. B. and Kelly, P. A. T. (1984) Intrahippocampal septal grafts ameliorate learning impairments in aged rats. Science 225:533-536.

10. Mudrick, L. A., Baimbridge, K. G. and Miller, J. J. (1987) Fetal hippocampal cells transplanted into the ischemically damaged CA1 region demonstrate normal characteristics of adult CA1 cells. Neuroscience Abstracts 13:514.

11. Woodruff, M. L., Baisden, R. H., Whittington, D. L., Shelton, N. L. and Wray, S. (1988) Grafts containing fetal hippocampal tissue reduce activity and improve passive avoidance in hippocampectomized or trimethyltin-exposed rats. Exp. Neurol. 102:130-143.

12. Arendash, G. W., Millard, W. J., Dunn, A. J. and Meyer, E. M. (1987) Long-term neuropathological and neurochemical effects of nucleus basalis lesions in the rat. Science 238:952-956.

13. Beninger, R. J., Jhamandas, K., Boegman, R.J. and El-Defrawy, S. R. (1986) Kynurenic acid-induced protection of neurochemical and behavioral deficits produced by quinolinic acid injections into the nucleus basalis of rats. Neuroscience Letters, 68:317-321.

14. Flicker, C., Dean, R. L., Watkins, D. L., Fisher, S. K. and Bartus, R. T. (1983) Behavioral and neurochemical effects following neurotoxic lesions of a major cholinergic input to the cerebral cortex in the rat. Pharmcol. Biochem. Behav. 18:973-981.

15. Segal, M. and Milgram, N. W. (1985) Can septal grafting facilitate recovery from physiological and behavioral deficits produced by fornix transections? In: Neural Grafting (ed: Bjorklund, A.), Elsevier, Amsterdam, pp. 627-637.

16. Tilson, H. A., McLamb, R. L., Shaw, S., Rogers, B.C. Pediaditakis, P. and Cook, L. (1988) Radial-arm maze deficits produced by colchicine administered into the area of the nucleus basalis are ameliorated by cholinergic agents. Brain Res. 438:83-94.

17. Wenk, G. L. and Olton, D. S. (1984) Recovery of neocortical choline acetyltransferase activity following ibotenic acid injection into the nucleus basalis Meynert in rats. Brain Res. 293:184-186.

18. Cotman, C. W. and Anderson, K. J. (1988) Synaptic plasticity and functional stabilization in the hippocampal formation: possible role in Alzheimer's disease. In: Advances in Neurology, Vol. 47, Functional Recovery in Neurological Disease (ed: Waxman, S.G.), Raven, New York, pp. 313-335.

19. Perry, E. K. and Perry, R. H. (1985) New insights into the nature of senile (Alzheimer-type) plaques. TINS 8:301-303.

20. Summers, W. K., Majovski, L. V., Marsh, G. M., Tachiki, K. and Kling, A. (1986) Oral tetrahydroaminoacridine in long-term treatment of senile dementia, Alzheimer type. NEJM 315:1241-1245.

21. Wilcock, G. K. and Esiri, M. M. (1982) Plaques, tangles and dementia: A quantitative study. J. Neurol. Sciences 56:343-356.

22. Bridges, R. J., Geddes, J. W., Monaghan, D. T. and Cotman, C. W. (1988) Excitatory amino acid receptors in Alzheimer's disease. In: Excitatory Amino Acids in Health and Disease (ed: Lodge, D.), John Wiley and Sons, New York, pp. 321-335.

23. Deutsch, S. I. and Morihisa, J. M. (1988) Glutamatergic abnormalities in Alzheimer's disease and a rationale for clinical trials with L-glutamate. Clinical Neuropharmacology 11:18-35.

24. Fagg, G. E., Foster, A. C. and Ganong, A. H. (1986) Excitatory amino acid synaptic mechanisms and neurological function. TIPS 7:357-363.

25. Greenamyre, J. T., Maragos, W. F., Albin, R. L., Penney, J. B. and Young, A. B. (1988) Glutamate transmission and toxicity in Alzheimer's disease. Prog. Neuro-Psychopharmacol. and Biol. Psychiat. 12:421-430.

26. Greenamyre, J. T., Penney, J. B., D'Amato, C. J. and Young, A. B. (1987) Dementia of the Alzheimer's type: changes in hippocampal L-[^{3}H] glutamate binding. J. Neurochem. 48:543-551.

27. Lester, R. A. J., Herron, C. E., Coan, E. J. and Collingridge, G. L. (1988) The role of NMDA receptors in synaptic plasticity and transmission in the hippocampus. In: Excitatory Amino Acids in Health and Disease (ed: Lodge, D.), John Wiley and Sons, New York, pp. 275-295.

28. Rothman, S. M. and Olney, J. W. (1987) Excitotoxicity and the NMDA receptor. TINS 10:299-302.

29. Simpson, M. D. C., Royston, M. C., Deakin, J. F. W., Cross, A. J., Mann, D. M. A. and Slater, P. (1988) Regional Changes in [^{3}H] D-aspartate and [^{3}H] TCP binding sites in Alzheimer's disease brains. Brain Res. 462:76-82.

30. Spencer, P. S., Nunn, P. B., Hugon, J., Ludolph, A. C., Ross, S. M., Roy, D. N. and Robertson, R. C. (1987) Guam amyotrophic lateral sclerosis-Parkinsonism-dementia linked to a plant excitant neurotoxin. Science 237:517-522.

31. Squire, L. R. (1986) Mechanisms of memory. Science 232:1612-1619.

32. Spencer P. S. (1987) Guam ALS/Parkinsonism-Dementia: A long-latency neurotoxic disorder caused by "slow toxin(s)" in food? Can. J. Neurol. Sci. 14:347-357.

33. Morris, R. G. M., Garrud, P., Rawlins, J. N. P. and O'Keefe, J. (1982) Place navigation impaired in rats with hippocampal lesions. Nature 297:681-683.

34. Morris, R. G. M., Anderson, E., Lynch, G. S. and Baudry, M. (1986) Selective impairment of learning and blockade of long term potentiation by an N-methyl-D-aspartate receptor antagonist, AP5. Nature 319:774-776.

35. Morris, R. G. M. (1988) Elements of a hypothesis concerning the participation of hippocampal NMDA receptors in learning. In: Excitatory Amino Acids in Health and Disease (ed: Lodge, D.), John Wiley and Sons, New York, pp. 297-320.

36. Nadler, J. V., Evenson, D. A. and Cuthbertson, G. J. (1981) Comparative toxicity of kainic acid and other acidic amino acids towards rat hippocampal neurons. Neuroscience 6:2505-2517.

37. Morris, R. G. M. (1984) Development of a water-maze procedure for studying spatial learning in the rat. J. Neuroscience Methods 11:47-60.

38. Bjorklund, A., Stenevi, U., Schmidt, R. H., Dunnett, S. B. and Gage, F. H. (1983) Intracerebral grafting of neuronal cell suspensions 1. Introduction and general methods of preparation. Acta. Physiol. Scand. 522:1-7.

39. Buzsaki, G., Czopf, J., Kondakor, I., Bjorklund, A. and Gage, F. H. (1987) Cellular activity of intracerebrally transplanted fetal hippocampus during behavior. Neuroscience 22:871-883.

40. Gash, D. M. (1987) Neural transplantation: potential therapy for Alzheimer's disease. J. Neural Transm.[suppl] 24:301-308.

41. Hounsgaard, J. and Yarom, Y. (1985) Intrinsic control of electroresponsive properties of transplanted mammalian brain neurons. Brain Res. 335:372-376.

42. Kimble, D. P., Bremiller, R. and Stickrod, G. (1986) Fetal brain implants improve maze performance in hippocampal-lesioned rats. Brain Res. 363:358-363.

43. Raisman, G. and Ebner, F. F. (1983) Mossy fibre projections into and out of hippocampal transplants. Neuroscience 9:783-801.

44. Sunde, N. A. and Zimmer, J. (1983) Cellular, histochemical and connective organization of the hippocampus and fascia dentata transplanted to different regions of immature and adult rat brains. Develop. Brain Res. 8:165-191.

45. Tonder, N., Sorensen, J. C., Bakkum, E., Danielsen, E. and Zimmer, J. (1988) Hippocampal neurons grafted to newborn rats establish efferent commissural connections. Exp. Brain Res. 72:577-583.

46. Lancaster, B. and Wheal, H. V. (1982) A comparative histological and electrophysiological study of some neurotoxins in the rat hippocampus. J. Comp. Neurol. 211:105-114.

47. Ransom, B. R., Neale, E., Henkart, M., Bullock, P. N. and Nelson, P. G. (1977) Mouse spinal cord in cell culture. I. Morphology and intrinsic neuronal electrophysiologic properties. J. Neurophysiol. 40:1132-1150.

48. Reece, L. J. and Schwartzkroin, P. A. (1987) Electrophysiology of morphologically identified septal neurons grafted into rat hippocampus. Neuroscience Abstracts 13:160.

49. Turner, D. A. (1988) Waveform and amplitude characteristics of evoked responses to dendritic stimulation in CA1 guinea-pig pyramidal cells. J. Physiology (London) 395:419-439.

50. Cotman, C. W., Monaghan, D. T., Ottersen, O. P. and Storm-Mathisen, J. (1987) Anatomical organization of excitatory amino acid receptors and their pathways. TINS 10:273-280.

51. Greenamyre, J. T., Young, A. B. and Penney, J. B. (1984) Quantitative autoradiographic distribution of L-[^{3}H]-glutamate-binding sites in rat central nervous system. J. Neurosci. 4:2133-2144.

52. Davies, P. (1988) Neurochemical studies: An update on Alzheimer's disease. J. Clin. Psychiatry 49:23-28.

53. Cowburn, R., Hardy, J., Roberts, P. and Briggs, R. (1988) Regional distribution of pre- and postsynaptic glutaminergic function in Alzheimer's disease. Brain Res. 452:403-407.

54. Danysz, W., Wroblewski, J. T. and Costa, E. (1988) Learning impairment in rats by N-Methyl-D-Aspartate Receptor Antagonists. Neuropharmacology 27:653-656.

EXCITOTOXIN MEDIATED NEURONAL LOSS AND THE REGULATION OF EXCITATORY AMINO

ACID RELEASE IN THE AGING BRAIN

Ralph Dawson Jr., Michael J. Meldrum and David R. Wallace

Department of Pharmacodynamics, College of Pharmacy
University of Florida, JHMHC Box J-487
Gainesville, FL 32610

INTRODUCTION AND OVERVIEW OF EXCITATORY AMINO ACIDS AND AGING

The aging brain is characterized by a decrease in weight and concomitant loss of neurons[1,2]. The exact causes and mechanisms for neuronal
loss in aging and age-related neurodegenerative diseases are largely
unknown. Recent studies have shown that in ischemic, hypoxic and hypogly-
cemic-induced neuronal loss, the necrotic changes are due to an excess
release of excitatory amino acids (glutamate, GLU: aspartate, ASP:
etc.)[3,4,5]. The ability of competitive and noncompetitive antagonists to
block or ameliorate neuronal cell death induced by excitatory amino acids
has further served to confirm the specificity and importance of receptor-
mediated excitotoxicity[6,7,8]. Therefore, in the central nervous system
excessive or unregulated release of excitatory amino acids appears to be a
predominate mechanism mediating neuronal death.

There are a number of endogenous compounds with excitotoxic potential
(GLU, ASP, cysteine, quinolinic acid, n-acetyl-ASP-GLU etc.)[9,10,11] and
several environmental excitotoxins (aspartame, ß-N-methylamino-L-alanine,
ß-N-oxalyamino-L-alanine)[12,13]. A number of recent review articles have
suggested a role for excitotoxins in neurodegenerative disorders such as
Huntington's disease, Alzheimer's disease (AD), amyotrophic lateral
sclerosis, Parkinson's disease and olivopontocerebellar degeneration[14-17].
AD has received particular attention since a number of markers for
glutaminergic function are decreased in postmortem tissues from AD
patients[18,19,20]. Reductions in GLU content, [^{3}H]-D-ASP uptake and n-methyl-
D-aspartate (NMDA) receptors have all been reported in AD patients most
notably in hippocampus and temporal cortex[18,19,20]. The recent data on the
role of GLU in long-term potentiation and memory function[21] draws further
intriguing parallels with the functional deficits seen in AD. Thus,
excitotoxin-mediated neuronal death may contribute to age-related neuronal
loss and could be an etiologic factor in age-related dementias such as AD.

GLU and ASP are the major excitatory neurotransmitters in the
mammalian brain. Therefore, a detailed understanding of their regulation
is important to our understanding of CNS function. GLU/ASP are thought to
be the transmitters utilized in cortical association pathways, the
corticostriate pathway, the perforant pathway and many other major
intrinsic and extrinsic cortical and subcortical projection systems[17]. The
release and reuptake mechanisms for GLU/ASP and other excitatory amino

acids are not completely understood but may differ among specific brain regions[22]. For example presynaptic modulation of GLU release by kainic acid is present in the cerebellum and hippocampus[23] but is absent in the frontal cortex[24]. Complete comparative data are not available on regional differences in the inhibitory modulation of glutamate release by adenosine (A_1) serotonergic, muscarinic (M_2), adrenergic (α_2), GABAergic, or dopaminergic (D_2) receptors although presynaptic modulation has been reported. It is also of interest that many of the presynaptic heteroreceptors that are known to inhibit GLU release are also decreased in the aged brain and Alzheimer's disease[25] which may suggest a link between the two. Moreover, calcium dependent release of neurotransmitters in general may be altered in the aged brain due to age-related deficits in calcium uptake and sequestration within the nerve terminal which are known to occur[26]. These age-related deficits point to the need for a careful examination of neurochemical mechanisms governing the release and modulation of excitatory amino acids in the aged brain, especially in light of their neurotoxic potential.

As previously mentioned, a number of different endogenous excitatory amino acids or small peptides may function as neurotransmitters. The relative amount or proportion of excitatory amino acids released from nerve terminals may change based on the energy demand of the neuron. For example, Szerb[30] has shown that ASP release increases and GLU release decreases under hypoglycemic conditions. Much work needs to be done to specifically identify the exact excitatory transmitter released from specific neuronal pathways. Thus, heterogeneity may exist in the type of excitatory amino acid released from nerve terminals (GLU, ASP, CYS, etc.), the specific transporter responsible for reuptake (Na^+ versus Cl^- dependent) and the degree or type of presynaptic modulation. This anatomical and biochemical heterogeneity is reflected by the multiple postsynaptic receptor subtypes that exist for the excitatory amino acids and the diversity of second messenger coupling for the various receptor subtypes[28,29]. In addition to the regional variation in receptor subtypes, transport processes and specific type of amino acid released, there are also multiple pools of excitatory amino acids. A neuronal pool and a glial pool of excitatory amino acids exist as well as the neurotransmitter and metabolic pools[30]. Our lack of knowledge of the control of excitatory amino acid neurotransmitters is at least in part due to the difficulties imposed by these same amino acids being involved in cellular metabolic activities. This can make the study of the various pools complicated since the metabolic and neurotransmitter pools are interrelated.

A number of biochemical alterations could lead to excitotoxin mediated neuronal death. Specific presynaptic and postsynaptic deficits in excitatory amino acid metabolism or neurotransmitter function are given in Table 1 that could lead to excess extracellular concentrations of excitatory amino acids. Most documented accounts of excitotoxin-induced neuronal loss involve conditions such as hypoxia, anoxia, hypoglycemia or metabolic alterations that result in greatly diminished intracellular ATP levels and the concomitant collapse of cellular ionic gradients[31]. These conditions may also favor the calcium-independent efflux of amino acids such as GLU and ASP[32]. Excessive depolarization of neurons induced by the release of excitatory amino acid neurotransmitters can also deplete ATP levels and initiate calcium-independent release of GLU which could further depolarize the neuron and decrease ATP levels that would create a vicious cycle resulting in neuronal death. This hypothesis needs investigation since one or more of the deficits listed in Table 1 must occur for these events to proceed and one must assume normal regulatory or feedback mechanisms are compromised.

TABLE 1. Neurochemical Mechanisms Contributing to or Potentiating
Excitatory Amino Acid Induced Neurotoxicity

Mechanism	Anatomic Localization of Deficit: Presynaptic	Postsynaptic
1. Decreased uptake	nerve terminal	glia
2. Decreased inactivation	neuronal GLU dehydrogenase	glial glutamine synthetase
3. Enhanced synthesis	neuronal glutaminase	glial glutaminase
4. Blood-Brain-Barrier deficit	------------	endothelium
5. Increased receptor number	neuronal kainic acid receptors	neuronal NMDA and/or quisqualate receptors
6. Increased excitatory amino acid coupling/efficacy	neuronal	neuronal
7. Decreased GLU growth factor function	neuronal	neuronal
8. Excess Release	a) decreased inhibitory neuronal presynaptic receptors b) increased facilitory neuronal presynaptic receptors c) neuronal calcium independent release d) neuronal calcium dependent release	a) glial release from metabolic pool b) neuronal release from metabolic pool

GLU is released by neuronal depolarization in a calcium dependent exocytotic process[32]. GLU can also be released by a calcium independent process from the cytoplasmic pool which may involve the high affinity GLU transporter operating in reverse[33]. This depolarization induced reversal of this GLU transporter may provide a unique mechanism for amino acid transmitter release[33]. Depletion of intracellular energy stores and/or the neuronal transmembrane sodium gradient has been shown to facilitate calcium independent GLU release[32] possibly through this transporter-reversal mechanism[33]. The neuronal-glial glutamine (GLN) cycle is thought to play a major role in regulating GLU release since GLN appears to be the predominant precursor to neurotransmitter GLU[30]. Inhibition of glutaminase inhibits GLU release whereas GLN precursor loading augments GLU release[30]. Therefore GLN appears to play a central role in regulating GLU synthesis although precursor dependence may shift during pathophysiological conditions[30,34]. Glucose and tricarboxylic acid cycle intermediates can also serve as precursors for transmitter GLU when GLN levels are depleted. Thus, neuronal energy metabolism and excitatory amino acid metabolism and release are intimately interrelated[35]. Age-related deficits in neuronal energy metabolism or calcium handling could lead to alterations in the release of excitatory amino acids[35]. Therefore, it is important to examine the mechanisms regulating excitatory amino acid release as well as those processes which may modulate this release.

STUDIES OF IN VIVO AND IN VITRO EXCITATORY AMINO ACID RELEASE IN THE AGED RAT BRAIN

Systemic or intracerebral administration of kainic acid has been shown to elicit severe convulsions and evoke significant depletions of brain monoamines[36,37]. These depletions in the stores of neurotransmitters are thought to reflect the excessive release of neurotransmitters induced by the excitatory actions of kainic acid[36]. We have explored this action of kainic acid in aged (30 month old) and adult (6 month) female Long-Evans rats. The neurochemical effects of 15 mg/kg of kainic acid administered i.p. are given in Table 2. This dose of kainic acid produced seizures in 7 out of 7 of the aged rats and no clonic-tonic seizures in the adult rats. All rats were terminated for neurochemical evaluation 2 hours after kainic acid administration. The data clearly indicate that transmitter and brain regional differences exist in the action of kainic acid. ASP and NE are markedly reduced in the entorhinal and frontal cortices of aged rats whereas this dose had no significant effect in the adult rats. Neurotransmitter content was not altered in the caudate of either adult or aged rats. This study suggests that the facilitory presynaptic mediation of ASP release by kainic acid may be altered in aging. It is of interest to note that GLU content was not altered by kainic acid in these brain regions. These data are in agreement with in vitro data that show preferential release of ASP by kainic acid in brain slices[23,38].

TABLE 2. Effects of Systemic Kainic Acid on Neurotransmitter Content in Adult and Aged Rats

Brain Region	ASP	GLN	GLU	NE	5-HT
Entorhinal Cortex					
Adult-Control	2.51±0.14	5.13±0.59	13.92±1.12	334±21	317±37
Aged-Control	2.32±0.14	6.05±0.69	12.37±0.87	349±23	386±99
Adult-Kainate	2.16±0.25	5.46±0.49	13.74±0.83	259±39	361±25
Aged-Kainate	1.34±0.12*	7.93±0.77	10.30±0.65	131±17*	307±63
Frontal Cortex					
Adult-Control	2.54±0.27	4.18±0.19	12.47±0.46	223±21	262±33
Aged-Control	2.72±0.18	5.07±0.71	12.30±0.82	231± 7	226±26
Adult-Kainate	2.18±0.22	4.65±0.23	13.70±0.63	194±25	244±21
Aged-Kainate	1.85±0.06*	7.33±0.42*	11.86±0.49	134±14*	209±19
Caudate+					
Adult-Control	2.10±0.13	3.43±0.38	8.26±0.99	337±54	465±29
Aged-Control	1.77±0.09	4.50±0.43	6.04±0.42	272±52	387±47
Adult-Kainate	1.89±0.15	3.30±0.36	8.32±0.84	283±39	453±41
Aged-Kainate	1.50±0.11	4.20±0.52	7.97±1.01	191±15	396±22

Amino acid data expressed as μmole/g tissue wt. ± SE (n=6-10 per group)
Monoamine data expressed as ng/g tissue wt. ± SE (n=6-10 per group)
*$p<0.05$ Aged-Control versus Aged-Kainate
+Dopamine content was not altered in either adult or aged rats by kainic acid.

Amino acid transmitter release has also been compared in frontal cortex slices of adult (6 month) and aged (20-24 month) male Fisher 344 rats[24]. Of the 11 amino acids measured only GLU showed significant reproducible levels of stimulation induced release above basal levels. Although in a pilot study using slices from these same animals ASP release appeared to be elevated by high potassium in the aged animals but not significantly in adult animals (Fig. 1). The ASP data support the above in vivo data but must be considered preliminary because of the small number of rats tested and the variability in the basal release data. In contrast, GLU was released in a calcium dependent manner by incubation in buffer containing high potassium (56 mM) in both aged and adult rats. Endogenous GLU levels were increased approximately 4-5 fold over the basal release samples during the stimulation period. GLU stimulated release was however not significantly different between the adult and aged animals[24]. Similar release patterns and results were also seen when a K^+ concentration of 40 mM was used to stimulate release in adult and aged animals (unpublished observations). ^3H-GLU uptake was also examined in adult and aged F344 rats and found not to be different in slices of frontal cortex[24]. Similar experiments used frontal cortex slices loaded with ^3H-D-ASP to compare potassium stimulated release in adult and aged Fisher 344 rats. Potassium (40 mM) induced significant release of ^3H-D-ASP, although it produced only about a 2 fold increase above basal release. The level of ^3H-D-ASP release is different than that seen with endogenous GLU, an effect also reported for hippocampal slices[38]. This difference in levels of release may suggest some differences in the pools from which these amino acids are being released. Similar to endogenous GLU release stimulated ^3H-D-ASP release was not different between adult and 28 month old male Fisher 344 rats (unpublished observations). Kainic acid (1 mM) also failed to significantly stimulate either endogenous GLU or ^3H-D-ASP release from these cortical slices.

It is also of interest that in these frontal cortex slices like that seen in hippocampal slices, endogenous stimulated GLU release is highly Ca^{++} dependent (>95%). This is in contrast to GABA release which shows much less Ca^{++} dependency of release[39-41]. The potassium activation of

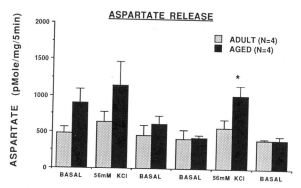

Fig. 1. Basal and KCl stimulated ASP release from slices of frontal cortex in adult (6 month) and aged (24 month) F344 rats. ASP release in aged rats was significantly (*p<0.05) higher than adults during the second KCl stimulation.

release is also of interest as relatively high concentrations of K⁺ are required to activate release from slices. In cortex (unpublished data), hippocampal[42] and cerebellar[43] slices the potassium activation response curves have shown that K⁺ concentrations of 20-30 mM show no significant release of GLU or ASP. KCl (40 mM) shows about a 3-4 fold increase in release and at 50-60 mM K⁺, amino acid release levels plateau. This level of K⁺ activation is in contrast to other neurotransmitter systems, like catecholamines, where significant activated release can be measured at 15-20 mM KCl. The significance of the high level of K⁺ required for amino acid transmitter release is not completely understood, although the data suggest more activation is required for amino acid transmitter release.

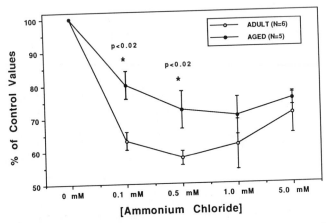

Fig. 2. Inhibition of PAG activity by ammonium chloride in adult (6 month) and aged (30 month) Sprague-Dawley rats. The inhibition of PAG by ammonium chloride was significantly (*p<0.02) attenuated in the aged rats relative to the adult control rats.

STUDIES OF GLUTAMINASE ACTIVITY IN AGED RATS

In addition to GLU release, the activity of glutaminase was assessed in both adult (6 month) and aged (30 month) male Sprague-Dawley rats. Glutaminase (L-glutamine amidohydrolase, EC 3.5.1.2) is the enzyme responsible for the formation of neurotransmitter GLU[44,45]. Glutaminase is strongly activated by phosphate, therefore it is referred to as phosphate-activated glutaminase, or PAG[46,47]. Ammonia is a potent inhibitor of PAG and it is also a product of the PAG hydrolysis of glutamine[48-51]. Ammonia inhibition of PAG activity was significantly attenuated in aged rats and this attenuation of PAG activity occurred within the physiological range of ammonia concentrations (100-500 μM) normally found within the brain (Fig. 2). This age-related deficit in PAG regulation may reflect an impaired ability of the aged brain to effectively remove ammonia from the CNS. Hence, these data suggest that the aged brain may have an increased production of both GLU and ammonia. This combination of increased GLU and increased ammonia may result in neuronal damage, or death, by a variety of mechanisms.

TABLE 3. Glutaminase Activity and GLU Content in Adult and Aged F-344
        Rats

Cortical Markers for GLU	Adult	Aged
GLU content	10.40 ± 0.43	8.89 ± 0.29*
Glutaminase Activity	26.64 ± 2.97	17.37 ± 2.36*

GLU content is expressed as μmole/g ± SE
Glutaminase activity is expressed as nmole GLU/mg protein/min ± SE.
n=7-8 per group

Current studies are underway to determine the regional activity of
PAG in 8 month and 28 month old Fischer-344 rats. Early indications are
that differences do exist between adult and aged rats. In the temporal
cortex, PAG activity in aged rats is significantly ($p<0.05$) reduced by 35%
which correlates well with decreased GLU content in the cortex (Table 3).
Further studies of PAG kinetics and regulation are currently being
performed in the cortex, striatum and hippocampus. The decreased PAG
activity may reflect a loss of glutamatergic neurons or a decrease in PAG
activity to compensate for the deficit in ammonia feedback inhibition on
PAG activity. If there is a loss of glutamatergic neurons, then the
surviving glutamatergic neurons must increase their GLU release capacity
since GLU release is not decreased in the cortex of aged F344 rats[24].
Further studies are needed to clarify the role of changes in PAG activity
and the relationship to the neurotransmitter pool of GLU in the aging
brain.

It has previously been reported that glutaminase activity is reduced
in whole brain preparation from 24 month old Wistar rats[52]. Significant
reductions in low affinity GLU uptake and GLU metabolism have also been
reported in cortical slices of aged rats[53]. Mitochondrial uptake of GLU is
decreased in the aged brain as well as glutamate driven mitochondrial
respiratory function[54]. Our current findings and those of others suggest
that alterations in the metabolic pool of GLU do occur in aging. Age
associated changes in PAG activity or regulation may also impact on the
neurotransmitter function of GLU or the neurotoxic potential of endogenous
GLU in the aged brain.

CONCLUSIONS

The present studies have been an attempt to examine age-associated
changes in excitatory amino acid function. These studies suggest that
age-associated differences do exist in seizure sensitivity to kainic acid,
cortical content of ASP and GLU, and cortical glutaminase activity.
However, age associated differences in glutamate release were not seen in
frontal cortex slices. These data suggest that while some parameters of
amino acid neurotransmission show age-related changes, not all responses
are altered. Our findings are in accord with Bowen and coworkers[55,56] who
found no differences in stimulated GLU release in AD patients, but found
evidence of metabolic changes that reflect an alteration in cortical
glutamatergic neurons in AD. Our data and those of others do however
provide the basis for much further study especially in the areas of
neurotransmitter release modulation. Other intriguing questions also need
study, for example: the significance of the high degree of potassium

activation required for amino acid release; the ability of potassium activation to significantly release ASP in aged animals but not in adult animals; the significance of changes in activity of glutaminase, the enzyme which produces neurotransmitter glutamate. The question of localization of these changes within the brain also needs to be addressed. These are all questions that need careful examination and clarification before one can completely understand the role of excitatory amino acids in the aging process.

REFERENCES

1. H. Brody, Organization of the cerebral cortex. III. A study of aging in the human cortex, J. Comp. Neurol., 102:511-445 (1955).
2. M.E. Scheibal and A.B. Scheibal, Structural changes in the aging brain, in: "Aging", Vol. 1, H. Brody et al., eds., Raven Press, New York, (1975).
3. S.M. Rothman and J.W. Olney, Glutamate and the pathophysiology of hypoxic-ischemic brain damage, Ann. Neurol. 19:105-111 (1986).
4. H. Benveniste, J. Drajer, A. Schousebor, and N.H. Diemer, Elevation of the extracellular concentrations of glutamate and aspartate in rat hippocampus during transient cerebral ischemia monitored by intracerebral microdialysis, J. Neurochem. 43:1369-1374 (1984).
5. T. Wieloch, Hypoglycemia-induced neuronal damage prevented by an N-methyl-D-aspartate antagonist, Science 230:681-683 (1985).
6. M.P. Goldberg, J.H. Weiss, P. Pham, and D. Choi, N-methyl-D-aspartate receptors mediate hypoxic neuronal injury in cortical culture, J. Pharmacol. Exp. Ther. 243:784-791, (1987).
7. M.P. Goldberg, V. Viseskul, and D.W. Choi, Phencyclidine receptor ligands attenuate cortical neuronal injury after n-methyl-D-aspartate exposure or hypoxia, J. Pharmacol. Exp. Ther. 245:1081-1087 (1988).
8. R.P. Simon, J.W. Schmidley, B.S. Meldrum, J.H. Swan, and A.G. Chapman, Excitotoxic mechanisms in hypoglycemic hippocampal injury, Neuropathol. Appl. Neurobiol. 12:567-576 (1986).
9. J.S. Kizer, C.B. Nemeroff, and W.W. Youngblood, Neurotoxic amino acids and structurally related analogs, Pharmacol. Rev. 29:301-318 (1978).
10. T.W. Stone and J.H. Connick, Quinolinic acid and other kynurenines in the central nervous system, Neuroscience 15:597-617 (1985).
11. K.J. Koller, R. Zaczek, and J.T. Coyle, N-Acetyl-aspartyl-glutamate: regional levels in rat brain and the effects of brain lesions as determined by a new HPLC method. J. Neurochem. 43:1136-1142 (1984).
12. J.W. Olney, Excitotoxic food additives-relevance of animal studies to human safety, Neurobehav. Toxicol. Teratol., 6:455-462 (1984).
13. P.S. Spencer, P.B. Nunn, J. Hugon, A.C. Ludolph, S.M. Ross, D.N. Roy, and R.D. Robertson, Guam Amyotrophic lateral sclerosis-Parkinsonism-dementia linked to a plant excitant neurotoxin, Science 237:517-522, (1987).
14. B. Engelsen, Neurotransmitter glutamate: its clinical importance, Acta Neurol. Scand. 74:337-355 (1986).
15. W.F. Maragos, J.T. Greenamyre, J.B. Penny, and A.B. Young, Glutamate dysfunction in Alzheimer's disease: an hypothesis, Trends Neurosci. 10:65-68 (1987).
16. J.T. Greenamyre, The role of glutamate in neurotransmission and in neurologic disease, Arch. Neurol. 43:1058-1063 (1986).
17. M.B. Robinson and J.T. Coyle, Glutamate and related acidic excitatory neurotransmitters: from basic science to clinical application, FASEB J. 1:446-455, (1987).
18. R. Cowburn, J. Hardy, P. Roberts, and R. Briggs, Presynaptic and postsynaptic glutamatergic function in Alzheimer's disease, Neurosci. Lett. 86:109-113, (1988).

19. J.T. Greenamyre, W.F. Maragos, R.L. Albin, J.B. Penney, and A.B. Young, Glutamate transmission and toxicity in Alzheimer's disease, Prog. Neuro-Psychopharmacol. & Biol. Psychiat. 12:421-430, (1988).

20. S.I. Deutsch and J.M. Morihisa, Glutamatergic abnormalities in Alzheimer's disease and a rationale for clinical trials with L-glutamate, Clin. Neuropharmacol. 11:18-35 (1988).

21. G. Lynch, J. Larson, U. Staubli, and M. Baudry, New Perspectives on the physiology, chemistry, and pharmacology of memory, Drug Dev. Res. 10:295-315, (1987).

22. J. Ferkany and J.T. Coyle, Heterogeneity of sodium-dependent excitatory amino acid uptake mechanisms in rat brain. J. Neurosci. Res. 16:491-503 (1986).

23. J.W. Ferkany and J.T. Coyle, Kainic acid selectively stimulates the release of endogenous excitatory acidic amino acids, J. Neurosci. Res. 16:491-503.

24. R. Dawson, Jr., D.R. Wallace, and M.J. Meldrum, Endogenous glutamate release from frontal cortex of adult and aged rats. Neurobiol. Aging in press, (1989).

25. P.J. Whitehouse, Neurotransmitter receptor alterations in Alzheimer's disease: A review, Alzheimer Disease Assoc. Disorders 1:9-18 (1987).

26. G.E. Gibson and C. Peterson, Calcium and the aging nervous system, Neurobiol. Aging 8:329-343 (1987).

27. J. Storm-Mathison and O.P. Otterson, Localization of excitatory amino acid transmitters, in: "Excitatory Amino Acids in Health and Disease", D. Lodge ed., John Wiley & Sons, New York (1988).

28. A.C. Foster and G.E. Fogg, Acidic amino acid binding sites in mammalian neuronal membranes: Their characteristics and relationship to synaptic receptors, Brain Res. Rev. 7:103-164 (1984).

29. E. Costa, A. Guidotti, H. Manev, A.M. Szekely and J.T. Wroblewski, Signal transduction at excitatory amino acid receptors: modulation by gangliosides in: "Frontiers in Excitatory Amino Acid Research" Alan R. Liss, New York (1988).

30. J.C. Szerb, Rate-limiting steps in the synthesis of GABA and glutamate, in: "Neurotransmitters and Cortical Function", M. Avoli, T.A. Reader, R.W. Dykes and P. Glour eds., Plenum, New York (1988).

31. A. Novelli, J.A. Reilly, P.G. Lysko and R.C. Henneberry, Glutamate becomes neurotoxic via the N-methyl-D-aspartic receptor when intracellular energy levels are reduced, Brain Res. 451:205-212 (1988).

32. D.G. Nicholls, Release of glutamate, aspartate, and gama-aminobutyric acid from isolated nerve terminals, J. Neurochem. 52:331-341 (1989).

33. M. Erecinska, The neurotransmitter amino acid transport systems: A fresh outlook on an old problem. Biochem. Pharmacol. 36:3547-3555 (1987).

34. R. Simantov, Glutamate neurotoxicity in culture depends on the presence of glutamine: implications for the role of glial cells in normal and pathological brain development. J. Neurochem. 52:1684-1699 (1989).

35. R.A. Kauppinen, H.T. McMahon and D.G. Nicholls, Ca^{2+}-Dependent and Ca^{2+}-independent glutamate release, energy status and cytosolic free Ca^{2+} concentration in isolated nerve terminals following metabolic inhibition: possible relevance to hypoglycemia and anoxia. Neuroscience 27:175-182 (1988).

36. M.F. Nelson, R. Zacek and J.T. Coyle, Effects of sustained seizures produced by intrahippocampal injection of kainic acid on noradrenergic neurons: evidence for local control of norepinephrine release. J. Pharmacol. Exp. Therap. 214:694-702 (1980).

37. H. Baran, H. Lassman, G. Sperk, F. Seitelberger and O. Hornykiewiez, Effect of mannitol treatment on brain neurotransmitters markers in kainic acid-induced epilepsy. Neuroscience 21:679-684 (1987).

38. J.W. Farkany and J.T. Coyle, Evoked release of aspartate and glutamate: disparities between prelabeling and direct measurements, Brain Research 278:279 (1983).

39. C. Arias and R. Tapia, Differential calcium dependence of gamma-aminobutyric acid and acetylcholine release in mouse brain synaptosomes, J. Neurochem. 47:396 (1986).

40. J.W. Haycock, W.B. Levy, L.A. Denner, and C.W. Cotman, Effects of elevated K on the release of neurotransmitters from cortical synaptosomes: Efflux or secretion?, J. Neurochem. 30:1113 (1978).

41. J.C. Szerb, Relationship between Ca-dependent and independent release of [^{3}H]-GABA evoked by high K, veratridine or electrical stimulation from rat cortical slices, J. Neurochem. 32:1565 (1979).

42. S.D. Burke and J.U. Nadler, Regulation of glutamate and aspartate release from slices of the hippocampal Ca, area: effects of adenosine and baclofen, J. Neurochem. 51:1541 (1988).

43. S. Barnes and J.A. Davies, The effects of calcium channel agonists and antagonists on the release of endogenous glutamate from cerebellar slices, Neuroscience Letters 92:58 (1988).

44. A.C. Hamberger, G.H. Chiang, E.S. Nylen, S.W. Schett, and C.W. Cotman, Glutamate as a CNS transmitter. I. Evaluation of glucose and glutamine as precursors for the synthesis of preferentially released glutamate, Brain Res. 168:513-530 (1979).

45. H.F. Bradford, H.K. Ward, and A.J. Thomas, Glutamine - a major substrate for nerve endings, J. Neurochem. 30:1453-1459 (1978).

46. H. Weil-Macherbe, Activators and inhibitors at brain glutaminase, J. Neurochem. 16:855-864 (1969).

47. H.F. Bradford, H.K. Ward, and M. Sandberg, Kinetic properties of glutaminase from cerebral cortex, Neurochem. Res. 9:751-757 (1984).

48. H.F. Bradford and H.K. Ward, On glutaminase activity in mammalian synaptosomes, Brain Res. 110:115-125 (1976).

49. A.M. Benjamin, Control of glutaminase activity in rat brain cortex in vitro: Influence of glutamate phosphate, ammonium, calcium, and hydrogen ions, Brain Res. 208:363-377 (1981).

50. E. Kvamme and K. Lenda, Regulation of glutaminase by exogenous glutamate, ammonia and ß-oxogluterate in synaptosomal enriched preparation from rat brain, Neurochem. Res. 7:667-677 (1982).

51. E. Kvamme, I.A. Torgner, and G. Svenneby, Regulation of phosphate-activated glutaminase in brain, Nordic Neurochem. Symposium 328-332 (1988).

52. T.S. Rajeswari and E. Radha, Metabolism of the glutamate group of amino acids in rat brain as a function of age, Mech. Aging Develop. 24:139-149 (1984).

53. H. Matsumoto, S. Kikuchi, and M. Ito, Age-related changes in the glutamate metabolism of cerebral cortical slices from rats. Neurochem. Res. 7:679-684 (1982).

54. J. Vitorica, A. Clark, A. Machado, and J. Satrustegui, Impairment of glutamate uptake and absence of alterations in the energy-transducing ability of old rat brain mitochondria, Mech. Aging Dev. 29:255-266 (1985).

55. C.C.T. Smith, D.M. Bowen, N.R. Sims, D. Neary, and A.N. Davison, Amino acid release from biopsy samples of temporal neocortex from patients with Alzheimer's disease, Brain Res. 264:138-141 (1983).

56. D.M. Bowen and A.N. Davison, Biochemical studies of nerve cells and energy metabolism in Alzheimer's disease, British Med. Bull. 42:75-80 (1986).

EEG POWER SPECTRA AND BRAIN FUNCTION

Jyunji Yamamoto

Section of Pharmacology
Research Laboratory, Taiho Pharmaceutical Co Ltd
224-2 Ebisuno, Hiraishi, Kawauchi-cho, Tokushima, Japan

INTRODUCTION

Research on brain function is one of the most important themes for the neurobiology of aging. While brain function declines in relation to aging, the assessment of the extent of decline is often difficult. Various methods involving behavior, neurochemistry, electrophysiology, image analysis and others are commonly employed for the study of CNS activity, and each has its particular strengths and caveats. The electroencephlogram (EEG) is one method of electrophysiological analysis that has a long and especially useful history in both experimental and clinical studies. Especially useful is its ability to assess the activity of the whole brain, unlike some of the other techniques. However, while EEG's can accurately measure changes in overall brain activity, they are often thought to reflect only simple changes in this activity, such as wakefulness or sleep.

Recently, various computer techniques for EEG analysis have been developed that create essentially new areas in electrophysiology, such as power spectral analysis. In this analysis, EEG signals are transformed from the electrical waves to spectra, which enables the quantification of subtle changes in EEG. If the analysis is employed to compare the relative power of each frequency, the assessment is almost the same as the visual assessment of EEG signals. It is expected that improved techniques for EEG analysis will yield even more information on brain function from EEG power spectra (1).

EEG power spectra could be useful in evaluating brain function in disease states in which brain functions are complex and not easily analyzed by other methods, such as aging, Alzheimer's disease or psychosis. However, it is important first to evaluate EEG power spectra responses to various drugs of potential use in these neurological disorders. We therefore investigated the relationship between changes in EEG power spectra and five important neuronal systems- acetylcholine (ACh), dopamine (DA), noradrenaline (NA), serotonin (5-HT) and gamma-aminobutyric acid (GABA)- using activating and blocking agents for each system. Next, the effects of various drugs, including psychotropic, cerebroactive and nootropic agents, on EEG power spectra were investigated (1, 2).

MATERIALS AND METHODS

Animals and surgical procedure

Male Japanese White rabbits, weighing 2.5-3.8 kg, were anesthetized with pentobarbital-sodium (30.0 mg/kg,i.v.), and bipolar stainless steel wire electrodes (0.25 mm diameter, insulated except for the last 0.5 mm of the tips; polar distance, 0.5-1.0 mm) were chronically implanted into the hippocampus (A:-4, L:4, H:5) according to the brain atlas of Sawyer et al. (3). Two stainless steel screw electrodes (1.0 mm diameter, silver-plated) were placed subdurally at an interval of 2 mm on the surface of the motor cortex. Each electrode was fixed with dental cement to a perforated hole in the skull and soldered to a connector socket. The socket itself was fixed by means of the cement together with screws driven into the skull, and all exposed parts of the electrodes were also covered with cement. Animals were allowed at least 1 week to recover from the surgery before commencing the experiments.

EEG recording and analysis

The animals were placed in a transparent plastic box (26x42x34 cm) in a sound-proof, shielded room. The EEGs of the cortex and hippocampus were recorded bipolarly on a polygraph (Nihondenki San-ei, 36.1) at a time constant of 0.1 sec and a low pass filter setting of 25Hz, concomitantly with observations of their freely moving behavior. While recording the EEG, power spectral analysis of the EEGs was performed simultaneously for 15 min with a signal processor (Nihondenki San-ei, 7T07), followed by Fast Fourie Transformation at frequencies of 0-25Hz.

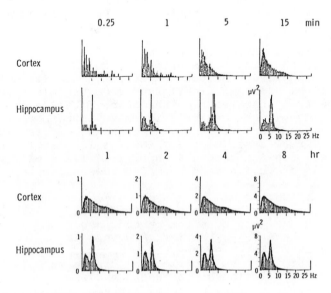

Fig. 1. Cortical and hippocampal EEG power spectra of rabbits for various analysis times.

The spectra were plotted on an X-Y recorder as histograms at
intervals of 0.22 Hz.

RESULTS AND DISCUSSIONS

1. EEG power spectra of cortex and hippocampus

The EEGs of the cortex and hippocampus were sampled and
analyzed during 0.25, 1, 5, 15, 30 min, 1, 2, 4 and 8 hr
periods (Fig. 1).

The EEG samples were taken for each time period from a given
animal and then analyzed. The histograms at a frequency of 0.22
Hz were not consistent for density at 15 sec or 1 min;
therefore, it was difficult to characterize their peaks and
features. However, 5 or 15 min histograms were consistent for
density, making definition of the peaks and features possible.
For longer periods (1 to 8 hrs), the peaks and features were
very clear. It is interesting to note that the peaks and
features became more defined as the analysis time increased.
This result suggests that each frequency of the EEG signals is
controlled at a regular power level to constitute the spectra,
and it seems to be the character of EEG.

EEG signals display voltage in the ordinate and time in the
abscissa, while power spectra consist of power in the ordinate
and frequency in the abscissa. It is important to set a suitable
time for EEG power spectral analysis. For our studies, the
analysis time was set at 15 min. This intermediate time interval
was chosen because, although some summation of EEG signals is
necessary, the spectra would change grossly over longer periods.

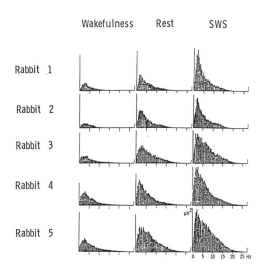

Fig. 2. Power spectra of cortical EEGs for 15 min during the
normal behavioral states of wakefulness, rest and slow wave
sleep (SWS) in rabbits.

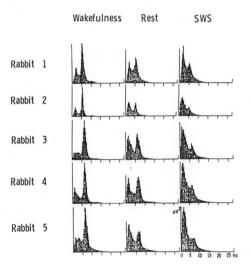

Fig. 3. Power spectra of hippocampal EEGs for 15 min during the normal behavioral states of wakefulness, rest slow wave sleep in rabbits.

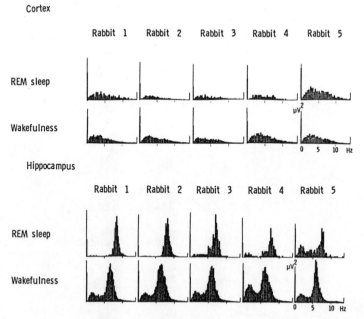

Fig. 4. Power spectra of cortical and hippocampal EEGs during the REM sleep in rabbits.

The EEG power spectra of the neocortex and hippocampus analyzed for 15 min periods during the normal behavioral states of wakefulness, rest, slow wave sleep (SWS) and rapid eye movement (REM) sleep are shown in Fig. 2, 3 and 4. The cortical spectra consisted of powers ranging from zero to frequencies higher than 20 Hz showing one peak at a delta wave band of about 2 Hz. Both peak and total powers are highest in the SWS state and lowest in the wakefulness state. The power during the rest state changes according to the level of consciousness; however, the values fall in any case between in the SWS and wakefulness states. On the other hand, the hippocampal spectra consist of powers ranging from zero to 15 Hz, and the spectra have two peaks at delta and theta wave bands. These two peaks alternate competitively with each other in correspondence to the level of consciousness. In the wakefulness states, the theta wave peak is higher and the delta wave peak is lower. In the SWS state, the opposite is true, with the delta wave peak being higher. In the rest state, the delta and theta wave peaks alternate according to the level of consciousness, but in any case the values fall between the SWS and wakefulness state powers. The features of the REM spectra are similar to those of the wakefulness states. However, in the hippocampal spectra, the frequency of the theta wave peak during REM sleep is about 1.5 Hz higher than in the wakefulness state.

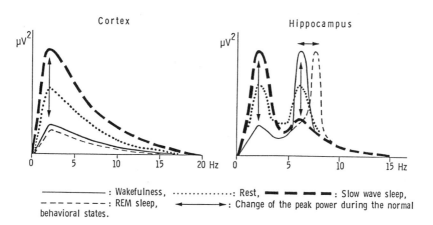

Fig. 5. Power spectral characterization of cortical and hippocampal EEGs and the alteration of their peak power densities during the normal behavioral states of wakefulness, rest, SWS and REM sleep in rabbits.

The alterations of the peaks of the cortical and hippocampal spectra during normal behavioral states are shown Fig. 5. These results suggest that power spectral analysis can transform the cortical and hippocampal EEGs corresponding to the level of consciousness into the alterations of spectra, most likely because the amplitude of each frequency of the EEG signals is regarded as more important for power spectral analysis than their appearence time. Thus, the power spectral analysis of EEG signals is distinctly different from the visual assessment of EEG's.

2. EEG power spectra and ACh, DA, NA, 5-HT and GABAergic systems

Since the EEG changes in relation to the level of consciousness, EEG signals can be very useful for studying the effects of drugs and other therapeutic treatments on brain function. These functions are considered to be controlled by the activating and inhibitory systems of the CNS, including the ACh, DA, NA, 5-HT and GABAergic systems. However, the role of each of these systems in the regulation of various components of EEG signals or brain function generally is not clear. Thus, the effects of the activating and blocking agents for these five neuronal systems were examined on the peak power and frequency in the cortical and hippocampal spectra (Fig. 6). The delta wave peak powers of the cortex and hippocampus

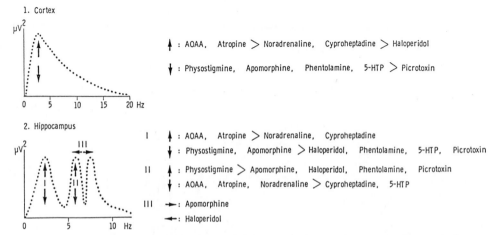

Fig. 6. Effects of cholinergic, dopaminergic, noradrenergic, serotonergic and GABAergic system activation and blockade on the cortical and hippocampal EEG spectra peak power and peak frequency in rabbits.

The alteration in the cortical and hippocampal EEG spectra during the normal behavioral states and the roles of ACh, DA, NA, 5-HT and GABA systems on the spectra are shown in Table 1 and Fig. 7. The peak powers were decreased by physostigmine, apomorphine, phentolamine, 5-HTP and picrotoxin. They were increased by atropine, noradrenaline, cyproheptadine, aminooxyacetic acid (AOAA) and haloperodol, but the last did not produce a marked increase. The peak power of the theta wave of hippocampus was increased by physostigmine, apomorphine, haloperidol, phentolamine and picrotoxin, while it was decreased by atropine, noradrenaline, 5-HTP, cyproheptadine and AOAA.

The cholinergic system agonist and blocking agents, physostigmine and atropine, produced a marked increase and decrease in each peak power, respectively, diametrically opposed to each other. However, the frequency and amplitude changes in the power spectra were in the range observed during normal

behavioral states. On the other hand, the DA, NA, 5-HT and GABA
system activating and blocking agents did not always produce
opposite spectral changes, as evidenced by the fact that the
spectra after administration of some of the agents were different
from the spectra observed during the normal behavioral states.
The dopaminergic agonists and blocking agents, apomorphine and
haloperidol, respectively increased the peak power of the theta
wave, while the 5-HT agonist and blocker, 5-HTP and
cyproheptadine, decreased it. The theta wave peaks after
administration of the NA and GABA receptor blockers, phentolamine
and picrotoxin, were sharp compared to those during the
wakefulness state.

From these results, it appears that the peak power of delta and
theta waves of the cortex and hippocampus are influenced by all
five neuronal systems, but ACh plays the most important role in
the regulation of the peak powers. The theta wave peak of hippocampus was shifted to higher frequencies by dopaminergic
agonist, apomorphine, and shifted to lower frequencies by the DA
receptor blocker, haloperidol. ACh, NA, 5-HT and GABAergic drugs
did not shift the peak. Therefore, DA seems to regulate the peak
frequency of the theta wave.of the cortical and hippocampal delta
waves decreased during the wakefulness state and increased during
the SWS state. The hippocampal theta wave increased during the
wakefulness state and decreased during the SWS state, and the peak
frequency of the latter was shifted to a higher value during the
REM sleep state.

When compared to the normal changes in the spectra, those
observed after intrathecal treatment with ACh, DA and 5-HT are
believed to activate the CNS, while NA and GABA are considered
to be suppressive. However, the spectral changes produced by
the ACh, DA and 5-HT system activation agents were not same.
The three drugs produced a marked decrease in the cortical
delta wave peak power, but the hippocampal spectral changes
caused by the three drugs were different, i.e., the theta wave
peak was markedly increased by physostigmine, shifted by
apomorphine and decreased by 5-HTP. Activation of the ACh, DA
and 5-HT systems thus seems to cause actions that are
different qualitatively.

ACh has been reported to produce psychological activations
that reverse or ameliorate cognitive impairment (4, 5). It is
known that apomorphine produces hyperactivity and stereotyped
behaviors (6, 7), while 5-HTP produces the abnormal behavior
head-twitching (8, 9). The difference in the hippocampal
spectra caused by the three drugs may reflect these and other
different drug-induced behavioral actions. At any rate, the
changes in the theta wave peak seems to be important for
differentiating the effects of drugs on the state of brain
function while the cortical EEG spectra alone does not.

Similarly, the relative changes in the cortex and
hippocampus spectra also seem to be important. Haloperidol and
5-HTP produced abnormal spectral changes, i.e. the changes in
cortex and hippocampus appeared dissociated when compared to
the normal patterns. As described above, the hippocampal theta
wave peak increases when the cortical delta wave peak
decreases during the normal behavioral states. While
haloperidol increased the theta wave peak but did not decrease
the delta wave peak, 5-HTP decreased both the delta and theta

Table 1. Alterations in the cortical and hippocampal EEG power spectra in rabbits during normal behavioral states and after administration of the cholinergic, dopaminergic, noradrenergic, serotonergic and GABAergic agonists and blocking agents.

	Cortex	Hippocampus		
	peak power	peak power		peak frequency
	delta wave	delta wave	theta wave	theta wave
Normal behavioral state				
Wakefulness	↓	↓	↑	—
Rest	—	—	—	—
Slow wave sleep	↑	↑	↓	—
REM sleep	↓	↓	↑	⇒
Cholinergic System				
Physostigmine	⬇	⬇	↑	—
Atropine	⬆	⬆	⬇	—
Dopaminergic System				
Apomorphine	⬇	⬇	↑	⇒
Haloperidol	↑	↓	↑	⇐
Noradrenergic System				
Noradrenaline	↑	↑	⬇	—
Phentolamine	⬇	↓	↑	—
Serotonergic System				
5-Hydroxytryptophan	⬇	↓	↓	—
Cyproheptadine	↑	↑	↓	—
GABAergic System				
AOAA	⬆	⬆	⬇	—
Picrotoxin	↓	↓	↑	—

—: No change, ↑: Increase, ⬆: Marked increase, ↓: Decrease
⬇: Mraked decrease, ⇒: Shift in higher frequencies,
⇐: Shift in lower frequencies.

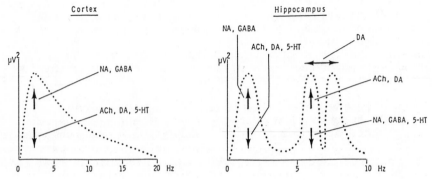

Fig. 7. Effects of acetylcholine, dopamine, noradrenaline, serotonin and GABA on cortical and hippocampal EEG power spectra in rabbits.

wave peaks. These results suggest that the controlling mechanisms for the cortex and hippocampus are different. Tokizane (10) reported that the neocortex was regulated by two control systems, one in the reticular formation and one in the hypothalamus, and that the limbic cortex was regulated only by the hypothalamic control system. The present results support the hypothesis that the control mechanisms of the neocortex and limbic cortex are different, and that brain DA and 5-HT may play some role in the differences between the control mechanisms for the cortex and hippocampus.

The activation state of the brain, the level of consciousness and the sleep-wakefulness cycle are regulated by the balance between the activation and inhibitory neurotransmitter systems of the CNS. Amines have been found to play an important role in this regulation, but their actions are not fully understood. The noradrenergic locus coeruleus has been reported to be involved in the ascending reticular activating system (11,12). However, data contrary to this hypothesis have been reported (13). Fuxe et al. (14) reported that clonidine, an alpha2-receptor stimulator, increased the state of SWS and that piperoxane, an alpha-receptor blocker, increased the state of wakefulness. The results of the present study are similar to their results in that they indicate that NA may play an inhibitory role in the CNS.

Jouvet et al. (15, 16) reported that 5-HT applied to the raphe nuclei produced sleep. However, the exact relationship between 5-HT and sleep is not clear (17, 18). It has been reported that quipazine, a 5-HT receptor agonist, produced suppression of SWS, that methysergide, a 5-HT receptor antagonist, blocked this suppression (19), while 5-HTP (a 5-HT substrate) was found to increase the degree of wakefulness in rats (20). The findings of the present study are similar to these results and indicate that 5-HT plays an activating role in the CNS. This hypothesis appears to be contrary to that of Jouvet et al. (15, 16).

DA has been reported to promote REM sleep (21, 22). As described above, apomorphine produced a shift in the theta wave peak, a phenomenon that is characteristic of a spectral change during REM sleep. However, it has also been reported that the promotion of REM sleep is controlled by ACh (23, 24) or NA (15, 16). Thus it appears that amines can play an important role in the regulation of brain activation and inhibitory systems, and that their roles differ both qualitatively and quantatively.

On the other hand, it has been reported that brain ACh is important for the regulation of the arousal state (25, 26) and that amines are modulators or regulators of ACh transmission (27, 28). The present results also suggest that ACh plays an important role in regulating the level of consciousness, because ACh played an important role in the changes of the cortical and hippocampal EEG spectra. However, unlike dopamine receptor stimulation, cholinergic activation did not shift the theta wave peak. Further, blocking the muscarinic system did not produce behavioral sleep, i.e., atropine produced dissociation between behavior and the EEG. Therefore, ACh seems to be limited to controlling the level of consciousness.

As described above, cholinergic transmission has an activating effect on the CNS, while NA is suppressive. ACh and NA are transmitters of the parasympathetic and sympathetic nervous systems, respectively. A difference in the mechanisms between the central and peripheral nervous systems may be involved in the dissociation, although it is difficult to draw any definite conclusions. Though ACh may not control all consciousness, the present data indicate that the role of ACh may be more important under these conditions than the other neurotransmitters studied. It may be concluded that ACh is important for the fundamental changes which occur between the wakefulness and SWS states, and that DA, NA, 5-HT and GABA play roles in the regulation of the delicate changes in consciousness, such as the role of DA in the production of REM sleep.

3. Effects of cerebroactive and psychotropic drugs on the EEG spectra

The effects of cerebroactive and nootropic drugs which are used in the treatment of Alzheimer's disease were investigated next. Tetrahydroaminoacridine (THA) at doses of 1,3 and 5 mg/kg, i.v. dose-dependently decreased the delta wave peak

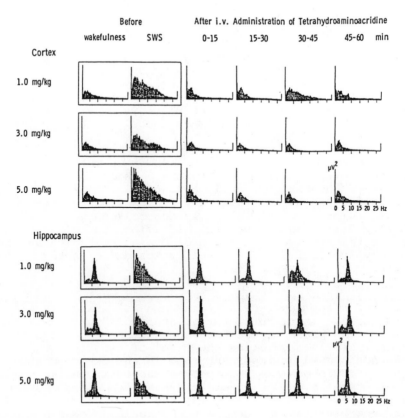

Fig. 8. Effects of THA on the power spectra of cortical and hippocampal EEGs in rabbits.

power of both cortical and hippocampal spectra. Although it
also increased the theta wave peak power of hippocampal
spectra, the frequency was not changed. During the 0-60 min
after administration of a dose of 5 mg/kg, the delta wave
peaks were significantly lower and the theta wave peaks were
higher than those observed in the wakefulness state (Fig. 8).
These effects of THA are similar to those of physostigmine.
Amantadine, a DA receptor agonist, and caffeine produced the
same spectral changes as did THA (Fig. 9, 10).

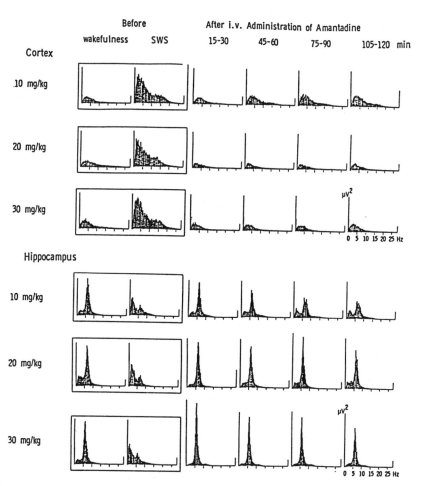

Fig. 9. Effects of amantadine on power spectra of cortical
and hippocampal EEGs in rabbits.

After administration of amantadine at a dose of 30 mg/kg,
i.v., and caffeine at a dose of 50 mg.kg, p.o., the delta wave
peaks were significantly lower and the theta wave peaks were
significantly higher than those observed during the
wakefulness state. Piracetam is a nootropic, cyclic GABA
analog, and it produced no significant changes in the cortical
and hippocampal spectra (Fig. 11).

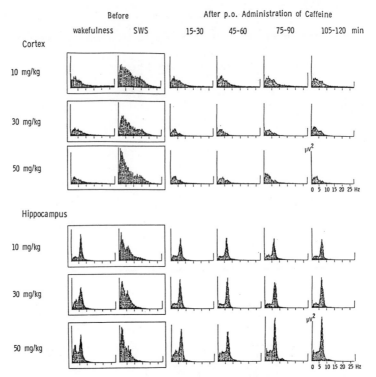

Fig. 10. Effects of caffeine on power spectra of cortical and hippocampal EEGs in rabbits.

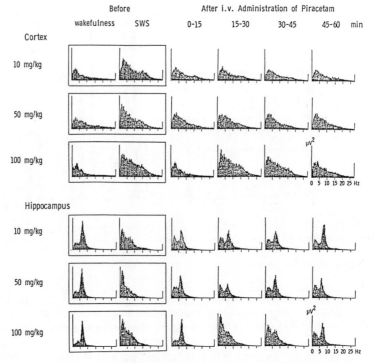

Fig. 11. Effects of piracetam on power spectra of cortical and hippocampal EEGs in rabbits.

Since these three cerebroactive drugs, THA, amantadine and
caffeine, have different pharmacological mechanisms of action,
yet show the same spectral changes, the decrease of delta wave
peak power and increase of theta wave peak power may be common
with cerebroactive drugs. A more detailed analysis of the
effect of the nootropics on the EEG spectra is clearly
warranted, however.

Antipsychotic drugs (chlorpromazine, reserpine), antianxiety
drugs (diazepam, chlordiazepoxide), antidipressants
(methanphetamine, amitriptyline), anesthesics (pentobarbital,
urethane) and narcotic analgesics (morphine, pentazocine) each
produced characteristic EEG spectra, and the alterations of
the cortical and hippocampal spectra caused by these
psychotropic drugs are shown in Fig. 12.

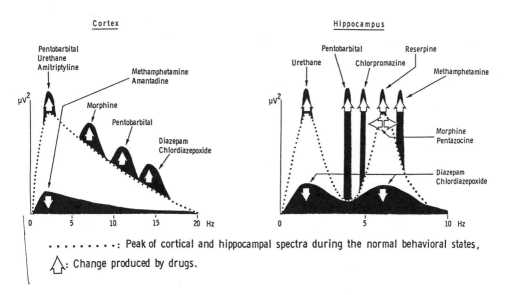

Fig. 12. Characteristic effects of psychotropic drugs on
power spectra of cortical and hippocampal EEGs in rabbits.

The characteristic alterations can be classified into three
patterns: 1) production of a new peak in the cortical spectra; 2)
shift of the theta wave peak in the hippocampal spectra; and 3)
change of the peak power. Morphine, pentobarbital, diazepam and
chlordioazepoxide produced the new peak at about 7, 11, 14 and 15
Hz in the cortical spectra, respectively. It was not easy to
identify the new peak produced by morphine, because it was near
the delta wave peak, and the productive effect differed between
individuals. But the new peaks produced by other drugs were
identified easily. Kareti et al. (29) reported that morphine
caused a few predominant peaks in the 2 to 8 Hz band in the

cortical EEG spectra of rats, but the peak EEG frequencies were not clear. Yamamoto et al. (30) reported that the power of the cortical EEG spectra of cats increased and the peak EEG frequency was found at about 13 Hz in the awake stage after administration of diazepam. Ishikawa et al. (31) reported that pentobarbital increased the power in the 8 to 16 Hz band in the cortical EEG spectra of rabbits. These results are similar to those in present study. Sterman and Kovalesky (32) reported that diazepam decreased the power in the 4 to 7 Hz band in the cortical EEG spectra of rhesus monkeys, and pentobarbital increased the power in the 16 to 24 Hz in the spectra. Conceivably, the drug effects on the EEG spectra may be different between rhesus monkeys and rabbits.

Both morphine and chlorpromazine shifted the theta wave peak of hippocampus to lower frequencies; however, chlorpromazine heightened the peak and morphine did not. On the other hand, the theta wave peak of the hippocampus was shifted to higher frequencies during the REM sleep. Moreover, psychological stress increased the power of the theta wave of the hippocampus to higher frequencies (33).

The frequency as well as the power of the theta wave peak may be related to the level of consciousness. Pentobarbital shifted the peaks of the delta and theta waves to about 4 Hz in the hippocampal spectra and produced a new high peak, and these spectra were not similar to that seen during the normal SWS state. Ishikawa et al. (31, 34) reported that chlorpromazine slightly decreased the total power of the hippocampal EEG spectra of rabbits, and pentobarbital increased the power in the 0 to 4 Hz band and decreased the power in the 4 to 16 Hz band in the spectra. However, they did not describe the alterations of the frequency and power of the theta wave peak, whose alterations cannot be shown by the alterations of the total power or the power in the 4 Hz band width.

Only diazepam of the drugs tested decreased the peak powers of both delta and theta waves in the hippocampal spectra. Yamamoto et al. (30) reported that diazepam decreased the power in the 2 to 6 Hz band in the hippocampal EEG spectra of cats, and the peak EEG frequency in the cat was not as clear as in rabbits, as seen presently.

Amitriptyline only increased the peak powers of delta waves in the cortical and hippocampal spectra. The spectra produced by amitriptyline were similar to those observed during the normal SWS state. Sakai and Matsui (35) reported that the cortical and hippocampal EEG spectra of rats at arousal and slow wave stages after administration of the antidepressants, mianserine or imipramine, were not different from that after treatment with vehicle. However, the increase in the peak power of the delta wave in the cortical spectra produced by amitriptyline tended to be more marked than that during the normal SWS state. Pentobarbital also produced a similar increase for a short time.

The present findings suggest that cerebroactive drugs and psychotropic drugs produced characteristic and different EEG spectra. The spectra produced by cerebroactive drugs were similar to those during the wakefulness state, and the spectra produced by psychotropic drugs were different from those during the normal behavioral states.

SUMMARY

1. EEG power spectra of cortex and hippocampus

Each frequency of the EEG signals is controlled at a regular power level to constitute the spectra, and the cortical and hippocampal EEGs produce characteristic spectra, respectively. The cortical spectra have one peak of delta wave, while the hippocampal spectra have two peaks of delta and theta waves. The peak power and peak frequency increase or decrease depending on the level of consciousness; therefore, the power spectral analysis of EEG signals is a more powerful analysis than simple visual assessment.

2. EEG power spectra and ACh, DA, NA, 5-HT and GABAergic systems

The activating and blocking agents for each of these five brain neuronal systems produced characteristic spectra, consistent with the different roles these neuronal systems play in the regulation of the level of consciousness. ACh appears to be important for the regulation of the level of consciousness between wakefulness and SWS, since cholinergic agents produced marked changes in the peak powers. DA transmission seems to be important for the regulation of the REM sleep because dopaminergic agents produced changes of the theta wave peak frequency.

3. Effects of cerebroactive and psychotropic drugs on the EEG spectra

Cerebroactive drugs produced spectra similar to those observed during wakefulness, but the decrease of delta wave peak and increase of theta wave peak were quite marked. The various psychotropic drugs (e.g., antipsychotics, antianxiety, antidepressant, anesthetics, and narcotic analgesics) produced characteristic spectra that were different from those seen during normal behavioral states. The characteristic alterations caused by these drugs were: 1)the production of a new peak; 2)the shift of the theta wave peak; and 3) the change in peak power. The effects of cerebroactive and psychotropic drugs on the EEG spectra were different.

EEG power spectra were found to reflect accurately subtle changes in the CNS activity; e.g., regulation of the level of consciousness, effects of psychotropic drugs on previously reported psychotic and emotional ststes. The use of EEG power spectra analysis to assess the effects of normal aging and Alzheimer's disease on power spectra is clearly warranted.

REFERENCES

1. Yamamoto, J. (1985) Characteristics of the cortical and hippocampal EEG power spectra of rabbits during normal behavioral states and after administration of CNS acting drugs. Japan. J. Pharmacol. 37:227-234.
2. Yamamoto, J. (1988) Roles of cholinergic, dopaminergic, noradrenergic, serotonergic and GABAergic systems in changes of the EEG power spectra and behavioral states in rabbits. Japan. J. Pharmacol. 47:123-134.

3. Sawyer, H.W,, Everret, J.W. and Green, J.D. (1954) The rabbit diencephalon in stereotaxic coordinates. J. Comp. Neurol. 101:801-824.
4. Whitehouse, P.J., Price, D.L., Clark, A.W., Coyle, J.T. and DeLong, M.R. (1981) Alzheimer disease, evidence for selective loss of cholinergic neurons in the nucleus basalis. Ann. Neurol. 10:122-126.
5. Friedman, E., Lerer, BN. and Kuster, J. (1983) Loss of cholinergic neurons in the rat neocortex produces deficits in passive avoidance learning. Pharmacol. Biochem. Behav. 19:309-312.
6. Ernst, A.M. (1967) Mode of action of apomorphine and dexampheamine on gnawing compulsion in rats. Psychopharmacologia 10:316-326.
7. Maj, J., Grabowska, M. and Gajda, L. (1972) Effect of apomorphine on motility in rats. Eur. J. Pharmacol. 17:208-214.
8. Corne, S.J. and Pickering, R.W. (1967) A possible corelation between drug-induced hallucination in man and a behavioral response in mice. Psychopharmacologia 11:65-78.
9. Boulton, C.S. and Handley, S.L. (1973) Factors modifying the head-twitch response to 5-hydroxytryptophan. Psychopharmacologia 31:205-214.
10. Tokizane, T (1965) Sleep mechanism, hypothalamic control of cortical activity. In: Aspects Anatomo Functionnels de la Physiologie du Sommeil, Coll Internat., C.N.R.S. No 127, pp. 151-185.
11. Jouvet, M. and Delorme, J. (1965) Locus coeruleus et sommmeil paradoxal. Compt. Rend. Soc. Biol. 159:895-899.
12. Lindbrink, P. (1974) The effect of lesions of ascending noradrenaline pathways on sleep and waking in the rats. Brain Res. 74:19-40.
13. Jones, B.E., Harper, S.T. and Halaris, A.E. (1977) Effects of locus coeruleus lesions upon cerebral monoamine content, sleep-wakefulness states and the response to amphetamine in the cat. Brain Res. 124: 473-496.
14. Fuxe, K., Lidbrink, P., Hokleft, T., P. and Goldstein, M. (1974) Effects of piperoxane on sleep waking in the rat. Evidence for increased waking by blocking inhibitory adrenaline receptorson the locus coeuleus. Acta Physiol. Scand. 91:566-567.
15. Matsumoto, J. and Jouvet, M. (1963) Effects de reserpine, DOPA et 5-HTP sur les deux etats de sommeil. Compt. Rend. Soc. Biol. 158: 2135-2139.
16. Jouvet, M. (1969) Biogenic amines and the state of sleep. Science 163:32-41.
17. McGinty, D.J. and Harper, R.M. (1976) Dorsal raphe neurons, depression of firing during sleep in cats. Brain Res. 101:569-575.
18. Adrien, J. (1976) Lesion of the anterior raphe nuclei in the new kitten and the effects on sleep. Brain Res. 103:579-583.
19. Fornal, D. and Radulovacki, M. (1982) Methysergide blocks the sleep suppressant action of quipazine in rats. Psychopharmacology 76:255-259.
20. Wojcik, W.J., Fornal, C. and Radulovacki, M. (1980) Effect of tryptophan on sleep in the rat. Neuropharmacology 19:163-167.
21. Kafi, S. and Gaillard, J.M. (1976) Brain dopamine receptprs and sleep in the rat. Effects of stimulation and blockade. Eur. J. Pharmacol. 38:357-363.

22. Radulovacki, M., Wojcik, W.J. and Fornal, C. (1979) Effects of bromocriptine and fluphentixol on sleep in REM sleep derived rats. Life Sci. 24:1705-1712.
23. Sitaram, N., Mendelson, W.B. Wyatt, R.J. and Gillin, J.C. (1977) The time-dependent induction of REM sleep and arousal by physostigmine infusion during normal human sleep. Brain Res. 122: 562-567.
24. Masserano, J.M. and King, C. (1982) Effects of sleep of acetylcholine perfusion of the locus coeruleus of cats. Neuropharmacology 69: 1163-1167.
25. Myers, R.D. (1974) Behavioral, pharmacological and physiological aspects, sleep and arousal. In: Handbook of Drug and Chemical Stimulation of the Brain. Van Nostrand Renhold Company, New York, pp. 429-468.
26. Giuditta, A. (1977) The biochemistry of sleep. In: Biochemical Correlation of Brain Structure and Function(ed:Davison, A.N.), Academic Press, New York, pp. 293
27. Grossland, J. (1963) In: The Clinical Chemistry of Monoamines (eds: Varley, H. and Gowenlock, A.H.), Elsevier, Amsterdam.
28. Carlson, A. (1964) Biogenic amines. Prog. Brain Res. 8:9
29. Kareti, S., Moreton, L.E. and Khazan, N. (1980) Effects of buprenorphine, a new narcotic agonist-antagonist on the EEG, power spectrun and behavior of the rat. Neuropharmacology 21:195-2012.
30. Yamamoto, K., Sawada, T., Utsumi, S., Naito, T. and Koshida, H. (1982) Behavioral and electrophysiological analysis of the effects of 2-o-chlorobenzoyl-4-chloro-N-methyl-N-glycylglycinanilide hydrate in the CNS in cats and monkeys. Neuropharmacology 21:413-421.
31. Ishikawa, T., Yamanouchi, K., Tanaka, Y., Yanagihashi, R. Nemoto, S. and Mochizuki, E. (1982) Electroencephalographical study on the central action of physostigmine and pentobarbital by quantitative analysis in freely moving rabbits. Folia Pharmacol. Japon. 79:73p
32. Sterman, M.B. and Kovalesky, R.A. (1983) Baseline studies and anticonvulsant drug effects on the sleep EEG power spectral profile. Electroencephalogr. Clin. Neurophysiol. 55:212-222.
33. Iwata, N. and Mikuni, N. (1982) EEG change in the conscious rats during immobility induced by psychological stress. Psychopharmacology 71:117-122.
34. Ishikawa, T., Yamanouchi, K., Tanaka, Y., Maruyama, R. and Mochizuki, E. (1983) Study of central action of some psychotropic drugs on the quantitatively analyzed EEG. Japan. J. Pharpacol. 33: Supp. 68p.
35. Sakai, Y. and Matsui, Y. (1980) Neurochemical and electroencephalographical studies on the central actions of mianserin. Folia Pharmacol. Japon. 76: 479-493.

POSTMORTEM STABILITY OF RNA METABOLISM IN HUMAN BRAIN: STUDIES OF THE

NONDEMENTED CONTROL AND ALZHEIMER'S DISEASE CASES

E.M. Sajdel-Sulkowska, H.J. Manz and C.A. Marotta

Department of Psychiatry, Harvard Medical School; Mailman
Research Center, McLean Hospital, Belmont, MA; Georgetown
University School of Medicine, Washington, DC;
Neurobiology Laboratory, Massachusetts General Hospital,
Boston, MA

INTRODUCTION

Neurochemical analyses of postmortem human brain tissue is
currently a challenging and expanding area of research. Many studies
are utilizing the autopsied brain material to probe the molecular
mechanism of neurological and psychiatric diseases that are uniquely
human and for which adequate animal models have not been developed.
Despite a logical misconception, the degeneration of some of the
cellular structures, enzyme activities, and macromolecules occurs
gradually in human brain. Since a number of enzymatic activities are
preserved during a period up to 24 hours, there is sufficient time to
carry out routine handling of autopsy material as well as specialized
procedures. Preservation of specific structures and functions allows
for direct examination of molecular changes that are characteristic of
the normal human aging process and changes that are unique to
pathological conditions such as Alzheimer's disease.

Of particular interest is the preservation of nucleic acid within
the cell, as was first demonstrated from this laboratory as early as
1980 (1,2,3,4,5,6). A number of studies have suggested an alteration at
the transcriptional and translational processes in the AD brain (6,7,8)
suggesting that the direct analyses of these mechanisms may be
informative. In addition to our earlier work on isolation of
translationally active mRNA from both nondemented control and
Alzheimer's disease cases (5,6,9), we have recently (10,11,12,13,14)
investigated a possibility that the RNA synthesis may be preserved in
postmortem human brain for a defined period following death. To our
knowledge RNA synthesis in postmortem human brain has not been
previously demonstrated.

Cellular processes preserved in the postmortem human brain

Results of studies of human autopsy material indicate remarkable
stability of a number of cellular functions in postmortem brain. Only
small changes occur in lysosomes during the first hours after death
(15). Synaptosomes survive for up to 24 hours (16,17). Dopamine,
glutamate decarboxylase and choline acetyltransferase show a remarkable

stability (18,19). Many enzymes involved in energy (glucose) and neurotransmitter metabolism remain stable for up to 72 hours postmortem (20,21,22) and muscarinic receptor retains activity for up to 51 hours postmortem (23). Cerebral cortical proteins show quantitative but not qualitative changes (24) and brain specific proteins are relatively unaffected by postmortem autolysis during defined periods (19). Membrane glycoproteins remain stable for up to 24 hours (25). Membrane associated enzymes such as succinate dehydrogenase are preserved for up to 100 hours postmortem (26). Although detailed discussion of postmortem changes is beyond the scope of this paper, our review of pertinent literature indicates several general findings: 1) Enzymatic activities appear more stable than cellular structures. 2) Different enzyme systems appear to change at different rates. 3) Individual enzymes in a given enzymatic system show a unique stability. An interesting observation has been made regarding respiratory enzymes implying that the disappearance of enzyme activityes is inversely related to their developmental expression (27).4)A specific enzyme activity may be different in different brain regions

Stability of RNA in postmortem human brain - changes observed in Alzheimer's disease

Detailed discussion of studies involving RNA metabolism is presented below. One could speculate that general findings regarding preservation of cellular functions in postmortem brain may be relevant to survival of RNA: 1) Structures involved in the synthesis and metabolism of RNA such as nuclei or polysomes may be less stable than nRNA activity. 2) Different classes of RNA such as ribosomal and mRNA may exhibit different stabilities. 3) Among mRNAs, individual species may show unique stability. 4) Individual mRNA species may show different stability in different brain regions. Postmortem changes must be viewed in the context of premortem and regional influences on RNA metabolism. Thus, complex issues must be addressed when designing experiments to examine possible changes in nucleic acid metabolism in the diseased brain.

Early investigations from this laboratory (3,4) demonstrated that polysomal mRNA could be extracted from postmortem brain tissue and translated in vitro. Subsequent direct extraction of postmortem human brain tissue with strong denaturing buffers by our group (5,6) resulted in increased yield and biological potency of RNA preparations from both control and Alzheimer brains. Total cellular RNA can be purified using oligo dT columns to obtain polyA containing mRNA (5). We routinely isolate mRNA from brain tissue up to 20 hours postmortem. In confirmation of our earlier studies, isolation of biologically active mRNA from human brain tissue with an 84 hour postmortem interval has been reported (28). Our studies have also been consistent with cytochemical analyses carried out by independent methods. Mann et al, (26) reported no significant changes in ribosomal RNA content within 100 hours postmortem. Others (29) examined nucleic acid content of several human brain regions and detected no changes up to 24 hours postmortem.

Using these procedures we have reported a decrease of 45% in total RNA and 64% in polyA containing mRNA in brain tissue from AD cases as compared to nondemented controls (30). A reduction in ribosomal RNA and polyA containing mRNA for preproenkephalin and preprosomatostatin in AD cases has been reported by Taylor et al., (31,32,33). A number of other laboratories have since reported a similar reduction in RNA in Alzheimer's disease (34,35,36,37,38,39).

Postmortem protein synthesis

Our laboratory has first demonstrated the ability of mRNA obtained from postmortem human brain to synthesize proteins in vitro (3,5,6). In early studies the postmortem time ranged from 0.5-20 hours. As mentioned above, other laboratories have since successfully translated mRNA isolated from autopsied human brains with postmortem time up to 84 hours (28). Several hundred individual proteins with moderately high molecular weights can be detected after in vitro protein synthesis in the rabbit reticulocyte system followed by polyacrylamide gel electrophoresis and autoradiography (3,4,5,6). Among the translation products one can identify major cytoskeletal proteins: tubulin, glial fibrillary acidic proteins (GFAP), and actin (3,4,5,6). In comparative studies the most striking difference between translation products of control and AD mRNA are quantitative rather than qualitative. There appears a general decrease in translational efficiency of mRNA isolated from AD brains. However, not all proteins are decreased; GFAP synthesis characteristically increases (9). A relative increase in glial specific mRNA has been observed by Oksova (40). There is wide variability in mRNA translational activity. This may partly reflect differences among brain regions and the extent of pathology with regard to both neuronal loss and astrocytosis.

Postmortem RNA as a template in preparation of human libraries

Based on the observations that mRNA prepared from both control and AD autopsied brains retains translational activity, initial trials were undertaken to prepare human brain libraries using the purified mRNA as a template for cDNA. In collaboration with S.B. Zain, W.-G. Chou and S. Salim, we reported the successful preparation of cDNA libraries for amyloid and glial fibrillary acidic proteins using AD mRNA as starting material (41,42). A segment of 1564 bases referred to as amy37 representing nearly one-half of the precursor amyloid protein mRNA included a substantial portion of the coding and 3' noncoding sequences. Sequence analysis revealed that the structure of non-AD and AD amyloid cDNA are identical (41). This indicates that factors other than an AD-specific amyloid structure must account for the overaccumulation of this protein in the AD brain. The complete structure of the precursor from AD mRNA is being completed; we have observed that even the amyloid variant containing the Kunitz type protease inhibitor is present in the AD brain, similar to non-AD sources (43).

In vitro uridine incorporation by postmortem human brain tissue

As an extension of our earlier studies, we have addressed the possibility that the postmortem tissue is capable of making the RNA. To date we have examined 29 cases with the age ranging from 56-91 years and the postmortem interval of 1.0 to 30 hours (manuscript submitted for publication). In order to quantitate RNA synthesis we measured the incorporation of radioactive uridine into an alkaline hydrolysed fraction of the homogenate that specifically reflects RNA. The cell homogenate was hydrolysed with alkali and the RNA was estimated by orcinol method; a portion of the digest was counted. The radioactivity was normalized to the amount of RNA in the sample and resulted in the specific activity value. Parallel aliquots of the homogenate were used for estimation of the DNA content. The amount of uridine incorporation could thus be normalized to DNA and expressed as synthetic capacity. When incubated under organotypic tissue culture conditions, autopsied tissue incorporated 3H uridine linearly for up to 90 min. The specific activity of RNA extracted with phenol from human samples ranged from 2.1 to 8.8×10^5 dpm/mg RNA. By comparison the fresh mouse tissues had specific activity value of 17.9×10^5.

To further verify that the incorporation of uridine was into RNA, we tested for the sensitivity of the product to the RNase. Computer degradation was observed after enzymatic treatment. We have observed that the synthesis was sensitive to ActinomycinD; however, there was considerable variability in the degree of inhibition. Electrophoresis of the radiolabeled RNA on agarose gels under denaturing conditions showed a peak of radioactivity in the 18S-28S region. Sucrose density analysis indicated similar size. Although it appears that the synthesized product may reflect DNA dependent RNA synthesis, it is our impression that terminal addition of uridine may have contributed to the overall incorporation. Further experiments are being carried out to more clearly define the contributing factors.

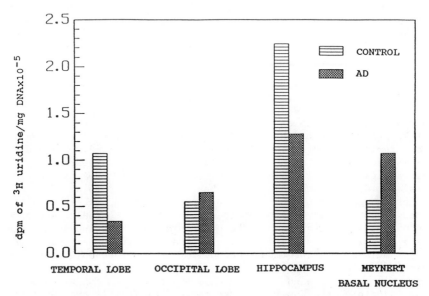

Fig. 1. Synthetic capacity (dpm ^{3}H uridine/mg DNAx10^{-5}) of different brain regions of postmortem human brain from control (82 yrs of age, 9 hrs) and AD (85 yrs of age, 23 hrs) cases.

RNA synthesis and the degree of pathology

In preliminary studies we have measured RNA synthesis in individual brain regions in slices that have been closely monitored for number of senile plaques. We observed some difference in the amount of ^{3}H uridine incorporation between different regions of both control and AD brains (Fig. 1). Control hippocampus was a most active brain region in RNA synthesis and also most affected in AD. We observed decreased RNA synthesis in AD hippocampus that coincided with the maximum number of amyloid plaques present in the region (13). In these preliminary studies we observed an indication of inverse relationship between RNA synthesis and number of plaques present.

RNA synthesis in the postmortem CSF

We have been interested in the relationship between CSF and brain tissue RNA metabolism and more specifically in the effect that the CSF cellular components may have on RNA synthesis in the brain tissue. CSF cells consist of three main types: 1) those of the lymphatic immune system, 2) the mononuclear phagocyte system, and 3) reticulohistocytic system (44). The functional expression of the cellular immune response in CSF remains little understood. In the preliminary studies we have examined ^{3}H uridine incorporation into cellular components of postmortem CSF from several AD cases. CSF was diluted (1:20) and incubated at 37°C for 90 min with an admixture of uridine at concentration of 50 μCi/ml. CSF cells were collected by centrifugation and the homogenate analyzed for uridine incorporation. The amount of uridine incorporation was as high as 8.04×10^6 dpm/mg RNA in some of the AD cases. These observations suggest that the RNA synthesis may be preserved in the other brain components in the postmortem stage. A defect in blood lymphocytes from AD cases to produce macrophage activating factor has been reported (45). Our preliminary observations suggest that postmortem CSF may prove useful in examining the immune competence of brain lymphocytes in AD.

SUMMARY

We focused on the capacity of human postmortem tissue to synthesize RNA because of the evidence suggesting impairment of the transcriptional process in the brains affected with Alzheimer's dementia (7,8). Evidence gained from biochemical studies using purified RNA is consistent with histochemical studies (46,47,48,49,50). The hypothesis of defect in AD brain at the transcriptional level is consistent with the relatively low level of protein synthesis in living patients with Alzheimer's disease (51). It can be hypothesized that reduced rates of transcription may contribute to the lower levels of cellular RNA and indirectly to a lower capacity to synthesize proteins.

CONCLUSIONS

Results derived from the studies discussed above suggest that future work on RNA metabolism in human postmortem brain and CSF are warranted and represent a suitable system for direct examination of cellular processes otherwise inaccessible to experimentation. At this point the variability observed in transcriptional and translational studies may make the system of limited usefulness for detailed comparisons between control and AD cases. However, using molecular biological approaches in postmortem brain tissue, one can address the questions regarding the regulation of RNA metabolism in human brain. More specifically, the effect of various hormonal and pharmacological substances on RNA synthesis can be explored. This research was supported by AHAF grant to EMSS and NIH grant AG02126 to CAM.

REFERENCES

1. Gilbert, J.M., Brown, B.A., Strocchi, P., Bird, E.D. and Marotta, C.A. (1980) The preparation of biologically active messenger RNA from human postmortem brain. Neurosci. Abst. (Society for Neuroscience), 263.5.

2. Marotta, C.A., Strocchi, P., Brown, B.A., Bonventre, J.A., Gilbert, J.M. (1981) Gel electrophoresis methods for the examination of human and rat brain fibrous proteins. Application to studies of human brain proteins from postmortem tissue. In: Genetic Research Strategies for Psychobiology and Psychiatry (eds: Gershon, E.S., Matthysse, S., Breakefield, X.O. and Ciaranello, R.D.), Boxwood Press, Pacific Grove, pp. 39-57.

3. Marotta, C.A., Brown, B.A., Strocchi, P., Bird, E.D. and Gilbert, J.M. (1981) In vitro synthesis of human brain proteins including tubulin and actin by purified postmortem polysomes. J. Neurochem. 36: 966-975.

4. Gilbert, J.M., Brown, B.A., Strocchi, P., Bird, E.D. and Marotta, C.A. (1981) The preparation of biologically active messenger RNA from human postmortem brain tissue. J. Neurochem. 36: 976-984.

5. Sajdel-Sulkowska, E.M., Coughlin, J.F. and Marotta, C.A. (1983) In vitro synthesis of polypeptides of moderately large size of poly (A) containing messenger RNA from postmortem human brain and mouse brain. J. Neurochem. 40: 670-680.

6. Sajdel-Sulkowska, E.M., Coughlin, J.F., Staton, D.M. and Marotta, C.M. (1983) Studies on the stimulation of protein synthesis by messenger RNA from Alzheimer's disease brain. In: Banbury Report 15 Biological Aspects of Alzheimer's Disease (ed: Katzman, R.), Cold Spring Harbor, New York, pp. 193-200.

7. Lewis, P.N., Lukiw, W.J., DeBoui, U. and Crapper McLachlan, D.R. (1981) Changes in chromatin structure associated with Alzheimer's Disease. J. Neurochem. 37: 1193-1202.

8. Marotta, C.A., Majocha, R.E., Coughlin, J.F., Manz, H.J., Davies, P., Ventosa-Michelman, M., Chou, W.-G., Zain, S.B. and Sajdel-Sulkowska, E.M. (1986) Transcriptional and translational regulatory mechanisms during normal aging of the mammalian brain and in Alzheimer's disease. Prog. Brain Res. 70: 303-320.

9. Sajdel-Sulkowska, E.M., Majocha, R.E., Salim, M., Zain, S.B. and Marotta, C.A. (1988) The postmortem Alzheimer brain is a source of structurally and functionally intact astrocytic messenger RNA. J. Neurosci. Methods 23: 173-179.

10. Sajdel-Sulkowska, E.M. and Marotta, C.A. Evidence for the preservation of transcription in postmortem brain of nondemented and Alzheimer's Disease cases. Manuscript in revision.

11. Sajdel-Sulkowska, E.M. and Marotta, C.A. (1987) Radioactive uridine incorporation into RNA by postmortem human brain tissue. Evidence for postmortem transcription in the Alzheimer brain. Soc. Neurosci. 13: abs. 366.7, p. 1326.

12. Sajdel-Sulkowska, E.M., Sulkowski, A. and Marotta, C.A. (1988) Evidence for the preservation of transcription in postmortem human brain. Neurochem. Intern. 13: 167.

13. Sajdel-Sulkowska, E.M., Manz, H., Burnside, E.S. and Marotta, C.A. (1989) RNA synthesis in distinct regions of postmortem Alzheimer brain. Transaction of the American Society of Neurochemistry 20: 107.

14. Sajdel-Sulkowska, E.M., Manz, H.J., Mandel, A., Sulkowski, A., Burnside, E.S. and Marotta, C.A. (1989) RNA synthesis in cortical and subcortical regions and CSF components of postmortem human brain. Suncoast Workshop on the Neurobiology of Aging, February, 1989.

15. McKeown, S.R. (1978) Postmortem autolytic response in rat brain lysosomes. J. Neurochem. 32: 391-396.

16. Dodd, P.R., Hardy, J.A., Bradford, H.F., Bennett, G.W., Edwardson, J.A., and Harding, B.N. (1979) Metabolic and secreting processes in nerve endings isolated from postmortem brain. Neurosci. Lett. 11: 87-92.

17. Hardy, J.A., Bateman, D.E., Kidd, A.M., Edwardson, J.A., Singh, G.B. and Dodd, P.R. (1984) Amino acid transport by synaptosomes isolated from postmortem human brain. J. Neural Transm. 60: 57-62.

18. Spokes, E.G. (1979) An analysis of factors influencing measurements of dopamine, noradrenaline, glutamate decarboxylase and choline acetylase in human postmortem brain tissue. Brain 102: 333-346.
19. Bowen, D.M., Smith, C.B., White, P. and Davison, A.N. (1976) Neurotransmitter-related enzymes and indices of hypoxia in senile dementia and other abiotrophies. Brain 99: 459-496.
20. Bird, E.D. and Iversen, L.L. (1974) Huntington's chorea. Postmortem measurement of glutamic acid decarboxylase, cholineacetyltransferase and dopamine in basal ganglia. Brain 97: 457-472.
21. Bird, E.D., Gale, J.S. and Spokes, E.G. (1977) Huntington's chorea: postmortem activity of enzyme involved in cerebral glucose metabolism. J. Neurochem. 29: 539-545.
22. Bird, E.D., Spokes, E.G., Barnes, J., MacKay, A.V., Iversen, L.L. and Shepherd, M. (1977) Increased brain dopamine and reduced glutamic acid decarboxylase and choline acetyl transferase activity in schizophrenia and related psychoses. Lancet 2: 1157-1158.
23. Uden, A., Meyerson, B., Winblad, B., Sachs, C. and Bartfai, T. (1983) Postmortem changes in binding to the muscarinic receptor from human cerebral cortex. J. Neurochem. 41: 102-106.
24. Narayan, R.K., Heydorn, W.E., Creed, G.J., Kornblith, P.L. and Jacobowitz, P.M. (1984) Proteins in normal, irradiated, and postmortem human brain quantitatively compared by using two-dimensional gel electrophoresis. Clin Chem. 30: 1989-1995.
25. Hukkanen, V. and Roytta, M. (1987) Autolytic changes of human white matter: an electron microscopic and electrophoretic study. Exp. Mol. Pathol. 46: 31-39.
26. Mann, D.M., Barton, C.M. and Davies, J.S. (1978) Post-mortem changes in human central nervous tissue and the effects on quantitation of nucleic acids and enzymes. Histochem. 10: 127-135.
27. Kozik, M.B. (1981) Postmortem activity of respiratory enzymes in human brain. Acta Histochem. 68: 79-90.
28. Perrett, C.W., Marchbanks, R.M. and Whatley, S.A. (1988) Characterisation of messenger RNA extracted postmortem from the brains of schizophrenic, depressed and control subjects. J. Neurol. Neurosurg. Psychiatry 51: 325-331.
29. Naber, D. and Dahnke, H.G. (1979) Protein and nucleic acid content in the aging human brain. Neuropathol. Appl. Neurobiol. 5:17-24.
30. Sajdel-Sulkowska, E.M. and Marotta, C.A. (1984) Alzheimer's Disease Brain: alterations in RNA levels and in a ribonuclease inhibitor complex. Science 225: 947-949.
31. Taylor, G.R., Carter, G.I., Crow, T.J., Perry, E.K. and Perry, R.H. (1985) Measurement of relative concentration of RNA in postmortem brains from senile dementia of the Alzheimer type (SDAT) and controls. J. Neurogenet. 2: 177.
32. Taylor, G.R., Carter, G.I., Crow, T.J., Johnson, J.A., Fairbairn, A.F., Perry, E.K. and Perry, R.H. (1986) Recovery and measurement of specific RNA species from postmortem brain tissue: a general reduction in Alzheimer's disease detected by molecular hybridization. Exp. Mol. Pathol. 44 : 111-116.
33. Taylor, G.R., Carter, G.I., Crow, T.J., Johnson, J.A., Fairbairn, A.F., Perry, E.K. and Perry, R.H. (1987) Recovery and measurement of RNA in Alzheimer's disease by molecular hybridization. J. Neurol. Neurosurg. Psychiatry 50: 356.
34. Guilemetti, J.G., Wong, L., Crapper McLachlan, D.R. and Lewis, P.N. (1986) Characterization of messenger RNA from cerebral cortex of control and Alzheimer-afflicted brain. J. Neurochem. 47: 987-997.
35. McLachlan, D.R., Lukin, W.J., Wong, L. and Beck-Hansen, N.T. (1987) Selective messenger RNA reduction in Alzheimer's disease. J. Cell Biochem. (Supplement 11D) UCLA Symposia on Molecular and Cellular Biology, abs. S407, p. 196.

36. Boyes, B.E., McGeer, P.L. and McGeer, E.G. (1986) Decreased hippocampal RNA in Alzheimer's disease brain. <u>Soc. Neurosci</u>. abs 12, 944.

37. Doebler, J.A., Markesbery, W.R., Anthony, A. and Rhoads, R.E. (1987) Neuronal RNA in relation to neuronal loss and neurofibrillary pathology in the hippocampus in Alzheimer's disease. <u>J. Neuropathol. Exp. Neurol</u>. 46: 28-39.

38. Neary, D., Snowden, J.S., Mann, D.M., Bowen, D.M., Sims, N.R., Northen, B., Yates, P.O. and Davison, A.N. (1986) Alzheimer's disease: A correlative study. <u>J. Neurol. Neurosurg Psychiatry</u> 49: 229-237.

39. Rhoads, R.E., Doebler, J.A., Markesbery, W.R. et al (1987) RNA levels and Alz50 immunoreactivity in Alzheimer's disease hippocampus. <u>J. Cell Biochem</u>. (Suppl. 11D) p. 198.

40. Oksova, E.E. (1975) Glio-neuronal relationship in cerebral cortex in senile dementia. <u>Zh. Neuropathol. Psikhiatr</u>. 75: 1026-1030.

41. Zain, S.B., Salim, M., Chou, W.-G., Sajdel-Sulkowska, E.M., Majocha, R.E. and Marotta, C.A. (1988) Molecular cloning of amyloid cDNA derived from mRNA of the Alzheimer brain. Coding and non-coding regions of the fetal precursor mRNA are expressed in the Alzheimer cortex. <u>Proc. Natl. Acad. Sci</u>. U.S.A. 85: 929-933.

42. Salim, M., Rehman, S., Sajdel-Sulkowska, E.M., Chou, W.-G., Majocha, R.E., Marotta, C.A. and Zain, S.B. (1988) Preparation of a recombinant cDNA library from poly(A+) RNA of the Alzheimer brain. Identification and characterization of a cDNA copy encoding a glial-specific protein. <u>Neurobiol. Aging</u> 9:163-171.

43. Chou, W.-G., Zhu, W., Salim, M., Rehman, S., Tate-Ostroff, B., Majocha, R.E., Sajdel-Sulkowska, E.M., Marotta, C.A. and Zain, S.B. Extracytoplasmic and A4 domains of the amyloid precursor protein: molecular cloning, genetically engineered cell lines and immunocytochemical investigations. In: <u>Alzheimer's Disease and Related Disorders</u> (eds: Iqbal, K., Wisniewski, H.M. and Winblad, B.), Alan R. Liss, Inc., New York, in press.

44. Schmidt, R.M. (1983) Classification of cells in the cerebrospinal fluid. <u>Schweiz. Arek. Neurol. Neurochim. Psychiat</u>r. 132: 309-314.

45. Cameron, D.J., Durst, G.G. and Majewski, J.A. (1985) Macrophage and polymorphonuclear leukocyte function in patients with Alzheimer's disease. <u>Biomed. Pharmacother</u>. 39: 310-314.

46. Dayan, A.D. and Ball, M.J. (1973) Histometric observations on the metabolism of tangle bearing neurons. <u>J. Neurol. Sci</u>. 19: 433-436.

47. Mann, D.M.A., Neary, D., Yates, P.O., Lincoln, F., Snowden, J.S. and Stanworth, P. (1981) Alterations in protein synthetic capability on nerve cells in Alzheimer's disease. <u>J. Neurol. Neurosurg. Psychiatry</u> 44: 97-102.

48. Mann, D.M.A. and Sinclair, K.G.A. (1978) The quantitative assessment of lipofuscin pigment, cytoplasmic RNA and nucleolar volume in senile dementia. <u>Neuropathol. Appl. Neurobiol</u>. 4: 129-135.

49. Mann, D.M.A. and Yates, P.O. (1981) The relationship between formation of senile plaques and neurofibrillary tangles and changes in nerve cell metabolism in Alzheimer type dementia. <u>Mech. Aging Dev</u>. 17: 395-401.

50. Watson, W.E. (1968) Observations on the nucleolar and total cell body nucleic acid of injured nerve cells. <u>J. Physiol</u>. 196: 655-676.

51. Bustany, P., Henry, J.F., Soussaline, F. and Comar, D. (1983) Brain protein synthesis in normal and demented patients - a study by positron emission tomography with [^{11}C]-L-methionine. In: <u>Functional Radionucleotide Imaging of Brain</u> (ed: Magistretti, P.S.), Raven Press, New York, pp. 319-326.

A MODEL SYSTEM DEMONSTRATING PARALLELS IN ANIMAL AND HUMAN AGING: EXTENSION TO ALZHEIMER'S DISEASE

Diana S. Woodruff-Pak, Richard G. Finkbiner, and Ira R. Katz

Department of Psychology
Temple University
Philadelphia, PA 19122

Philadelphia Geriatric Center
Philadelphia, PA 19141

INTRODUCTION

The model system, classical conditioning of the eyeblink response in rabbits and humans, has a number of advantages for research on the neurobiology of learning and memory in normal aging. This model system may also have application to the study of senile dementia of the Alzheimer's type (SDAT). Useful features of this model system for the study of learning and memory and its neurobiological substrates have been elaborated by Gormezano (1966) and Thompson et al. (1976). Woodruff-Pak and Thompson (1985) have highlighted the potential of this model system for research on the neurobiology of learning, memory, and aging. Among the advantages of classical conditioning of the eyeblink response in rabbits and humans are that:

1. Dramatic parallels in acquisition of this simple form of learning exist between humans and rabbits.

2. The neural circuitry underlying classical conditioning of the eyeblink response has been almost completely identified. The essential site of the plasticity for learning resides in the ipsilateral cerebellum, and the hippocampus plays a modulatory role.

3. Large age differences in the rate and level of acquisition exist in both humans and rabbits.

THE BASIC PARADIGM

The techniques involved in classical conditioning of the eyeblink response in rabbits and humans have been described extensively (e.g., Gormezano, 1966; Gormezano and Kehoe, 1975; Gormezano, Kehoe, and Marshall, 1983; Moore and Gormezano, 1977; Patterson and Romano, 1987). Until recently, a mechanical measure of blinking was used in both humans and rabbits. Infrared eyeblink detectors are commonly used in human classical conditioning research, at present (Solomon, Pomerleau, Bennett, James, and Morse, 1989; Woodruff-Pak and

Thompson, 1988b) and are being used increasingly with rabbits (Deyo, Straube, and Disterhoft, 1989).

In the rabbit, the movement of the nictitating membrane (NM) or third eyelid is typically measured instead of the actual eyeblink. The NM and eyeblink response are highly correlated (r = .95; McCormick, Lavond, and Thompson, 1982). Consequently, because we are discussing research with humans and rabbits, we will use the term eyeblink as inclusive of studies in which the rabbit NM was measured.

The standard format for the presentation of stimuli in eyeblink conditioning is called the delay paradigm. A neutral stimulus such as a tone or light is called the conditioned stimulus (CS). It is presented for a duration of around half a second. While it is still on, the unconditioned stimulus (US) is presented, and the CS and US coterminate 50 to 100 msec later. In humans, the US is a corneal airpuff, usually around 3 psi in intensity. In rabbits, the US which elicits an eyeblink unconditioned response (UR) is either a shock infraorbital region of the eye or a corneal airpuff. In our laboratory, we use an airpuff US for both rabbits and humans. The timing in the delay paradigm which we have used with both humans and rabbits involves a 500 msec, 80 dB SPL tone CS followed 400 msec after its onset by a 100 msec, 3 psi corneal airpuff. In this stimulus configuration, the CS-US interval is 400 msec.

The interval between CS and US onset plays a significant role in the rate of acquisition. CS-US intervals of less than 100 msec result in little or no conditioning, and CS-US intervals exceeding 500 msec make acquisition more difficult for rabbits. For humans, the CS-US interval must exceed 1 second before acquisition rate becomes significantly slower. Our unpublished observations along with those of Paul Solomon and his associates indicate that the CS-US interval which is optimal for young adult subjects is shorter than the CS-US interval which is optimal for adults over the age of 50 years.

A variation of the classical conditioning procedure is called the trace paradigm. The CS turns on and then is turned off, a blank period ensues, followed by the US. We typically use a 250 msec CS, a 500 msec blank interval, and a 100 msec US. This means than the CS-US interval is 750 msec. It takes rabbits about five times as long to attain a learning criterion of 8 conditioned responses (CRs) in 9 successive trials in these conditions (Woodruff-Pak, Lavond, & Thompson, 1985).

EARLY RESEARCH INVOLVING THE HIPPOCAMPUS

The hippocampus and septo-hippocampal (ACh) system proved to be much involved in basic associative learning of the sort represented by eyeblink conditioning in the rabbit (see Berger, Berry, and Thompson, 1986). This provides a point of contact with current interest in the possible role of the forebrain cholinergic system in human memory and in SDAT (Coyle, Price, and DeLong, 1983; Sitaram, Weingartner, and Gillin, 1978; Hyman, Van Hoesen, Damasio, and Barnes, 1984). In rabbit eyeblink conditioning, the involvement of the hippocampal system is profound but modulatory in nature.

Neuronal unit activity in the hippocampus increases markedly within trials early in the classical conditioning process. Activity recorded in the CA1 region of the hippocampus forms a predictive "model" of the amplitude-time course of the learned behavioral response, but only under conditions where behavioral learning occurs (Berger, Alger, and Thompson, 1976; Berger and Thompson, 1978b; Thompson et al., 1980). This response is generated largely by pyramidal neurons (Berger and Thompson, 1978a; Berger, Rinaldi, Weisz, and Thompson, 1983). Figure 1 illustrates the "modeling" of CA1 pyramidal cells after classical conditioning has occurred in a young rabbit.

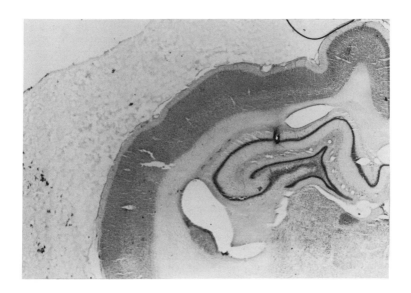

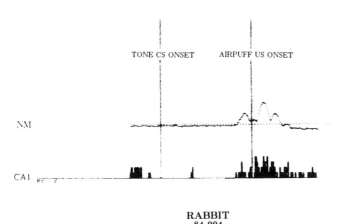

RABBIT
84-004

Fig. 1. Above: Section of the dorsal hippocampus in a 3-month-old rabbit showing marking lesion in left CA1. Bottom: Recording from electrode shown above during the overtraining session which occurred one day after the rabbit had attained a criterion of 8/9 conditioned responses (CRs) in the trace classical conditioning paradigm. The trial shown is number 8-2; the second trial of the eighth block which is trial 65 in that overtraining session. The hippocampal units recorded in left CA1 model the nictitating membrane (NM) response which is labeled NM and shown above the CA1 neuronal units. Vertical lines mark the onset of the tone conditioned stimulus (CS) and corneal airpuff unconditioned stimulus (US). The CS-US interval is 750 msec, and the entire tracing represents 1150 msec. (From Woodruff-Pak, Lavond, Logan, and Thompson, 1987).

In addition to neural "modeling" correlates of conditioning, the ongoing, spontaneous activity in the rabbit hippocampus predicted rate of acquisition (Berry and Thompson, 1978). The degree to which the hippocampal EEG showed theta (8 Hz waves) just prior to learning was highly predictive of how fast an animal would subsequently learn the conditioned eyeblink response. Furthermore, small lesions of the medial septum (the principle source of cholinergic projections to the hippocampus) made prior to training markedly impair acquisition of the conditioned eyeblink response (Berry and Thompson, 1979). This lesion destroys the septo-hippocampal ACh system and also abolishes hippocampal theta. Another consequence of the medial septal lesion is a significant impairment of the learning-induced increase in hippocampal unit activity.

The role of the hippocampus in classical conditioning of the eyeblink response is called "modulatory" because manipulations of the hippocampus can impair or enhance the rate of acquisition. Berger (1984) enhanced acquisition by establishing long-term-potentiation (LTP) in the hippocampus before classically conditioning the rabbits. Moore, Goodell, and Solomon (1976) interfered with the septo-hippocampal cholinergic system by administering scopolamine, and acquisition in the delay paradigm was markedly impaired. However, if the hippocampus is removed prior to training, learning proceeds normally (Solomon and Moore, 1975). An abnormally functioning hippocampus impairs learning, but the absence of a hippocampus does not. The memory trace itself is not in the hippocampus, but the hippocampus can markedly influence the storage process. We feel that this modulatory role for the hippocampus is particularly significant in SDAT.

A striking experiment which argues strongly for a modulatory role of the hippocampus in eyeblink classical conditioning was conducted by Solomon, Solomon, Vander Schaaf, and Perry (1983). Rabbits were given hippocampal ablations, ablations of the overlying cortex, or no lesions, and they were trained after administration of scopolamine or saline. Replicating previous research, hippocampal ablation had no effect on acquisition of the conditioned eyeblink response, but scopolamine severely retarded acquisition in the cortically lesioned and in the non-lesioned control animals. Significantly, in animals with hippocampal ablations, scopolamine had no effect on conditioning. The scopolamine-treated, hippocampal ablation group conditioned at about the same rate (165.4 versus 182.4 trials to criterion, $t(8) < 1$; $p > .05$). These results suggest that altered neuronal activity in the hippocampus is more detrimental to conditioning than removing the structure.

The Hippocampus and Classical Conditioning in Aging Rabbits

Research in the laboratories of Donald Powell in South Carolina and Paul Solomon in Massachusetts demonstrated age differences in acquisition of the conditioned eyeblink response in the trace classical conditioning paradigm (Graves and Solomon, 1985; Powell, Buchanan, and Hernandez, 1981). Because the hippocampus is a structure clearly affected by the histopathology of aging, our initial hypothesis was that age differences in rate of acquisition of the conditioned eyeblink response involved changes in the hippocampus.

In rabbits ranging in age from 3 to 50 months, we recorded hippocampal neuronal unit activity in the CA1 region and hippocampal EEG. Rabbits were trained first in the trace classical conditioning paradigm and then in the delay paradigm. Hippocampal neuronal activity modeling the eyeblink response took longer to develop in older animals, but once it developed, the "model" in the older hippocampus was indistinguishable from the "model" in the younger hippocampus. (Woodruff-Pak et al., 1987). Figure 2 presents hippocampal modeling data for a 45-month-old rabbit in the delay conditioning paradigm. As shown in Figure 3, hippocampal theta frequency was virtually identical for all age groups of rabbits (Woodruff-Pak and Logan, 1988). While much remains to be explored in hippocampal correlates of eyeblink conditioning in normal aging rabbits, we made the decision to examine other brain structures which might be associated with age differences in classical conditioning of the eyeblink response. A logical structure to explore was the cerebellum.

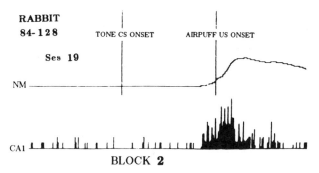

Fig. 2. Example of hippocampal neuronal unit activity modeling the conditioned eyeblink response (called NM for nictitating membrane response) in a 45-month-old rabbit. The average represents 9 trials presented in the delay classical conditioning paradigm. The NM response shown in the top tracing is an average of 9 trials. The hippocampal unit response shown below is a summation of activity in those same 9 trials. The first vertical line is the onset of the tone conditioned stimulus (CS), while the second vertical line represents the onset of the corneal airpuff unconditioned stimulus (US). The CS-US interval is 250 msec, and the total time period represented by the average is 750 msec. (From Woodruff-Pak et al., 1987).

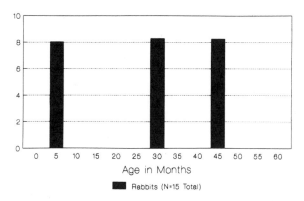

Fig. 3. Mean EEG frequency recorded in the left dorsal hippocampus during a 2-minute epoch before classical conditioning began in 3-, 30-, and 45-month-old rabbits. (From Woodruff-Pak and Logan, 1988).

ESSENTIAL ROLE OF CEREBELLUM IN EYEBLINK CLASSICAL CONDITIONING

There is mounting evidence that the neural circuitry involved in the essential plasticity for classical conditioning of the eyeblink response resides in the cerebellum (e.g., McCormick and Thompson, 1984a, 1984b; Thompson, 1986; Thompson, McCormick and Lavond, 1986; Woodruff-Pak et al., 1985). Data from stimulating, recording, and lesion studies suggest that the ipsilateral cerebellum is the site of the primary memory trace for the classically conditioned eyeblink response. To date, evidence is most consistent with storage of the memory traces in localized regions of cerebellar cortex and interpositus nucleus.

A hypothetical scheme or model has been developed of the neuronal system that could serve as the essential memory trace circuit for discrete, adaptive, learned somatic motor responses (Thompson, 1986). This model is presented in Figure 4. The feature of the model which may be particularly significant for understanding how aging affects eyeblink conditioning involves Purkinje cells. The site of the memory trace in the model is assumed to be at the principal cells of the interpositus nucleus and perhaps also at Purkinje cells. Purkinje cells serve as a central, integrating cell, receiving mossy fiber CS input and climbing fiber US input. Damage to Purkinje cells could interrupt the integration of CS and US information.

Woodruff-Pak and Sheffield (1987) examined Purkinje cells in sections of rabbit cerebellar cortical areas including left and right HVI and vermis. Comparisons of the total number of Purkinje cells counted for 12 rabbits ranging in age from 3 to 50 months revealed a significant decline in Purkinje cell number in older rabbits. The correlation between age and number of Purkinke cells was -.77 ($p < .005$). Cell counts in the molecular layer of the same animals indicated no age differences. This result suggests that differential tissue shrinkage in young and old brains was not the cause of the age difference in Purkinje cell number.

The correlation between trials to criterion and Purkinje cell number was -.79 ($p < .005$). A partial correlation was computed removing the variance due to age, and the resulting relationship between Purkinje cell number and trials to criterion was r = -.61 ($p < .025$). Multiple regression analysis indicated that Purkinje cell number accounted for a significant amount of the variance in acquisition, and no significant variance was attributable to age. It was the number of Purkinje cells rather than age, per se, which accounted for the learning deficits. Thus, the differences in Purkinje cell numbers in younger and older rabbits may be related to age differences in rate of classical conditioning.

There is evidence for Purkinje cell loss in many mammalian species, including humans. Hall, Miller, and Corsellis (1975) found a 25% reduction in the number of Purkinje cells over the human adult life span. Thus, Purkinje cell loss could be responsible for some of the age differences in eyeblink conditioning observed over the human life span.

The ipsilateral cerebellum may be essential for eyeblink classical conditioning in humans as well as rabbits. Lye, O'Boyle, Ramsden and Schady (1988) reported on classical conditioning of the eyeblink response in a patient with a right unilateral cerebellar lesion. They trained the patient repeatedly on the right and the left eye. In rabbits, cerebellar lesions affect conditioning in the eye ipsilateral to the lesion.

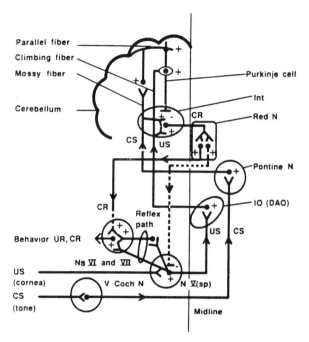

Fig. 4. Simplified schematic of hypothetical memory trace circuit for discrete behavioral responses learned as adaptations to aversive events. The corneal airpuff US pathway seems to consist of somatosensory projections to the dorsal accessory portion of the inferior olive (DAO) and its climbing fiber projections to the cerebellum. The tone CS pathway seems to consist of auditory projections to pontine nuclei (Pontine N) and their mossy fiber projections to the cerebellum. The efferent (eyelid closure) CR pathway projects from the interpositus nucleus (Int) of the cerebellum to the red nucleus (Red N) and via the descending rubral pathway to act ultimately on motor neurons. The red nucleus may also exert inhibitory control over the transmission of somatic sensory information about the US to the inferior olive (IO), so that when a CR occurs (eyelid closes), the red nucleus dampens US activation of climbing fibers. Evidence to date is most consistent with storage of the memory traces in the interpositus nucleus and possibly in localized regions of cerebellar cortex as well. Pluses indicate excitatory and minuses inhibitory synaptic action. Additional abbreviations: N V (sp), spinal fifth cranial nucleus; N VI sixth cranial nucleus; N VII, seventh cranial nucleus; V Coch N, ventral cochlear nucleus. (From Thompson, 1986).

This result occurred in the cerebellar patient as well. He demonstrated few CRs in the right eye and never attained learning criterion in 396 trials. However, he conditioned well in the left eye. This pattern of good left eye conditioning and no right eye conditioning was maintained throughout four sequential reversals of the side of training. Neurological, audiometric, and electrophysiological examinations of the subject tended to rule out primary sensory or motor deficits as the cause of the absence of conditioning in the right eye.

Behavioral data demonstrate striking parallels between the effects of aging on human and rabbit eyeblink conditioning. The data on the cerebellar patient suggest that the underlying brain circuitry for eyelid conditioning as well as the behavior are similar in rabbits and humans.

HUMAN EYELID CONDITIONING AND NORMAL AGING

The age differences in acquisition of the classically conditioned eyeblink response are large, and they first appear in the decade of the 40s (Woodruff-Pak and Thompson, 1988b). Early studies of eyeblink conditioning and aging compared the performance of young adults to adults over the age of 60 and found large age differences (Braun and Geiselhart, 1959; Gakkel and Zinina, reported in Jerome, 1959; Kimble and Pennypacker, 1963; Solyom and Barik, 1965). In older adults, the process of conditioning was markedly prolonged.

More recent studies of eyeblink conditioning in adulthood spanned the entire adult age range from the late teens to the mid-80s and found increasingly prolonged acquisition in each decade (Solomon et al., 1989; Woodruff-Pak and Thompson, 1988b). The robust nature of these age differences in human eyeblink conditioning is confirmed by the remarkable consistency of the data collected independently in Solomon's laboratory in Williamstown, Massachusetts and Woodruff-Pak's laboratory in Philadelphia, Pennsylvania. The correlation between age and the number of trials to learning criterion (8 CRs out of 9 consecutive trials) in the 60 subjects ranging in age from 18-85 in Williamstown was -.58 ($p < .001$), and in 44 subjects with normal UR amplitude ranging in age from 18-83 in Philadelphia was -.58 ($p < .001$). Controls for hearing acuity, eyeblink rate, level of alertness, and voluntary responding were carried out in these studies, and the results suggest that the age differences involved the associative learning capacities of the various cohorts rather than peripheral, non-associative factors. We suspect that the age differences in associative learning capacities may be caused by age differences in the cerebellum.

A number of changes occur in the aging cerebellum to decrease the efficiency of mossy fiber-granule cell-parallel fiber input to Purkinje cells and to impair or eliminate the Purkinje cells themselves. We have described these changes and discussed how such loss could impair eyeblink classical conditioning as conceptualized in the model presented in Figure 4 (Woodruff-Pak and Thompson, 1988a). We have also demonstrated in rabbits that mossy fiber stimulation as a CS results in an acquisition rate five times longer in older than in younger rabbits (Woodruff-Pak, Steinmetz, and Thompson, 1988). Our working hypothesis is that the documented decrease in the number of Purkinje cells in the human cerebellum along with changes affecting the mossy fiber-granule cell-parallel fiber input to Purkinje cells result in a slower rate of acquisition in normal aging humans.

HUMAN EYELID CONDITIONING AND SENILE DEMENTIA OF THE ALZHEIMER'S TYPE (SDAT)

We have indicated previously in this chapter that the involvement of the hippocampus in classical conditioning of the eyeblink response is profound, but modulatory in nature. If the hippocampus is ablated, rabbits learn normally (Schmaltz and Theios, 1972; Solomon and Moore, 1975; Solomon et al., 1983). However, if the septo-hippocampal cholinergic system is altered so that it functions abnormally, acquisition is seriously impaired. Alterations in hippocampal neuronal activity such as systemic scopolamine administration (Moore et al., 1976), microinjections of scopolamine into the medial septum (Solomon and Gottfried, 1981), and medial septal lesions (Berry and Thompson, 1979) all impair acquisition. Other manipulations producing altered hippocampal neuronal activity also retard acquisition. For example, producing hippocampal seizures with local penicillin injections to the hippocampus (Berger, Clark, and Thompson, 1980) impairs acquisition. Thus, an abnormally functioning hippocampus impairs acquisition while the removal of a hippocampus does not.

SDAT appears to profoundly alter hippocampal neuronal function. A major disruption of the brain cholinergic system occurs, impairing cortical and hippocampal cholinergic neurons (Coyle et al., 1983). Experimental procedures disrupting hippocampal cholinergic function such as microinjections of scopolamine to the medial septum (Solomon and Gottfried, 1981) and lesions of the medial septum (Berry and Thompson, 1979) prolong the rate of acquisition of the classically conditioned eyeblink response in rabbits. These data from the animal model would lead to the prediction that SDAT patients, having hippocampal dysfunction, should show poorer acquisition of the classically conditioned eyeblink response than normal adults.

Hyman et al. (1984) examined hippocampal tissue at autopsy in 5 patients confirmed as having SDAT and 5 normal old control patients. They observed a specific cellular pattern of pathology such that the affected cells were essentially the input and output of the hippocampus. These investigators argued that SDAT effectively isolates the hippocampus from the rest of the brain. They also observed significant loss of the CA1 pyramidal cells in SDAT. In rabbits, these are the hippocampal cells which model the eyeblink response as shown in Figures 1 and 2 (Berger and Thompson, 1978a; Berger et al., 1983). If the abnormally functioning hippocampus was completely isolated from the rest of the brain in SDAT, it might be analogous to an ablated hippocampus in rabbits. Our prediction for classical conditioning in SDAT in the case of a totally isolated hippocampus would be acquisition similar to age-matched controls.

We have focused on the hippocampus in SDAT because there is such widespread agreement that profound hippocampal impairment exists in this disease. For example, Bird et al. (1989) reported that neurofibrillary tangles and senile plaques were common and most frequently seen in hippocampus and temporal cortex in 45 autopsy reports on SDAT. Damage to the cerebellum in these patients was relatively rare. Although there are not many studies of the cerebellum in SDAT, it appears that the cerebellum of SDAT patients is roughly similar to the cerebellum of age-matched controls. What distinguishes SDAT patients with regard to the two brain structures (cerebellum and hippocampus) most involved in the rabbit in classical conditioning of the eyeblink response is the major damage to the hippocampus. It was our assumption that SDAT patients would have Purkinje cell loss that accompanies normal aging, and they would have abnormal hippocampal neuronal activity associated with cell loss and cholinergic neural dysfunction. We suspected that abnormalities in both of the brain structures invloved with eyeblink classical conditioning might dramatically impair acquisition of the conditioned eyeblink response. We predicted that the degree of classical conditioning in patients with probable SDAT would be minimal.

Eyeblink Conditioning in Patients Diagnosed with SDAT

The resources of the NIMH Clinical Research Center for the Study of the Psychopathology of the Elderly at the Philadelphia Geriatric Center (PGC) served to identify a group of patients from among the Center's 1100 residents who met NINCDS-ADRDA criteria for the diagnosis of probable Alzheimer's disease. The initial sample of 7 patients had a mean score of 15.2 on the Blessed Memory-Information-Concentration test (range of 13 to 17) and a mean age of 82.6 years (range of 76 to 88). Though moderately impaired, these patients all were maintaining themselves in the Center's congregate housing facility, living either independently, or with companion care. Eight age-matched control subjects who were also residents of PGC were classically conditioned. The control subjects had a mean Blessed score of 2.6 (range of 0 to 6) and a mean age of 84.1 years (range of 72 to 93).

The classical conditioning laboratory was on the premises of PGC, so patients were classically conditioned in their own apartment building. The methods and equipment were identical to those used for normal aging adults and reported by Woodruff-Pak and Thompson (1988b). Briefly, the subject sat in a chair and wore an adjustable headgear. This headgear held an infrared photocell transducer which measured the eyeblink. Also attached to the headgear was a tube resting 1 cm from the subject's left cornea that delivered a 5-psi airpuff of medical grade oxygen as the US. Voltage changes from the photocell transducer were input to an Apple IIe computer that stored and analyzed the data. A speaker presented the CS which was a 1-KHz-tone CS of 80 dB SPL. All subjects stated that they could hear the tone very clearly.

The timing and presentation of the stimuli was controlled by an Apple IIe computer. A CR was scored if the response was an eyeblink of .5 mm or larger and occurred in the period between 25-399 msec after the onset of the CS. The UR was scored as any response at 400-600 msec after CS onset (which was also after US onset).

After adjusting the headgear, a video recorder placed in front of the subject was turned on and the subject was invited to watch a silent film (Charlie Chaplin in *Gold Rush*). When the subject was engaged in that activity, the computer-controlled sequence of tone-CS and airpuff-US was initiated. The CS-US interval was 400 msec, and all parameters were identical to those used in the normal aging study (Woodruff-Pak and Thompson, 1988b). There were a total of 90 trials in the delay classical conditioning paradigm, with 80 trials being paired CS and US and 10 trials being tone-CS alone. The tone CS-alone trial occurred every 9th trial. The entire session lasted about 45 minutes.

Results indicated very striking differences between patients diagnosed with probable SDAT and normal age-matched controls. While age-matched normal control subjects produced a total of 45.2% CRs, probable SDAT patients produced only 16.7% CRs. This difference was statistically significant ($t[13]$ = 3.19; $p < .01$).

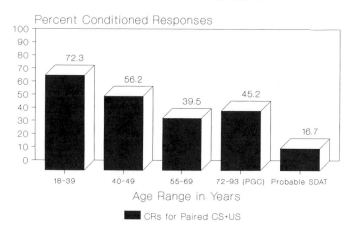

Normal Adults and Probable SDAT

Fig. 5. Total percentage of conditioned responses (CRs) for five groups of adults. Total percent CRs in paired trials in the delay classical conditioning paradigm for 88 men and women ranging in age from 18 to 93 years. The age range in the youngest group was 18-39 years (N=40), and for the older groups was 40-49 (N=20), 55-69 (N=13), 72-93 (N=8), and probable SDAT (N=7). The first three groups were tested on a university campus, and the last two groups were tested at the Philadelphia Geriatric Center (PGC). In one day of training shown in these data, there were a total of 80 paired CS-US trials for those tested at PGC and 96 paired trials for those tested at the university. The delay classical conditioning paradigm was used with a CS-US interval of 400 msec.

With normal aging there is a difference in the degree to which individuals classically condition. Subjects in the decade of the 50s and older condition more poorly than subjects in the 20s and 30s. In the 40s, age differences in amplitude of the conditioned response begin to be significantly lower than the CR amplitude of younger adults (Woodruff-Pak and Thompson, 1988). Nevertheless, all age groups of normal adults show clear evidence of associative learning. This is not the case in patients diagnosed with probable SDAT. Figure 5 presents a comparison of classical conditioning in normal adults in various age groups and patients with probable SDAT.

A one-way ANOVA revealed that the age differences in total percent CRs were statistically significant ($F[4,83] = 9.97$; $p < .01$). A Tukey-Kramer modification of the HSD test for unequal sample sizes indicated that probable SDAT patients conditioned significantly more poorly than normal subjects of all ages ($q[5,83] = 6.15$; $p < .01$). Differences in percent CRs between the 55-69 age group and the 72-93 age group were not statistically significant ($q[5,83] = 0.61$).

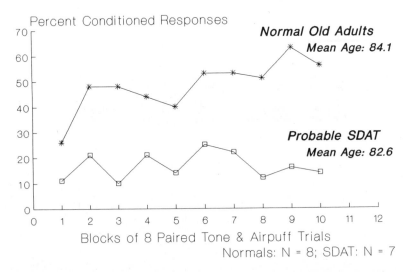

Fig. 6. Acquisition over 10 conditioning blocks for patients diagnosed with probable SDAT and normal age-matched Philadelphia Geriatric Center residents. Each block represents eight paired trials of 500 msec, 80 dB SPL, 1 Khz tone conditioned stimulus (CS) coterminating with a 100-msec, 5-psi corneal airpuff unconditioned stimulus (US) presented 400 msec after the onset of the CS.

While acquisition in normal age-matched control subjects shows a clear incremental function, acquisition is not evident in patients diagnosed with probable SDAT. A 2 by 10 repeated measures ANOVA comparing the performance of normal controls and probable SDAT patients on percent CRs revealed a statistically significant group effect ($F = 10.2$; $p < .01$). The other effects were not statistically significant ($F[9, 117] = 1.59$ and $.995$ for acquisition over blocks and the group times acquisition over blocks effects, respectively).

These results with human patients with a diagnosis of probable SDAT parallel the observation in rabbits that an abnormally functioning hippocampus impairs acquisition of the classically conditioned eyeblink response. Control rabbits injected with scopolamine show less than 10% CRs for 400 learning trials and did not attain a learning criterion of 5 consecutive CRs until 532 trials (Solomon et al., 1983). We ran patients diagnosed as probable SDAT for 90 trials, and they showed no signs of associative learning.

Our data do not support the contention of Hyman et al. (1984) that a consequence of SDAT is to isolate the hippocampus. To support that hypothesis, patients diagnosed with probable SDAT should have conditioned like normal, age-matched control subjects. However, our patients with probable SDAT had moderate cognitive impairment and were still living in residential apartments (alone or with the assistance of caretakers). Perhaps by the time of death, the disease has progressed to effectively isolate the hippocampus from its input and output. Interestingly, if this isolation of the hippocampus were to occur at some point late in the progression of SDAT, we would predict that very late probable SDAT patients would be able to produce conditioned responses at a higher level than they would have at the early stages of the disease.

The above discussion contrasting predictions from Hyman et al.'s model of the isolated hippocampus in SDAT to Coyle et al.'s model of general cholinergic neuronal dysfunction which would create an abnormal hippocampus requires some qualifications. We have found classical conditioning of the eyeblink response in rabbits and humans to have great potential for the study of the neurobiology of learning and memory in normal aging and SDAT (Thompson and Woodruff-Pak, 1987; Woodruff-Pak, 1988; Woodruff-Pak and Thompson, 1985). However, there is no animal model which mimics all aspects of SDAT. There are so many brain structures and neurotransmitter systems adversely impacted in SDAT that classical conditioning could be abolished in patients diagnosed with probable SDAT for many different reasons. We have attempted to control for some of the peripheral phenomena which might account for the failure of SDAT patients to condition (e.g., hearing impairment, loss of eyeblink reflex, insensitive cornea). However, we will continue to test hypothesis about non-neural and non-hippocampal phenomena which might prevent patients with SDAT from producing conditioned responses.

There are major difficulties involved in applying an animal model with controlled and experimentally altered brain function to aging humans with a progressive, degenerative disease. In that sense, it is remarkable that our predictions from the animal model were so clearly supported in the behavior of patients diagnosed with probable SDAT. Additional neurobiological and behavioral data in rabbits and humans diagnosed and confirmed as having SDAT are required to assess the usefulness of classical conditioning of the eyeblink response as a behavioral assessment of SDAT and as an index of the degree of underlying hippocampal dysfunction.

SUMMARY AND CONCLUSIONS

Classical conditioning of the eyeblink response in rabbits and humans is a useful model system for the study of the neurobiology of learning, memory, and aging which has implications for research and assessment in SDAT. Parallels exist between rabbits and humans in the way they condition behaviorally and in the manner in which aging affects behavioral conditioning. The neural circuitry underlying this behavior is almost completely understood in rabbits, and there are indications that the circuitry is similar in humans.

The brain structures involved in eyeblink classical conditioning are the hippocampus, which plays a modulatory role, and the cerebellum, which is essential for learning and retention. A consequence of normal aging is loss of Purkinje cells in cerebellar cortex. Purkinje cell loss may be at least partially responsible for poorer conditioning in older organisms. In rabbits, the correlation between Purkinje cell number and learning trials to criterion was -.79 which was highly significant.

In addition to the Purkinje cell loss which accompanies normal aging, patients with probable SDAT have an abnormally functioning hippocampus, including dysfunction of the septo-hippocampal cholinergic system. In rabbits, impairment in the septo-hippocampal cholinergic system seriously impairs classical conditioning. Results with 7 patients diagnosed as probable SDAT indicated very low levels of classical conditioning (16.9% CRs) compared with normal, age-matched conrtol subjects (48.4% CRs).

Eyeblink classical conditioning may serve as a useful assessment technique in SDAT. With the close parallels between the animal model and human behavior, the model system has potential usefulness for testing pharmacological agents which may optimize learning and retention in animals, normal aging humans, and patients with SDAT.

REFERENCES

Berger, T. W. (1984). Long-term potentiation of hippocampal synaptic transmission affects rate of behavioral learning. Science, 224, 627-630.

Berger, T. W., Alger, B. E., & Thompson, R. F. (1976). Neuronal substrate of classical conditioning in the hippocampus. Science, 192, 483-485.

Berger, T. W., Berry, S. D., & Thompson, R. F. (1986). Role of the hippocampus in classical conditioning of aversive and appetitive behaviors. In R. L. Isaacson & K. H. Pribram (Eds.), The hippocampus, (Vol. IV, pp. 203-239). New York: Plenum.

Berger, T. W., Clark, G. A., & Thompson, R. F. (1980). Learning-dependent neuronal responses recorded from limbic system brain structures during classical conditioning. Physiological Psychology, 8, 155-167.

Berger, T. W., Rinaldi, P., Weisz, D. J., & Thompson, R. F. (1983). Single unit analysis of different hippocampal cell types during classical conditioning of the rabbit nictitating membrane response. Journal of Neurophysiology, 59, 1197-1219.

Berger, T. W. & Thompson, R. F. (1978a). Neuronal plasticity in the limbic system during classical conditioning of the rabbit nictitating membrane response. I. The hippocampus. Brain Research, 145, 323-346.

Berger, T. W. & Thompson, R. F. (1978b). Identification of pyramidal cells as the critical elements in hippocampal neuronal plasticity during learning. Proceedings of the National Academy of Science, 75, 1572-1576.

Berry, S. D. & Thompson, R. F. (1978). Prediction of learning rate from the hippocampal EEG. Science, 200, 1298-1300.

Berry, S. D. & Thompson, R. F. (1979). Medial septal lesions retard classical conditioning of the nictitating membrane response in rabbits. Science, 205, 209-211.

Bird, T. D., Sumi, S. M., Nemens, E. J., Nochlin, D., Schellenberg, G., Lampe, T. H., Sadovnick, A., Chui, H., Miner, G. W., & Tinklenberg, J. (1989). Phenotypic heterogeneity in familial Alzheimer's disease: A study of 24 kindreds. Annals of Neurology, 25, 12-25.

Braun, H. W., & Geiselhart, R. (1959). Age differences in the acquisition and extinction of the conditioned eyelid response. Journal of Experimental Psychology, 57, 386-388.

Coyle, J. T., Price, D. L., & DeLong, M. R. (1983). Alzheimer's disease: A disorder of cortical cholinergic innervation. Science, 219, 1184-1190.

Deyo, R. A., Straube, K. T., & Disterhoft, J. F. (1989). Nimodipine facilitates associative learning in aging rabbits. Science, 243, 809-811.

Gendreau, P., & Suboski, M. D. (1971). Intelligence and age in discrimination conditioning of the eyelid response. Journal of Experimental Psychology, 89, 379-382.

Gormezano, I. (1966). Classical conditioning. In J. B. Sidowski (Ed.), Experimental methods and instrumentation in psychology (pp. 385-420). New York: McGraw-Hill.

Gormezano, I. & Kehoe, E. J. (1975). Classical conditioning: Some methodological-conceptal issues. In W. K. Estes (Ed.), Handbook of learning and cognitive processes. Vol. 2. Conditioning and behavior theory (pp. 143-179). New Jersey: Lawrence Erlbaum Associates.

Gormezano, I., Kehoe, E. J., & Marshall, B. S. (1983). Twenty years of classical conditioning research with the rabbit. In J. M. Sprague & A. N. Epstein (Eds.), Progress in psychobiology and physiological psychology, Vol. 10 (pp. 197-275). New York: Academic Press.

Graves, C. A. & Solomon, P. R. (1985). Age related disruption of trace but not delay classical conditioning of the rabbit's nictitating membrane response. Behavioral Neuroscience, 99, 88-96.

Hall, T. C., Miller, K. H., & Corsellis, J. A. N. (1975). Variations in the human Purkinje cell population according to age and sex. Neuropathology and Applied Neurobiology, 1, 267-292.

Hyman, B., Van Hoesen, G. W., Damasio, A., & Barnes, C. (1984). Alzheimer's disease: Cell specific pathology isolates the hippocampal formation. Science, 225, 1168-1170.

Jerome, E. A. (1959). Age and learning -- Experimental studies. In J. E. Birren (Ed.), Handbook of aging and the individual (pp. 655-699). Chicago: University of Chicago Press.

Kimble, G. A. (1961). Pavlovian conference on higher nervous activity: Discussion: Part IV. New York Academy of Sciences, 92, 1189-1192.

Kimble, G. A., & Pennypacker, H. S. (1963). Eyelid conditioning in young and aged subjects. Journal of Genetic Psychology, 103, 283-289.

Lye, R. H., O'Boyle, D. J., Ramsden, R. T., & Schady, W. (1988). Effects of a unilateral cerebellar lesion on the acquisition of eye-blink conditioning in man. Journal of Physiology (London), 403, 58P.

McCormick, D. A., Lavond, D. G., & Thompson, R. F. (1982). Concomitant classical conditioning of the rabbit nictitating membrane and eyelid responses: Correlations and implications. Physiology and Behavior, 28, 769-775.

McCormick, D. A., & Thompson, R. F. (1984a). Cerebellum: Essential involvement in the classically conditioned eyelid response. Science, 223, 296-299.

McCormick, D. S. & Thompson, R. F. (1984b). Neuronal responses of the rabbit cerebellum during acquisition and performance of a classically conditioned nictitating membrane/eyelid response. Journal of Neuroscience, 4, 2811-2822.

McKhann, G., Drachman, D., Folstein, M., Katzman, R., Price, D., & Stadlan, E. M. (1984). Clinical diagnosis of Alzheimer's disease: Report of the NINCDS-ADRDA work group under the auspices of Department of Health and Human Services Task Force on Alzheimer's disease. Neurology, 34, 939-944.

Moore, J. W., Goodell, N. A., & Solomon, P. R. (1976). Central cholinergic blockage by scopolamine and habituaation, classical conditioning, and latent inhibition of the rabbit's nictitating membrane response. Physiological Psychology, 4, 395-399.

Moore, J. W. & Gormezano, I. (1977). Classical conditioning. In M. H. Marx & M. Bunch (Eds.), Fundamentals and applications of learning (pp. 87-120). New York: Macmillan.

Patterson, M. M. & Romano, A. R. (1987). The rabbit in Pavlovian conditioning. In I. Gormezano, W. F. Prokasy, & R. F. Thompson (Eds.), Classical conditioning (3rd ed., pp. 1-36). New Jersey: Lawrence Erlbaum Associates.

Powell, D. A., Buchanan, S. L., & Hernandez, L. L. (1981). Age related changes in classical (Pavlovian) conditioning in the New Zealand albino rabbit. Experimental Aging Research, 7, 453-465.

Schmaltz, L. W. & Theios, J. (1972). Acquisition and extinction of a classically conditioned response in hippocampectomized rabbits (Oryctolagus cuniculus). Journal of Comparative and Physiological Psychology, 79, 328-333.

Sitiram, N., Weingartner, H., & Gillin, J. C. (1978). Human serial learning: Enhancement with arecoline and choline, and impairment with scopolamine. Science, 201, 274-276.

Solomon, P. R. & Gottfried, K. E. (1981). The spetohippocampal cholinergic system and classical conditioning of the rabbit's nictitating membrane response. Journal of Comparative and Physiological Psychology, 95, 322-330.

Solomon, P. R. & Moore, J. W. (1975). Latent inhibition and stimulus generalization of the classically conditioned nictitating membrane response in rabbits (Oryctolagus cuniculus) following dorsal hippocampal ablations. Journal of Comparative and Physiological Psychology, 89, 1192-1203.

Solomon, P. R., Pomerleau, D., Bennett, L., James, J., & Morse, D. L. (1989). Acquisition of the classically conditioned eyeblink response in humans over the life span. Psychology and Aging, 4, 34-41.

Solomon, P. R., Solomon, S. D., Vander Schaaf, E., & Perry, H. E. (1983). Altered activity in the hippocampus is more detrimental to classical conditioning than removing the structure. Science, 220, 329-331.

Solyom, L., & Barik, H. C. (1965). Conditioning in senescence and senility. Journal of Gerontology, 20, 483-488.

Thompson, R. F. (1986). The neurobiology of learning and memory. Science, 233, 941-947.

Thompson, R. F., Berger, T. W., Berry, S. D., Hoehler, F. K., Kettner, R. E., & Weisz, D. J. (1980). Hippocampal substrate of classical conditioning. Physiological Psychology, 8, 262-279.

Thompson, R. F., Berger, T. W., Cegavske, C. F., Patterson, M. M., Roemer, R. A., Teyler, T. J., & Young, R. A. (1976). A search for the engram. American Psychologist, 31, 209-227.

Thompson, R. F., McCormick, D. A., & Lavond, D. G. (1986). Localization of the essential memory trace system for a basic form of associative learning in the mammalian brain. In S. Hulse (Ed.), One hundred years of psychological research in America (pp. 125-171). Baltimore: Johns Hopkins University Press.

Thompson, R. F., & Woodruff-Pak, D. S. (1987). A model system approach to age and the neuronal bases of learning and memory. In M. W. Riley, J. D. Matarazzo, & A. Baum (Eds.), The aging dimension. (pp. 49-76). Hillsdale, NJ: Erlbaum.

Woodruff-Pak, D. S. (1988). Aging and classical conditioning: Parallel studies in rabbits and humans. Neurobiology of Aging, 9, 511-522.

Woodruff-Pak, D. S., Lavond, D. G., Logan, C. G., & Thompson, R. F. (1987). Classical conditioning in 3-, 30-, and 45-month-old rabbits: Behavioral learning and hippocampal unit activity. Neurobiology of Aging, 8, 101-108.

Woodruff-Pak, D. S., Lavond, D. G., & Thompson, R. F. (1985). Trace conditioning: Abolished by cerebellar nuclear lesions but not lateral cerebellar cortex aspirations. Brain Research, 348, 249-260.

Woodruff-Pak, D. S. & Logan, C. G. (1988). No apparent age differences in hippocampal theta frequency in rabbits aged 3-50 months. Comprehensive Gerontology, 2, 24-28.

Woodruff-Pak, D. S., & Sheffield, J. B. (1987). Age differences in Purkinje cells and rate of classical conditioning in young and older rabbits. Society for Neuroscience Abstracts, 13, 441.

Woodruff-Pak, D. S., Steinmetz, J. E., & Thompson, R. F. (1988). Classical conditioning of rabbits 2-1/2 to 4 years old using mossy fiber stimulation as a CS. Neurobiology of Aging, 9, 187-193.

Woodruff-Pak, D. S., & Thompson, R. F. (1985). Classical conditioning of the eyelid response in rabbits as a model system for the study of brain mechanisms of learning and memory in aging. Experimental Aging Research, 11, 109-122.

Woodruff-Pak, D. S., & Thompson, R. F. (1988a). Cerebellar correlates of classical conditioning across the life span. In P. B. Baltes, R. M. Lerner, & D. M. Featherman (Eds.), Life-span development and behavior (Vol. 9) (pp. 1-37). Hillsdale, NJ: Erlbaum.

Woodruff-Pak, D. S. & Thompson, R. F. (1988b). Classical conditioning of the eyeblink response in the delay paradigm in adults aged 18-83 years. Psychology and Aging, 3, 219-229.

COMPUTER-SIMULATED EVERYDAY MEMORY TESTING FOR CLINICAL TRIALS IN MEMORY DISORDERS OF AGING

Glenn J. Larrabee and
Thomas H. Crook III

Memory Assessment Clinics, Inc.
Sarasota, FL and Bethesda, MD

Clinical trials in Alzheimer's disease and Age-Associated Memory Impairment (AAMI)[1] frequently employ memory tests as major dependent variables. Accurate assessment of memory is critical in selecting patients for geriatric drug trials and for measurement of drug response. In the past, memory tests have included visual reproduction of geometric designs, story recall and tests of word list learning which frequently bear little relationship to the memory demands of everyday life. Additionally, the majority of these traditional memory tests are available in only one or two alternate forms, presenting a serious limitation in clinical trials employing repeated measurements designs.[2]

Another important consideration in selecting dependent measures of memory function is the overall process of development of candidate treatments for memory disorders of aging. As highlighted in the current volume, this process typically begins with preclinical animal models, ultimately leading to clinical trials in humans. Hence, tests which incorporate research paradigms that are effective in measuring animal memory should have enhanced potential sensitivity in measuring pharmacologic effects on memory in human subjects.[2,3] Spatial memory, object location recall, and tasks requiring responding after varying periods of delay, in particular, delayed non-match to sample paradigms, are particularly sensitive to age related memory change in both animals and man. Consequently, memory tests employing these procedures allow evaluation of comparable memory processes across species.[2,3,4]

In addition to issues of face validity, and similarity of memory paradigms across species, several other issues are related to selection of memory tests for clinical trials. These factors include the psychometric properties of particular tests (reliability, validity, and alternate form availability), and the relationship of test parameters to current theoretical approaches and experimental learning and memory paradigms. Larrabee and Crook[2] discuss these issues in greater detail. Leber[5] had highlighted the need for multiple measures of legitimate symptoms and signs which are truly related to psychogeriatric conditions, in order to maximize the chance of detecting treatment effects when they are actually present. Clearly, measurement approaches which integrate face validity with experimental, theoretical, and psychometric constructs should have greater sensitivity in the detection of potential treatment response. The computer-simulated everyday memory battery described in the remainder of this chapter is an attempt at such an integration.

A COMPUTERIZED EVERYDAY MEMORY BATTERY FOR CLINICAL TRIALS

Over the past several years, Crook, Ferris, and colleagues have been investigating measurement of various everyday memory functions including memory for names, faces, grocery list items, object location, and telephone numbers.[6,7,8,9,10] Recently, a number of these earlier tasks have been refined further utilizing customized computer graphics and laser disk technology.[11,12] Although the battery is computerized, research subjects do not encounter a keyboard, joystick, or other potentially unfamiliar manipulanda. Rather, persons respond either verbally, by pressing a video touchscreen, or by operating familiar objects such as a touchtone telephone.

Six of the tests in the computerized battery are technologically advanced modifications of tasks developed previously and found in prior studies to be of particular utility in studies of aging and dementia. These include a verbal learning and memory task requiring grocery list learning,[10] a facial recognition test employing a signal detection paradigm,[8] a name-face learning and delayed recall task,[9] a facial recognition test employing a delayed non-matching to sample paradigm,[13] and a misplaced objects task requiring subjects to place computer-generated representations of common objects within the representation of a house and later, recall the locations chosen.[6] Three additional measures in the battery include a narrative recall test in which the subject is tested for recall of factual information after viewing an abbreviated television news broadcast, a measure of reaction time based on a simulated automobile driving task, and paired associate learning for first and last names.

The computerized tests are administered in a standardized manner in a controlled clinical setting. The subject is seated in front of a large color monitor and the other manipulanda required for testing while the tester, who is present throughout the session, operates the computerized equipment behind, and generally out of view of, the subject. Tests are administered with an AT&T 6300 computer equipped with a 20 megabyte hard-disk drive and customized computer graphic hardware, a Pioneer LDV-6010 laser-disk player, a Sony 19 inch PVM 1910 color monitor with a Personal Touch touchscreen, and various customized peripheral hardware and manipulanda. Subject responses are recorded and stored for later data analysis during the actual testing session. Responses involving a motor component (e.g., touching the screen for object placement, dialing the telephone) are automatically scored and stored. Subject verbal responses (e.g., to verbal selective reminding) are entered by the tester. Description of the various tasks follows. Each is available in 5 alternate forms in English, French, German, Italian, Swedish, Danish, Finnish, and Dutch. Preliminary data suggest comparability of performance, in relation to age, gender, and education effects between the American, Italian, and Belgian (French) versions (M. Salama and G. Zappala, personal communication, May, 1988).

Name-Face Association - Immediate Recall

In this test subjects are shown live color video recordings (stored on laser disk) of individuals (actors) introducing themselves by common first names. After a series of introductions, recall is assessed by showing the same individuals in a different order and asking the subject to provide the name of each person. To provide the subject with expressive, acoustical, and other cues available in daily life, individuals who appear on the screen during the recall phase of the test indicate the city where they reside with the statement "I'm from _____." Following this statement, subjects are asked to provide the individual's name. In Phase I of the test, subjects are shown three different series of introductions consisting of two, four, and six individuals and recall occurs following each series. In Phase 2, subjects are shown the same 14 individuals (in a different order) for 3 consecutive trials (to measure acquisition). Scoring is based on the total correct for each recall condition.

Name-Face Association - Delayed Recall

This phase of the test is administered approximately 40 minutes after the third acquisition trial described above. For a fourth time subjects are shown the 14 individuals introduced in the acquisition paradigm. No introductions are provided for the delayed recall trial; rather, the subject's task is to recall the individual's name when presented with the "I'm from _____" portion of the video. Scoring is for total names correctly recalled.

Selective Reminding

This test follows the standard selective reminding paradigm using common grocery list items as the stimuli to be recalled. On the first trial, subjects are shown a list of 15 items, appearing individually on the video screen. Following the recall attempt, the words which subjects have not recalled reappear on the screen, and subjects must then attempt to recall the entire list, having been selectively reminded of the words they omitted on the previous trial. Scoring is for the following aspects of performance: total recall, summed across all five test trials; long-term storage or LTS (i.e., words that have been recalled at least once without reminding are assumed to remain in LTS on successive trials, even if the subject does not mention

them subsequently); consistent long-term retrieval or CLTR
(consistent recall of a word in LTS, to the end of the test
trials); and half-hour delayed free recall. Scores for LTS
and CLTR are cumulative over the five continuous learning
trials. The test is terminated prior to five trials if the
subject recalls the entire list on two successive trials.

First-Last Names

This is a test of associative learning and memory of
verbal stimuli. On each of five trials, subjects are
presented with a series of six paired first and last names,
followed by a presentation of the last names only. The
subject's task is to recall the first name which was paired
with each last name. As in Selective Reminding, the test
does not extend to five trials if a subject correctly
recalls the first names on two successive trials prior to
the fifth trial. The score is the total of first names
correctly identified for each trial.

Narrative Recall

This test follows the design of older narrative recall
tests in which subjects are required to recall the content
of a paragraph read to them by the tester. In this case,
however, subjects watch a 6-minute television news
broadcast. They are then given a series of 25 factual,
multiple-choice questions on the touchscreen and asked to
select the correct answer by touching a corresponding box
on the screen. There are no time limits for response and
the score is simply the number of correct responses.

Misplaced Objects

In this test, subjects are shown computer
representations of 20 common objects that are frequently
misplaced (for example, eyeglasses) and the detailed
interior of a 12-room house. During the first phase of the
test the house remains displayed on the screen and subjects
are asked to place each object, one at a time, in a
location where it can later be recalled. The only
limitation is that no more than two objects can be placed
in a single room. After all objects are placed, the
subject goes on to other tests. Approximately 40 minutes
later, recall is tested. In this phase, the rooms are
again displayed and the subject's task is to recall the
room in which each object was placed. They do so by
touching the correct room and, if the response is correct,
the object appears briefly in the room. Subjects are
allowed two attempts to recall each object and the two
attempts are scored separately. There are no time limits
on either placement or recall of objects.

Recognition of Faces - Signal Detection

In this test, subjects are shown 156 actual facial
photographs, each displayed on a touchscreen monitor for
2.6 seconds. The task of subjects is to touch a "YES" or
"NO" box displayed in color on the screen to indicate
whether they have or have not seen the photograph earlier
in the test session. Fifty of the faces are shown twice;

the remainder are shown only once. Of those shown twice, the interval between first and second presentation is varied systematically from 0 to 4 minutes. Signal detection methods are employed to control for differing response criteria among subjects and the statistic d' is calculated at each delay interval.

Recognition of Faces - Signal Detection, Delayed

This test is a delayed version of the test described above. Approximately 40 minutes after the initial recognition test, subjects are shown 20 photographs, 10 of which were shown (only once) in the earlier phase of the test and 10 of which are being shown for the first time. The subject's task is to identify those faces which are repeated by pressing the appropriate box ("YES" or "NO") on the touchscreen and, again, signal detection methods are used in scoring.

Recognition of Faces - Delayed Nonmatching to Sample

On the first trial of this test, subjects are shown a single facial photograph on the touchscreen monitor and asked to touch the face. On each of 24 subsequent trials a "new" face is added to the array, and the subject's task is to identify the new face added by touching it on the monitor. Each trial is separated from the preceding trial by an 8-second interval, during which the screen is black. Subjects receive feedback for their responses on each trial in the form of a red square that appears momentarily around the photograph if it is correctly identified. Two scores are computed. The first is the number correctly identified until subjects make their first error. The second is the total number correctly identified.

Telephone Dialing (Without Interference)

This task is a variation on the standard digit-recall test and is intended to provide greater ecologic validity. Subjects are shown a series of 7- or 10-digit numbers (as in local or long distance numbers) on the monitor screen and asked to read the series aloud. Immediately after the final digit is read and disappears from the screen, subjects are instructed to dial the total number on a touchtone phone interfaced with the computer. Numbers dialed by the subject are automatically displayed on the screen, but no other feedback is provided. Eight trials are conducted, four at each of the two series lengths. In scoring, credit is given for each digit dialed in the correct position regardless of errors made elsewhere in the sequence.

Telephone Dialing (With Interference)

This proceeds in the same manner as the previously described dialing task, with the exception that after subjects have completed dialing, they hear either a busy signal or a ring. If they hear a busy signal, "Please Redial" appears on the video screen, and they are then asked to redial. Scoring is the same as in telephone dialing without interference.

Reaction Time - Noninterference

This is a variation on a standard information-processing paradigm in which the task of driving a car and responding appropriately to changing traffic signals is simulated. On the screen, subjects are shown a representation of a traffic light and representations of brake and accelerator pedals. Subjects are instructed to change pedals appropriately and as quickly as possible when the light changes colors (using the dominant hand). The light changes colors at varying intervals of 3, 4, and 5 seconds, and both lift and travel time are recorded in milliseconds at each of these intervals.

Reaction Time - Divided Attention

This follows the same format as the previously described task, with the exception that the simulated driving task is performed while subjects listen to simulated radio weather and traffic reports. Subjects are asked to recall as much information as possible from the weather and traffic reports in a free-recall format. The number of facts correctly recalled in each of the two reports is scored.

TEST BATTERY CHARACTERISTICS

Performance on the battery is significantly associated with age in normal subjects ages 18 to 88.[11,12] Normative data exceed 1000 normal subjects for each test. Additional data are available on over several hundred persons manifesting AAMI.

Previous research on clinical memory tests and batteries has demonstrated performance dimensions of verbal and visual memory, and attention/concentration/psychomotor speed.[14,15,16,17,18] Consequently, the factor structure of the computerized everyday memory battery was investigated to determine if similar dimensions were represented. In the first study, four factors were elicited including general everyday memory (defined by Name-Face Association, Narrative Recall, Misplaced Objects-First Try, and both facial recognition tests), complex attention and vigilance (defined by Misplaced Objects-Second Try and Reaction Time - lift component), psychomotor speed (Reaction Time - lift and travel components), and simple attention (Name-Face Association, 6 Faces and Telephone Dialing, 3 Digits).[11] The factor structure was not affected by age, since the same basic results were obtained when raw scores were factored, and when scores which had been adjusted for age were factored. This indicates that while level of performance on the computerized everyday tests changes with age, the pattern of performance does not. Consequently, clinicians and researchers can be confident that they are measuring the same constructs or clusters of abilities regardless of the age of the adult subject.

In the Crook and Larrabee study,[11] separate verbal and visual memory factors were not obtained; rather, a general (verbal and visual) factor was obtained. Others have reported similar findings for standard memory tests.[18] However, the set of computerized procedures analyzed by Crook and Larrabee did not contain sufficient purely verbal measures. A follow-up factor analysis was conducted, incorporating the Selective Reminding and First-Last Names everyday verbal memory procedures. With the inclusion of these measures, Larrabee and Crook[19] demonstrated a verbal everyday memory factor (defined by Name-Face Association, Incidental Memory, First-Last Names, and Selective Reminding), as well as a visual everyday memory factor (defined by both facial recognition memory procedures). Additionally, Larrabee and Crook factored the set of computerized everyday memory tasks combined with WAIS Vocabulary, Wechsler Memory Scale Logical Memory (LM) and Paired Associate Learning (PAL), and the Benton Visual Retention Test (BVRT).[20] Concurrent validity was established, with WMS Hard Associates loading with the everyday verbal memory factor, WMS LM loading with both Incidental recall and WAIS Vocabulary, and BVRT loading with two factors: everyday visual memory and psychomotor speed and vigilance.

In summary, these two factor analytic studies support the factorial and concurrent validity of the computerized everyday memory battery. The multidimensional structure, similar to that obtained in standard memory batteries, allows for assessment of differential treatment effects and differential patterns of impairment in terms of processing speed, vigilance, and verbal and visual memory functions. The stimulation of tasks of everyday memory suggests that generalization from test performance to performance in a natural setting would appear to be more accurate than may be the case with more traditional paper and pencil tests.

Additional research on the validity of the computer-simulated everyday memory battery has focused on the relationship of self-rated memory function[21,22] with performance on the battery, as well as on subtypes of memory performance patterns. Larrabee and colleagues,[23] investigated the relationship of memory self-report on the MAC-S, a memory self-rating questionnaire,[21,22] to computerized test performance. These authors found a significant canonical correlation of .528 between objective performance factor scores and MAC-S self-rated everyday memory factor scores.

Larrabee and Crook have reported data on subgroups of persons with different profiles of everyday strengths and weaknesses.[24] Subgroups were identified manifesting overall superior general performance, inferior general performance, superior everyday visual memory (with inferior everyday verbal-visual memory) and superior everyday verbal-visual memory (with inferior visual memory). Additional data were presented suggesting that AAMI is composed of at least two groups of subjects: Those with age-related performance decline relative to young adult controls and those with performance decline relative to their own age peers, suggestive of senescent forgetfulness.

In the past 3 years, the computerized everyday memory battery has been employed as the major dependent variable

in numerous clinical trials in the United States and
Europe. At present, the battery is being employed in more
than a dozen clinical trials at over 30 sites in the United
States and Europe for evaluation of the efficacy of a
variety of candidate pharmacologic compounds for treatment
of early stage Alzheimer-type Dementia, and AAMI. In these
clinical trials, measurement follows a multicomponent
model, including: objective performance on the
computerized battery, objective performance on standard
memory tests for definition of AAMI,[1] patient self report
of memory function,[21,22] and affective status,[25] family
report of patient's memory function, and investigator
ratings of memory function and global deterioration.[26]

CONCLUSION

     We have presented a computer-simulated everyday memory
battery designed for measurement of treatment response in
the investigation of candidate pharmacological treatments
for age-related memory disorders. The suitability of the
battery for this purpose is enhanced by a high degree of
everyday face validity, five alternate forms for multiple
trial testing, theoretical and paradigmatic links with
human and animal research (in particular, delayed response
and object location testing), and the presence of multiple
dimensions of verbal, visual, and attentional factors of
memory and memory-related skills.

REFERENCES

1.   T. Crook, R.T. Bartus, S.H. Ferris, P. Whitehouse,
        G.D. Cohen, and S. Gershon, Age-Associated
        Memory Impairment: Proposed diagnostic criteria
        and measures of clinical change--Report of a
        National Institute of Mental Health work group,
        Developmental Neuropsychology, 2:261-276
        (1986).
2.   G.J. Larrabee and T. Crook, Assessment of drug
        effects in age-related memory disorders:
        Clinical, theoretical, and psychometric
        considerations, Psychopharmacology Bulletin,
        24:515-522 (1988).
3.   R.T. Bartus, T.H. Crook, and R.L. Dean. Current
        progress in treating age-related memory
        problems: A perspective from animal
        preclinical and human clinical research, in:
        "Geriatric Clinical Pharmacology and the Aging
        Individual," W.G. Wood, ed., Raven Press, New
        York, NY, (1987)
4.   C. Flicker, R.Dean, R.T. Bartus, S.H. Ferris, T.
        Crook, Animal and human memory dysfunctions
        associated with aging, cholinergic lesions, and
        senile dementia, Annals of the New York Academy
        of Sciences: Vol 444. Memory Dysfunction: An
        Integration of Animal and Human Research from
        Preclinical and Clinical Perspectives. New
        York: The New York Academy of Sciences (1985).
5.   P. Leber, Establishing the efficacy of drugs with
        psychogeriatric indications, in: "Treatment

Development Strategies for Alzheimer's Disease," T. Crook, R.T. Bartus, S. Ferris, and S. Gershon, eds., Mark Powley Associates, Inc., Madison, CT (1986).

6. T. Crook, S. Ferris, and M. McCarthy, The misplaced-objects task: A brief test for memory dysfunction in the aged, <u>Journal of American Geriatric Society</u>, 27:284-287 (1979).

7. T. Crook, S.H. Ferris, M. McCarthy, and D. Rae, The utility of digit recall tasks for assessing memory in the aged, <u>Journal of Consulting and Clinical Psychology</u>, 48:228-233 (1980).

8. S.H. Ferris, T. Crook, E. Clark, M. McCarthy, and D. Rae, Facial recognition memory deficits in normal aging and senile dementia, <u>Journal of Gerontology</u>, 35:707-714 (1980).

9. S.H. Ferris, T. Crook, C. Flicker, B. Reisberg, and R.T. Bartus, Assessing cognitive impairment and evaluating treatment effects: Psychometric performance tests, <u>in</u>: "Handbook for Clinical Memory Assessment of Older Adults,", pp. 139-148, L.W. Poon, T. Crook, K.L. Davis, C. Eisdorfer, B.J. Gurland, A.W. Kaszniak, and L.W. Thompson, eds., American Psychological Association, Washington, DC (1986).

10. M. McCarthy, S.H. Ferris, E. Clark, and T. Crook, Acquisition and retention of categorized material in normal aging and senile dementia, <u>Experimental Aging Research</u>, 7:127-135 (1981).

11. T. Crook and G.J. Larrabee, Interrelationships among everyday memory tests: Stability of factor structure with age, <u>Neuropsychology</u>, 2:1-12 (1988).

12. T. Crook, M. Salama, and J. Gobert, A computerized test battery for detecting and assessing memory disorders, <u>in</u>: "Senile Dementias: Early Detection," pp. 79-85, A. Bes, J. Cohn, S. Hoyer, J.P. Marc-Vergenes, and H.M. Wisniewski, eds., John Libbey Eurotext, London-Paris (1986).

13. C. Flicker, S.H. Ferris, T. Crook, and R. Bartus, A visual recognition memory test for the assessment of cognitive function in aging and dementia, <u>Experimental Aging Research</u>, 13:127-132 (1987).

14. G.J. Larrabee, R.L. Kane, and J.R. Schuck, Factor analysis of the WAIS and Wechsler Memory Scale: An analysis of the construct validity of the Wechsler Memory Scale, <u>Journal of Clinical Neuropsychology</u>, 5:159-168 (1983).

15. G.J. Larrabee, R.L. Kane, J.R. Schuck, and D.E. Francis, The construct validity of various memory testing procedures, <u>Journal of Clinical and Experimental Neuropsychology</u>, 7:239-250 (1985).

16. G.J. Larrabee and H.S. Levin, Memory self-ratings and objective test performance in a normal elderly sample, <u>Journal Clinical and Experimental Neuropsychology</u>, 8:275-284 (1986).

17. G.P. Prigatano, Wechsler Memory Scale: A selective review of the literature, <u>Journal of Clinical</u>

Psychology (Special Monograph Supplement), 34:816-832 (1978).

18. D.A. Wechsler, "Wechsler Memory Scale-Revised: Manual," The Psychological Corporation, Harcourt, Brace Jovanovich, Inc., San Antonio (1987).

19. G.J. Larrabee and T. Crook, Dimensions of everyday memory in Age-Associated Memory Impairment, Psychological Assessment, A Journal of Consulting and Clinical Psychology, In press (1989).

20. A.L. Benton, "Revised Visual Retention Test: Clinical and Experimental Applications," The Psychological Corporation, New York (1974).

21. T. Crook and G.J. Larrabee, A Self-Rating Scale for Evaluating Memory in Everyday Life, Psychology and Aging, In press (1989).

22. D. Winterling, T. Crook, M. Salama, and J. Gobert, A self-rating scale for assessing memory loss, in: "Senile Dementias: Early Detection," pp. 482-486, A. Bes, J. Cohn, S. Hoyer, J.P. Marc-Vergenes, and H.M. Wisniewski, eds., John Libbey Eurotext, London-Paris (1986).

23. G.J. Larrabee, R.L. West, and T. Crook, The association of memory complaint with everyday memory performance, Paper presented at the 17th annual meeting of the International Neuropsychological Society, Vancouver, B.C., Canada (1989, February).

24. G.J. Larrabee and T.H. Crook, Performance subtypes of everyday memory function, Developmental Neuropsychology, Paper presented at the Annual Meeting of the American Psychological Association, New Orleans, LA, August, 1989.

25. J. Yesavage, T. Brink, T. Rose, O. Lum, O. Huang, V. Adey, and V. Leirer, Development and validation of a geriatric depression scale: A preliminary report, Journal of Psychiatric Research, 17:37-49 (1983).

26. B. Reisberg, S.H. Ferris, M.J. de Leon, and T. Crook, The Global Deterioration Scale for assessment of primary degenerative dementia, American Journal of Psychiatry, 139:1136-1139.

Acetylcholine, (ACh) 11, 12, 25-36,53-59, 71, 72, 87, 103, 107, 108,110, 156-159, 173, 185, 191, 205, 213, 244, 246, 247, 250, 251, 255-265, 273-275, 300, 329, 334-337, 343, 356, 358

Acetylcholinesterase, (ACHE) 11, 26, 74,76, 81-83, 87, 173, 174, 176, 177, 255, 256

ACh, (see acetylcholine)

ACHE, (see acetylcholinesterase)

ACPD, (see amino-cyclopentyl-1,3-dicarboxylate)

ACTH, 221, 222, 228-231

Actinomycin, D 127-130

Adenosine receptors, 186

Adenylate cyclase, 6, 12, 34, 272

Adrenergic receptors, 299

Adrenocorticotropic hormone, (see ACTH)

AF102B, 4, 11-14

Aging, 112, 113, 130, 133, 168, 280, 343, 356, 358, 360, 364, 373
   brain 71, 119,-121, 247, 248, 250, 251, 273-275, 293, 297, 298-300, 319, 322, 325, 326, 329
   human brain 13, 120, 294, 295, 374
   human 39, 213, 215, 345, 354, 355, 362, 365, 368
   and color preference 43

Aluminum, 185, 213

Amantadine, 338, 339, 341

Amino-cyclopentyl-1,3-dicarboxylate (ACPD), 294

Aminopyridine, 11, 173, 175

Amitriptyline, 341, 342

Amygdala, 50, 234, 237, 242, 244, 249, 255, 294

Amyloid plaques, 350

Anoxia, 188, 193, 194, 295, 320, 327

Apomorphine, 334, 335

Arecoline, 58

Aspartate, 185, 191, 195, 299, 319-323

Astrocytes, 99, 134, 135, 137, 139, 140, 142-145, 214, 299

Atropine, 1, 55, 272, 334, 337

Autoimmunity, 213, 215

Autopsied brains, 245, 349

Basal forebrain, 5, 11, 64, 71, 75, 80, 88, 91, 97, 103, 107, 110, 111, 118-121, 127, 133, 135, 159, 173, 205, 222, 231, 255, 280

Benzstigmine, 174, 177

Beta-endorphin, 214

Bethanechol, 11, 58

Caffeine, 338, 341

Calcium, 20, 21, 34, 55, 95, 215, 294, 295, 299, 314, 321, 323
   calcium dependent release 320, 321
   calcium-dependent potassium current 17
   calcium dependent release 273

Carbachol, 12, 17-22

Caudate, 294, 299, 322

Cell culture, 71, 73, 130

Cerebellum, 12, 13, 54, 75, 135, 155, 168, 299, 304, 307, 355, 360-363, 370

Cerebral artherosclerosis, 214

ChAT, (see choline acetyltransferase)

Choline, 244, 255, 257, 259, 265, 274

Choline acetyltransferase (ChAT), 26, 53-57, 64, 79, 80, 85-90, 103, 104-113, 118, 121, 185, 244, 249, 255-259, 262-265, 270, 273, 348

Cortex, 50, 53-55, 72, 75, 103, 121, 134, 139, 155, 165, 185, 205, 206, 244, 255, 262, 264, 265, 313, 323, 325, 331, 333-337, 343, 358

adrenal cortex, 221

cerebral cortex, 3, 11-13, 26, 34, 105, 113, 155, 158, 165, 204, 205, 212, 255, 263

cingulate cortex, 98, 106, 139, 225, 295

entorhinal cortex, 135, 234, 235, 243, 244, 248-250, 275, 294, 295, 310, 322

frontal cortex, 12, 25,-27, 30-37, 49, 53-59, 105, 109, 110, 112, 154, 155, 229, 231, 245, 254, 290, 319, 322, 323

occipital cortex, 164, 280

motor cortex, 330

parietal cortex, 104, 105, 109, 135, 222, 231, 237, 23-241, 246, 248, 256, 257, 269-275, 280, 290, 295-297

piriform cortex, 295

prefrontal cortex, 231

somatosensory cortex, 225

temporal cortex, 106, 109, 110, 280, 319, 325, 363

visual cortex, 167, 168, 170

Creutzfeldt-Jacob disease, 213

Cyclic AMP, 4, 6, 8, 17, 244, 272

Cyclic GABA, 185, 190

Cyclosporin A, 218

Cyproheptadine, 334, 335

Delivery system, 65, 71, 174, 179, 197, 199-203, 207, 208

Delta wave, 331, 333, 334, 336, 338, 341, 342, 343

Dentate gyrus, 295-297

Depression, 43, 58, 206

Diazepam, 341, 342

DNA, 3,78, 84, 88, 95, 349, 350

Dopamine, 10, 72, 73, 96, 175, 199, 213, 299, 322, 329, 335, 337, 347

Dopamine, receptors 299

Dopaminergic, 120, 135, 293, 320

EEG, 329, 330, 331, 333, 334, 335, 336, 337, 338, 341, 342, 343, 358, 359

Elongation Factor-2, 128

Estradiol, 175, 195-208

Estrogens, 202, 204, 206

Excitotoxins, 319

FC receptors, 214

FGF, (see fibroblast growth factor)

Fibroblast growth factor (FGF), 65, 88, 89,98, 159

GABA, 120, 135, 185-193, 320, 323, 329, 334-336, 338, 343

GH, (see growth hormone)

Glutamate, 21, 185, 184, 192, 195, 246, 295, 297, 298, 299, 303, 304, 310, 313, 314, 319, 320, 325, 324, 348

Glutaminase, 321, 324, 326, 327

Glycine, 6, 8, 294, 295

Grafts, 94, 95, 98, 99, 290, 304, 305, 305, 308, 311, 313

Growth hormone, (GH)154, 215

Guam ALS-Parkinson's Dementia, 304, 312

Hippocampal, 333

Hippocampus, 11, 13, 17, 17, 21, 22, 25-27, 33-37, 50, 53-58, 71-83, 95, 103, 105, 104, 109, 110, 112, 113, 118, 121, 133-142, 144,154, 155, 157, 158, 185, 205-207, 222, 230, 234, 235, 244, 246, 249, 273, 280, 290, 295, 398, 300, 303-314, 319, 320, 325, 330, 331, 333-339, 342, 343, 350, 355-359, 363, 364, 365, 368

Huntington's disease, 319

Hypoglycemia, 294, 295, 320

Hypothalamus, 139, 202, 204, 205, 269, 300, 334

Hypoxia, 320

Ia antigens, 214

IGF, (see insulin-like growth factor)

Immune system, 131, 153, 213, 214, 215, 216

Inferior olive, 361

Insulin, 63, 65, 133, 143, 148

Insulin-like growth factor (IGF) 63, 65, 133, 143, 153-158

Interleukin-1, 65, 70, 75, 131, 133, 214, 219
Interleukin-2, 130, 214
Ischemia, 118, 142, 195, 294, 295

Kainic acid, 155, 156, 256, 294, 295, 298, 304, 305, 307, 309, 311, 320, 322, 323, 325

Lymphocytes, 214, 215, 351
Lymphokines, 75, 153, 158
Lysosomes, 345

Membrane fluidity, 215
Methylcarbamylcholine 54-56
Mossy fiber, 295, 360, 361, 362
mRNA, 128, 129
　Alzheimer's disease (continued)
　　brain levels, 345-349
　for FGF, 135, 139, 140, 142, 144
　for IGF, 153
　for m1 and m3 (continued)
　　muscarinic receptors, 20
　for NGF 64, 75, 77-79, 84, 85-89, 112, 115, 118, 122
　for NPY, 245, 249, 270-275
Multiple sclerosis, 215
Muscarinic receptor mRNA, 16
Muscarinic receptors, 1, 3, 4, 5, 11, 13, 17, 20, 21, 26, 35, 36, 37, 53, 58, 89, 244, 255, 272, 300
Myelin, 214, 216, 217

N-methyl-D-aspartate receptors, (see NMDA receptors)
N-methylscopolamine, 3, 6
Nerve growth factor, (NGF) 63-67, 72, 74, 75, 77-84, 85-91, 95, 97-99, 103-113, 115-125, 127-135, 142, 142, 153, 158, 159, 218, 273
Neurofibrillary tangles, 174, 214, 245, 363
Neuropeptide Y (NPY), 204, 207, 244-251, 269-272, 274, 275
NGF, (see nerve growth factor)
Nicotine, 25, 28, 33-37, 39, 40, 42-51, 54, 59, 265
Nicotinic acid, 174, 175, 180, 186
Nicotinic receptors, 26, 36, 37, 39, 40, 48, 50, 52, 53-58, 255, 265
NMDA, 21, 22, 195, 293, 294, 295, 296, 297, 298, 299, 300, 303, 304, 305,

307, 309, 310, 311, 312, 313, 314, 319
Nootropics, 11, 191, 341
Noradrenaline, 329, 334, 335
NPY, (see Neuropeptide Y)
Nucleus accumbens, 294
Nucleus basalis, 51, 269-275, 279
Nucleus basalis of Meynert, 34, 53, 280
Nucleus basalis magnocellularis, 72, 235-250, 255, 280

Oligodendrocytes, 99, 134, 214
Olivopontocerebellar, 319
Oxotremorine, 5, 6, 8, 11, 12, 13, 17, 18, 19, 20, 21, 22, 25, 28, 32, 33, 35, 36, 37, 55, 272, 275

Parkinson, 94, 99, 293, 304, 312, 319
Passive avoidance, 13, 188, 194, 195, 224, 232, 236, 245, 269, 279, 280, 281, 282, 289, 290
Pentobarbital, 26, 188, 189, 190, 223, 281, 330, 341, 342
Perirhinal, 295
Periventricular, 305, 310
Phosphatidyl inositide, 17, 34
Phospholipase C 20, 21
Physostigmine (eserine), 11, 27, 28, 173, 174, 176, 259, 334, 336, 338
PI hydrolysis, 4, 6, 8, 12, 14, 17, 22, 34
Picrotoxin, 334, 335
Piracetam, 11, 191, 338
Pirenzepine, 3, 4, 8, 12, 20, 22, 53, 55, 89
Plaques, 120, 159, 174, 185, 245, 312, 350, 363
Polyacrylamide gel, 349
Polyacrylamide gel electrophoretic, 88
Polysomes, 348
Power Spectra, 329, 330, 331, 333, 335, 338, 343
Pro-opiomelanocortin, 222, 230
Proteases, 63, 134, 135, 138, 140, 143, 349
Protein Kinase, (C) 21, 272
Protein Kinases, 128
Putamen, 294, 299
Pyridostigmine, 176
Pyrrolidinone, 185, 186, 187, 190, 191

Rapid eye movement, 331
Red nucleus, 361
REM, 333, 335, 337, 338, 342, 343
Reserpine, 341

Scopolamine, 13, 25, 28, 30, 31, 32, 35,
    36, 89, 175, 188, 194, 358, 363,
    365, 370
Septal-Hippocampal Cholinergic
    System, 71-83, 104, 112, 118, 356,
    358, 363, 368
Septum, 34, 71-90, 95, 98, 103, 106, 118,
    119, 121, 133, 135, 141, 155, 222,
    280, 290, 296, 297, 303, 304, 310,
    312, 313, 358, 363
Serotonin, (5-HT) 11, 59, 72, 120, 185,
    213, 329, 334, 335
Serotonin receptors, 320, 335
Shuttle box avoidance paradigms,
    221, 223, 224, 226, 231, 280,-282,
    286, 289, 290
Slow wave sleep, 331
Somatostatin, 11, 72, 154, 204, 205,
    213, 214, 244, 245, 246, 247, 249,
    251, 254, 269, 348
Spatial memory, 159, 304, 308, 312,
    313, 373

Stroke, 294, 295
Subiculum, 295
Substance, P 213, 214
Substantia nigra, 73, 96
Succinate dehydrogenase, 349

T cells, 128, 132, 214, 216
Thalamus, 49, 135, 154-156, 222, 223,
    225, 296, 300
Theta wave, 333-338, 341-343
Thy-1, 214
Thyroid hormones, 66
Transfer Factor (TF), 215, 218
Trigonelline, 175, 177
Trimethyltin, 303 315
Tubulin, 349

Uridine, 349-351

Viral gene transduction, 84
Viral genomes, 95
Viral RNA, 129

WAIS vocabulary, 379
Wechsler memory scale, 379